REGENSBURGER BEITRÄGE
ZUR GENDER-FORSCHUNG
Band 7

Herausgegeben von
Rainer Emig
Anne-Julia Zwierlein

Gender and Disease in Literary and Medical Cultures

Edited by
ANNE-JULIA ZWIERLEIN
IRIS M. HEID

Universitätsverlag
WINTER
Heidelberg

Bibliografische Information der Deutschen Nationalbibliothek

Die Deutsche Nationalbibliothek verzeichnet diese Publikation
in der Deutschen Nationalbibliografie;
detaillierte bibliografische Daten sind im Internet
über *http://dnb.d-nb.de* abrufbar.

COVER ILLUSTRATION
Hogarth, William. "VI: The Lady's Death." *Marriage à-la-mode.* c. 1743.

ISBN 978-3-8253-6376-5

© 2014 Universitätsverlag Winter GmbH Heidelberg
Imprimé en Allemagne · Printed in Germany
Druck: Memminger MedienCentrum, 87700 Memmingen

Gedruckt auf umweltfreundlichem, chlorfrei gebleichtem
und alterungsbeständigem Papier

Den Verlag erreichen Sie im Internet unter:
www.winter-verlag.de

Contents

Anne-Julia Zwierlein and Iris M. Heid

Preface: Gender and Disease in Literary and Medical Cultures

This collection responds to recent developments in several vibrant inter-disciplinary fields that have kept expanding over the last decades: Gender Medicine, the Medical Humanities, and the cultural history of medicine. Not only do literary and cultural studies increasingly integrate insights from the history of medicine but medical faculties are also, in their turn, starting to employ methodologies from the fields of cultural studies or narratology. The Program in Narrative Medicine at Columbia University, founded in 1996, incorporates narrative competence into medical practice in order to enhance connections between medical practitioners and patients,[1] and indeed, as the British Council observes, "in the UK, there are now paid bibliotherapists, and in some clinics and surgeries a recommended reading list is offered to patients suffering from depression […] or even breast cancer".[2] The complex relations between "Gender and the Language of Illness" have been analysed from a linguistic point of view in 2010,[3] and Centres for Gender Medicine, which enhance the role of sociocultural aspects in medical research, were founded in New York in 2001 or in 2003 at the Charité in Berlin. The journal *Gender Medicine: Journal for the Study of Sex & Gender Differences* ran between 2004-2012; since then its areas of specialization have been incorporated by other, established medical journals. Simultaneously, numerous Medical Humanities Centres have sprung up around the US, the UK, and on the European continent, such as the Medical Humanities Centre at King's College, London, with the support of the Wellcome Centre for the Humanities & Health, and the various Medical Humanities Centres at Aberdeen, Durham, Edinburgh, Exeter, Glasgow, Leeds, Leicester, and Sheffield, to name but a few.

It has now become possible to investigate the impact of gender differences and gender constructions within various branches of the medical field, and "the influence of gender on the creation of medical knowledge" (Laflen 2010: xxxvi).

[1] See also the preface by Rita Charon, Director of the Program in Narrative Medicine at Columbia, to Block and Laflen 2010.

[2] The British Council, Walberberg Literature Seminar, 27-30 January 2011, "Literature and Health", advertisement.

[3] See Charteris-Black and Seale 2010.

One central concern is to readdress (sex and) gender difference for concrete therapeutic purposes, since men have long represented the "medical norm" even though specific diseases affect males and females in different ways, and they also diverge in their response to treatment. Due to their – statistically significant – differences in terms of medical histories and disease trajectories, males and females also require different doses of medication for optimal effect. Even in the field of "personalized medicine" which "aims at considering all individual risk factors of a human being", it is now acknowledged that "it seems mandatory to construct individualized clinical care algorithms based on individual risk profiles on top of gender-based assessment" (Regitz-Zagrosek 2012: 4). As Vera Regitz-Zagrosek maintains, gender medicine started around the year 2000, when the "medical community discovered that 'women are not small men'" (ibid.: 1).[4] In current medical practice, the dosage of medication, for example, is based exclusively on body weight, with women (and children) allocated lower doses simply because of their statistically lower relative weight. However, dosage re-commendations do not sufficiently take into account that sex differences may impact dose response independent of mere body size. Yet in medical studies as elsewhere, gauging interactions between sex and gender is complex, for instance where the perception of pain is concerned: do women and men have different biological pain profiles, or are sensitivities to pain, and ways of communicating about pain, different because of diverging gender-specific expectations and role modeling? Gender Medicine has reimported a female-specific dimension into medicine in many areas while also addressing gender aspects for males such as the 'invisibility' of clinical depression in male patients.[5]

In the early years of gender medicine, researchers targeted endocrine and reproductive systems, yet other diseases such as diabetes and cardiovascular syndromes were also soon recognized to have different trajectories for women and men (see Regitz-Zagrosek 2012: 1). Certain diseases have been stereotyped as 'male' or 'female', as with lung cancer or cardiovascular diseases for men, even though in the case of female obesity, heart attacks can be even more frequent and more frequently fatal for females than for males (while they go undiagnosed more frequently in females due to gendered preassumptions). It has now been recognized that "cardiovascular disease, long defined as primarily a male disease, is the number one killer of adult women" (Schiebinger 2012: 5). Indeed, geneticists have established that the double copy of the X-chromosome carried by women is silenced across most stretches of the additional X. So for

[4] The 'environmental justice movement' agitating against chemical waste disposal sites in the living areas of minority populations have argued similarly that "Women and children are not considered in the determination of safe levels of exposure because pathology testing is normalized based upon the reaction of the average 150-180-pound white male" (Collins, 2006: 6).

[5] See Möller-Leimkühler 2008. See also Segal and Demos 2003.

most areas of chromosome X, only one of the two female copies contributes to gene expression. More recently, evidence of sex-specific genetic constructs has emerged, which highlights sex differences in gene expression and gene regulation beyond the influence of the sex chromosomes.[6] Thus, genetic research is still facing challenges in terms of understanding gene expression differences between men and women and their potential role in disease development.

It has also been acknowledged in the field of gender medicine that "sex is not a dichotomous variable", i.e. that we can observe "intersex syndromes" or "hormonal or gene expression profile[s] [that are] close to the other sex" (Regitz-Zagrosek 2012: 1). Medical studies are now increasingly taking into account that there are environmentally determined variations in physiological response to disease and treatment, and they also increasingly base their investigations on an acknowledgement that the distinction between biologically- or life style-induced types of disease can be nearly impossible to make. In the area of epigenetics, it has been demonstrated that the process of DNA methylation introduces experiential factors into individual gene expression, and indeed, "epigenetic mechanisms are affected by estrogen receptors and therefore their effect may differ in male and female fetuses" (ibid.: 3). As Regitz-Zagrosek summarizes:

> Gender is associated with behaviour, with stress and life style associated diseases. It determines access to health care, help-seeking behaviour and individual use of the health care system. [...] In the medical field it is not easy to separate the influence of sex and gender. On the one hand, sex influences gendered medical roles, i.e. testosterone determines aggressive behaviour that may be associated with risk seeking and neglect of prevention. On the other hand, gender roles, e.g. professional exposure to stress, poor nutrition, environmental toxins, or endocrine disrupters may lead to genetic or epigenetic modifications that differ in women and men. DNA repair and epigenetic modifications are modified by sex hormone receptors. Genetic or epigenetic modifications can affect adults, but also the DNA of a developing fetus. Simpler, gender roles like exercise behaviour or training will interact with sex hormones to influence physical functions, for example bone density and the likelihood of osteoporosis.

(Regitz-Zagrosek 2012: 2)

Still, as Jonathan Metzl and Suzanne Poirier have pointed out in a special issue of *Literature and Medicine* (2004), "difference is often defined through disease" (Metzl and Poirier 2004: vi), i.e. within medical culture and the history of medicine, gender difference itself was often pathologized. Diane Price Herndl

[6] "[...] recent studies suggest that sex-specific genetic architecture also influences human phenotypes, including reproductive, physiological and disease traits. It is likely that an underlying mechanism is differential gene regulation in males and females, particularly in sex steroid-responsive genes. Genetic studies that ignore sex-specific effects in their design and interpretation could fail to identify a significant proportion of the genes that contribute to risk for complex diseases" (Ober, Loisel and Gilad 2008).

maintains that masculine privilege was perpetuated by medical thought and the larger culture "defining women as ill and enforcing that definition" (Price Herndl 1993: 6). Cultural gender norms arguably continue to influence therapeutic decisions as well as patient-doctor interaction. Thus put more simply, "If narratives by and about female medical professionals challenged the linking of women to illness, narratives focused on male patients inherently question the attribution of health and virility to masculinity" (Laflen 2010: xli).

In British and American literary and cultural studies, the narrative representation of diseases, of medical knowledge and practice, has long been a thriving area of research. Attention has been given in recent years to new bio-fictional, biographical or autobiographical modes of 'writing' or 'communicating' disease, to narrative representations of life trajectories and the scripts of epidemics, or cinematic versions of pathology and pathologists. A recent collection, Carmen Birkle and Johanna Heil's *Communicating Disease: Cultural Representations of American Medicine* (2013), highlights transatlantic and transnational readings of the intersections between literature and medicine while also intermittently addressing questions of gender norms and scripts. In the fields of history of medicine and cultural studies, attention has been given for decades to the cultural history of specific diseases or culturally divergent conceptualizations of specific organs or body parts;[7] gender-specific constructions of diseases have also been addressed. Thus Juliana Schiesari in *The Gendering of Melancholia: Feminism, Psychoanalysis, and the Symbolics of Loss in Renaissance Literature* (1992) has analysed early modern ideas about melancholia as a disease promoting and advancing male genius and uniqueness, while female melancholia was constructed as debilitating. Consumption has a similar history as the disease of the (male) Romantic genius, and gout has been demonstrated by Roy Porter and G.S. Rousseau (2000) to have been conceived almost exclusively as a male, and an upper-class, 'gentleman's' disease. Hysteria, of course, has its own long history as a specifically female, physiologically grounded psychological deviation, recounted, for instance, in Charles Bernheimer and Claire Kahan's collection *In Dora's Case: Freud, Hysteria, Feminism* (1985), Elaine Showalter's *The Female Malady: Women, Madness, and English Culture, 1830-1980* (1987), and Janet Beizer's *Ventriloquized Bodies: Narratives of Hysteria in Nineteenth-Century France* (1994). Linked to hysteria, but with their own more variegated ramifications, are the multiple nineteenth-century theories of nervous disease documented by Athena Vrettos in *Somatic Fictions: Imagining Illness in Victorian Culture* (1995), Peter Melville Logan in *Nerves and Narratives: A Cultural History of Hysteria in Nineteenth-Century British Prose* (1997), and Helen Small in *Love's Madness: Medicine, the Novel, and Female Insanity, 1800-1865* (1998). Erin O'Connor in *Raw Material: Producing*

---

[7] See the various examples in 'Selected Further Reading'.

Pathology in Victorian Culture (2000) has combined the strands of medical history and disability studies to offer new insights into cultural constructions of the body's materiality as a site of disease, while Alison Bashford in *Purity and Pollution: Gender, Embodiment and Victorian Medicine* (1998) has traced some of the same questions from an anthropological and gender perspective. Taken together, these cultural histories of specific diseases have advanced the work of rewriting reductive narratives about gender difference in medical studies and Western cultures at large.

In terms of literary genres, there has been a remarkable surge of dramatic work engaging with the cultural scripts of disease, as assembled, for instance, in Angela Belli's collection *Bodies and Barriers: Dramas of Dis-Ease* (2008). While gender questions are not at the forefront of Belli's enterprise, a considerable number of plays in her collection explicitly discuss conceptions of the female body as a physiological site, like Margaret Edson's 1999 play *Wit*, or Arthur Kopit's *Wings* (1997). Comparing both plays, indeed, can help to highlight how the crisis of disease is represented as a moment when gendered visions of physiology and the doctor-patient relationship are reexamined, irrespective of whether the disease is ovarian cancer (Edson) or a cerebral stroke (Kopit). In both cases, the patient's own language and narrative constructions are integrated formally and thematically into the play's development, as when the professor of English literature Vivian in *Wit*, who learns about her terminal-stage cancer at the outset, 'directs' the play through immediate audience address and the metaphorical language and "wit" of John Donne's *Holy Sonnets*, or when Kopit follows the fragmentation of perception through brain damage by using as one of his major sources besides medical research, neurologist A.R. Luria's 1972 *The Man with a Shattered World*, which presents a narrative of brain damage in the language of the patient – while Kopit in the process also re-examines the gendered assumptions of that prior account. Other, feminist plays addressing gender aspects in medicine have in their majority been concerned with female forms of cancer, or with reproduction. Examples of the latter are assembled in Jozefina Komporaly's *Staging Motherhood: British Women Playwrights, 1956 to the Present* (2007), which includes plays addressing Down's Syndrome and antenatal examinations (Claire Luckham's *The Choice*, 1992) or infertility and medically assisted reproduction (Anna Furse's *Yerma's Eggs*, 2003); examples of the former are analysed by Mary K. Deshazer in "Fractured Borders: Women's Cancer and Feminist Theatre".[8]

Irrespective of the patient's gender, however, medical and cultural historians have long recognized that the patient-doctor binary itself, and the cultural scripts about how we respond to disease, partake of underlying, and always-already gendered, cultural patterns. Such patterns, usually invisible as a result of hege-

[8] See Deshazer 2003.

monization,[9] become visible again when they are disturbed or disrupted, as in the various examples of gender confusion described in this collection, for instance by Clark Lawlor in his account of eighteenth-century 'melancholy', by Ingrid Gessner in her discussion of "He-Nurses and She-Doctors" in postbellum American literature, by Martin Decker's investigations of cases of endangered masculinity in Sean O'Casey, or by the images of sexual excess in Spanish cinema which, as Ralf Junkerjürgen demonstrates, disrupt both established norms of sexuality as well as heteronormative gender classifications. This volume analyses the medical, social and cultural construction of both gender and disease in a diachronic perspective, reexamining some of the cricial *ideés reçues*, such as Thomas Laqueur's diagnosis of the eighteenth-century shift from a one-sex model to a two-sex model in human biology and medicine (*Making Sex: Body and Gender from the Greeks to Freud*, 1990), or the idea of the increasing medicalization of life from the nineteenth century onwards. Our contributors also examine the ideological work of 'disease' (as a metaphorical marker of social or political difference) as well as the question how to 'make visible the invisible' – raised on the one hand in the field of medical symptommatology and on the other in terms of changing literary techniques for representing disease. For Michel Foucault, famously, the origins of modern medicine at the end of the eighteenth century can be linked to a change in the relation between what is visible and what is invisible (Foucault 1973: 120),[10] yet no epistemic shift is ever complete, and the relations between the visible and the invisible, in ideological terms as well, keep changing. Bringing together scholars from both the Humanities and the Medical Departments at the University of Regensburg and other experts from Germany, the UK and the US, the volume also profited by a lecture series and workshop held at Regensburg in 2012 where contributions by the Medical faculty alternated with those of Humanities researchers, and where central methodological questions of Gender Medicine and the Medical Humanities were addressed.[11]

As a whole, the volume engages with some of the following questions (and many others besides): What is a symptom, how is it represented in medical and literary studies? What are the medical and literary strategies for narrating disease? How is disease represented and visualized? How does the rise of statistical science, the technologizing of the medical profession, but also initiatives towards a "personalized medicine" influence the relationship between practitioner and patient, and how do questions of gender shift the balance in all of these

[9] On the idea of hegemonization, originally developed by Marxists such as Antonio Gramsci and others, see Abercrombie and Turner 1978.

[10] See also Zwierlein on "the doctor and the detective" in Zwierlein 2005.

[11] We thank all contributors for making possible this joint enterprise; thanks are also due to Martin Decker, MA, Julia McIntosh-Schneider, MA, and Francesca Palitzsch, MA, for their valuable assistance in bringing the edited volume to fruition.

settings? Investigating the construction, diagnosis and perception of diseases from the perspective of gender studies and in a cultural-historical framework, the volume proceeds chronologically to highlight neuralgic moments of gendered perceptions of disease through the ages, from medieval times until today. It includes individual chapters on the link between disease and redemption in medieval literature (Edith Feistner), on humanist women authors and early modern medical constructions of the female soul (Dorothea Heitsch), fashionable diseases and gender during the long eighteenth century (Clark Lawlor), childbed and child-birth during the nineteenth century (Felix Sprang), hysteria and the construction of the 'surplus female' in nineteenth-century literature and medical discourse (Anne-Julia Zwierlein), puerperal insanity and child murder in late-Victorian British literature (Anna Farkas), gendered accounts of yellow fever in postbellum American literature (Ingrid Gessner), masculinity and the maimed body in Irish playwright Sean O'Casey (Martin Decker), gendered images of sexual addiction in Spanish cinema (Ralf Junkerjürgen), gender and medical realism in the poetry of Donald Hall (Katharina Boehm), boys, 'masculinity' and representations of illness in contemporary children's and juvenile literature (Anita Schilcher), and contemporary artists' representations of the complex links between disease and gender (Barbara Oettl). Together, they produce a panorama of historically grounded analyses of cultural constructions of gender and disease which, in spite of all historical specificity, also offers insight into the striking resemblances of cultural scripts across the centuries – as in the recurring image of woman as 'agent of healing' and as (voluntary) sacrificial victim, encountered in very different ways both in medieval continental and nineteenth-century American cultural manifestations. All contributions also offer insights into how national stereotypes and antagonisms were and are played out via gendered narratives about disease (in plots turning around 'redemption', 'separation', or 'romance'). Individual chapters also demonstrate how disease could become 'heroic', or indeed a 'spectacle', in various cultural settings. While such narratives have been working towards enhancing stereotypical gender scripts in many respects, their analysis and strategic redeployment can also counteract the 'blind spots' created by the workings of hegemony. And even though the metaphor risks repeating the meliorism of nineteenth-century medical and cultural narratives about technological advances, such critical investigations can indeed contribute towards 'making visible the invisible'.

List of Works Cited

Abercrombie, Nicholas and Bryan S. Turner. "The Dominant Ideology Thesis." *The British Journal of Sociology* 29.2 (1978): 149-70.

Bashford, Alison. *Purity and Pollution: Gender, Embodiment and Victorian Medicine.* Houndmills: Palgrave, 1998.

Beizer, Janet. *Ventriloquized Bodies: Narratives of Hysteria in Nineteenth-Century France.* Ithaca, NY: Cornell UP, 1994.

Belli, Angela (ed.). *Bodies and Barriers: Dramas of Dis-Ease.* Kent: Kent State UP, 2008.

Berkenkotter, Carol. *Patient Tales: Case Histories and the Uses of Narrative in Psychiatry.* Columbia: U of South Carolina P, 2008.

Bernheimer, Charles and Claire Kahan (eds.). *In Dora's Case: Freud, Hysteria, Feminism.* New York: Columbia UP, 1985.

Birkle, Carmen and Johanna Heil (eds.). *Communicating Disease: Cultural Representations of American Medicine.* Heidelberg: Winter, 2013.

Block, Marcelline, and Angela Laflen (eds.). *Gender Scripts in Medicine and Narrative.* Newcastle: Cambridge Scholars, 2010.

British Council, Walberberg Literature Seminar, 27-30 January 2011, "Literature and Health", advertisement.

Bußmann, Hadumod and Renate Hof (eds.). *Genus: Zur Geschlechterdifferenz in den Kulturwissenschaften.* Stuttgart: Kröner, 1995.

Charon, Rita. "Preface." *Gender Scripts in Medicine and Narrative.* Ed. Marcelline Block and Angela Laflen. Newcastle: Cambridge Scholars, 2010. xiv-xviii.

Charteris-Black, Jonathan and Clive Seale. *Gender and the Language of Illness.* Basingstoke: Palgrave, 2010.

Collins, Robin Morris. "The Apocalyptic Vision, Environmentalism, and a Wider Embrace." *Interdisciplinary Studies in Literature and Environment* 13 (2006): 1-11.

Deshazer, Mary K. "Fractured Borders: Women's Cancer and Feminist Theatre." *NWSA Journal* 15.2 (2003): 1-26.

Foucault, Michel. *Die Geburt der Klinik: Eine Archäologie des ärztlichen Blicks.* 1963. Trans. München: Hanser, 1973.

Frantz, Andrea B. *Redemption and Madness: Three Nineteenth-Century Feminist Views on Motherhood and Childbearing.* Las Colinas: Ide House, 1993.

Gehlbach, Stephen H. *Interpreting Medical Literature.* New York: McGraw-Hill, 1993.

Hawkins, Anne Hunsaker and Marilyn Chandler McEntyre (eds.). *Teaching Literature and Medicine.* New York: MLA, 2000.

Herndl, Diane Price. *Invalid Women: Figuring Feminine Illness in American Fiction and Culture, 1840-1940.* Chapel Hill: U of North Carolina P, 1993.

---."Disease versus Disability: The Medical Humanities and Disability Studies." *PMLA* 120.2 (2005): 593-98.

Komporaly, Jozefina. *Staging Motherhood: British Women Playwrights, 1956 to the Present.* Basingstoke: Palgrave Macmillan, 2007.

Kravitz, Bennett. *Representations of Illness in Literature and Film.* Newcastle: Cambridge Scholars, 2010.

Laflen, Angela. "Introduction: Gender at the Intersections of Medicine and Narrative." *Gender Scripts in Medicine and Narrative.* Ed. Marcelline Block and Angela Laflen. Newcastle: Cambridge Scholars, 2010. xxxvi-xlix.

Laqueur, Thomas. *Making Sex: Body and Gender from the Greeks to Freud.* Cambridge: Harvard UP, 1990.

Lawlor, Clark. *From Melancholia to Prozac: A History of Depression.* Oxford: Oxford UP, 2012.

Logan, Peter Melville. *Nerves and Narratives: A Cultural History of Hysteria in Nineteenth-Century British Prose.* Berkeley: U of California P, 1997.

Luria, Alexander R. *The Man with a Shattered World: The History of a Brain Wound.* 1972. Repr. New Haven: Harvard UP, 1987.

Metzl, Jonathan M. and Suzanne Poirier. "Editors' Preface: Difference and Identity in Medicine." *Literature and Medicine* 23.1 (2004): i-xiii.

Möller-Leimkühler, Anne Maria. "Depression – überdiagnostiziert bei Frauen, unterdiagnostiziert bei Männern?" *Der Gynäkologe* 41.5 (2008): 381-88.

Ober, Carole, Dagan A. Loisel and Yoav Gilad. "Sex-Specific Genetic Architecture of Human Disease." *Nature Reviews Genetics* 9 (2008): 911-22.

Oertelt-Prigione, Sabine and Vera Regitz-Zagrosek (eds.). *Sex and Gender Aspects in Clinical Medicine.* London: Springer, 2012.

O'Connor, Erin. *Raw Material: Producing Pathology in Victorian Culture.* Durham: Duke UP, 2000.

Porter, Roy, and G.S. Rousseau. *Gout: The Patrician Malady.* New Haven: Yale UP, 2000.

Regitz-Zagrosek, Vera. "Why Do We Need Gender Medicine?" *Sex and Gender Aspects in Clinical Medicine.* Ed. Sabine Oertelt-Prigione and Vera Regitz-Zagrosek. London: Springer, 2012. 1-4.

Rothfield, Lawrence. *Vital Signs: Medical Realism in Nineteenth-Century Fiction.* Princeton: Princeton UP, 1992.

Schiebinger, Londa. "Gendered Innovations in Biomedicine and Public Health Research." *Sex and Gender Aspects in Clinical Medicine.* Ed. Sabine Oertelt-Prigione and Vera Regitz-Zagrosek. London: Springer, 2012. 5-8.

Schiesari, Juliana. *The Gendering of Melancholia: Feminism, Psychoanalysis, and the Symbolics of Loss in Renaissance Literature.* Ithaca: Cornell UP, 1992.

Segal, M. Texler and Vasilikie Demos (eds.). *Gender Perspectives on Health and Medicine: Key Themes.* Oxford: Elsevier, 2003.

Showalter, Elaine. *The Female Malady: Women, Madness and English Culture, 1830-1980.* New York: Penguin, 1987.

Small, Helen. *Love's Madness: Medicine, the Novel, and Female Insanity, 1800-1865.* New York: Oxford UP, 1998.

Sontag, Susan. *Illness as Metaphor.* New York: Farrar, 1978.

Vrettos, Athena. *Somatic Fictions: Imagining Illness in Victorian Culture.* Stanford: Stanford UP, 1995.

Zwierlein, Anne-Julia. "Der medizinische Diskurs in der viktorianischen Literatur." *Eine Kulturgeschichte der englischen Literatur: Von der Renaissance bis zur Gegenwart.* Ed. Vera Nünning. Tübingen: A. Francke, 2005. 182-95.

Selected Further Reading

Medieval and Early Modern

Anselment, Raymond A. *The Realms of Apollo: Literature and Healing in Seventeenth-Century England.* Newark: U of Delaware P, 1995.

Bishop, Louise M. *Words, Stones, and Herbs: The Healing Word in Medieval and Early Modern England*. Syracuse, NY: Syracuse UP, 2007.

Boehrer, Bruce Thomas. "Early Modern Syphilis." *Journal of the History of Sexuality* 1.2 (1990): 197-214.

Dawson, Lesel. *Lovesickness and Gender in Early Modern English Literature*. Oxford: Oxford UP, 2008.

Enterline, Lynn. *The Tears of Narcissus: Melancholia and Masculinity in Early Modern Writing*. Stanford: Stanford UP, 1995.

Green, Monica. "Bodies, Gender, Health, Disease: Recent Work on Medieval Women's Medicine." *Studies in Medieval and Renaissance History* 17.2 (2005): 1-46.

Healy, Margaret. *Fictions of Disease in Early Modern England: Bodies, Plagues and Politics*. Basingstoke: Palgrave, 2001.

Hellwarth, Jennifer Wynne. *The Reproductive Unconscious in Medieval and Early Modern England*. New York: Routledge, 2002.

Jose, Laura. "Monstrous Conceptions: Sex, Madness and Gender in Medieval Medical Medical Texts." *Comparative Critical Studies* 5.2-3 (2008): 153-63.

Kerwin, William. *Beyond the Body: The Boundaries of Medicine and English Renaissance Drama*. Amherst: U of Massachusetts P, 2005.

Laroche, Rebecca. *Medical Authority and English Women's Herbal Texts: 1550-1650*. Farnham: Ashgate, 2009.

Marland, Hilary and Anne Marie Rafferty (eds.). *Midwives, Society and Childbirth: Debates and Controversies in the Modern Period*. London: Routledge, 1997.

Moss, Stephanie and Kaara L. Peterson (eds.). *Disease, Diagnosis, and Cure on the Early Modern Stage*. Aldershot: Ashgate, 2004.

Neely, Carol Thomas. *Distracted Subjects: Madness and Gender in Shakespeare and Early Modern Culture*. Ithaca, NY: Cornell UP, 2004.

Peterson, Kaara L. *Popular Medicine, Hysterical Disease, and Social Controversy in Shakespeare's England*. Farnham: Ashgate, 2010.

Seargeant, Philip. "Discursive Diversity in the Textual Articulation of Epidemic Disease in Early Modern England." *Language and Literature: Journal of the Poetics and Linguistics Association* 16.4 (2007): 323-44.

Siena, Kevin (ed.). *Sins of the Flesh: Responding to Sexual Disease in Early Modern Europe*. Toronto: Centre for Reformation and Renaissance Studies, 2005.

Taavitsainen, Irma (ed.). *Medical Writing in Early Modern English*. Cambridge: Cambridge UP, 2011.

Vaught, Jennifer C. *Rhetorics of Bodily Disease and Health in Medieval and Early Modern England*. Farnham: Ashgate, 2010.

Eighteenth Century

Beatty, Heather. *Nervous Disease in Late Eighteenth-Century Britain: The Reality of a Fashionable Disorder*. London: Pickering & Chatto, 2012.

Bewell, Alan. *Romanticism and Colonial Disease*. Baltimore: Johns Hopkins UP, 1999.

Byrd, Max. *Visits to Bedlam: Madness and Literature in the Eighteenth Century*. Columbia: U of South Carolina P, 1974.

Foucault, Michel. *Madness and Civilization: A History of Insanity in the Age of Reason*. Trans. Richard Howard. New York: Pantheon, 1965.

Grinnell, George C. *The Age of Hypochondria: Interpreting Romantic Health and Illness*. Basingstoke: Palgrave Macmillan, 2010.

Ingram, Allan and Michelle Faubert. *Cultural Constructions of Madness in Eighteenth-Century Writing*. Basingstoke: Palgrave Macmillan, 2005.

Kipp, Julie. *Romanticism, Maternity, and the Body Politic*. New York: Cambridge UP, 2003.

Kopans, Dana Gliserman. "'With the Affection of a Parent': The Invention of the Patriarchal Mad-Doctor." *The English Malady: Enabling and Disabling Fictions*. Ed. Glen Colburn. Newcastle: Cambridge Scholars, 2008. 124-52.

Lee, Debbie. "Yellow Fever and the Slave Trade: Coleridge's The Rime of the Ancient Mariner." *English Literary History* 65.3 (1998): 675-700.

Meek, Heather. "Medical Women and Hysterical Doctors: Interpreting Hysteria's Symptoms in Eighteenth-Century Britain." *The English Malady: Enabling and Disabling Fictions*. Ed. Glen Colburn. Newcastle: Cambridge Scholars, 2008. 223-47.

Merians, Linda E. (ed.). *The Secret Malady: Venereal Disease in Eighteenth-Century Britain and France*. Lexington: UP of Kentucky, 1996.

Sedlmayr, Gerold. "Insular Insanities: Going Mental in Early Eighteenth-Century Britain." *Insular Mentalities: Mental Maps of Britain*. Ed. Jürgen Kamm, Gerold Sedlmayr and Bernd Lenz. Passau: Stutz, 2007. 39-52.

Vidal, Fernando. *Nymphomania and the Gendering of the Imagination in the Eighteenth Century*. Berlin: Max Planck Institut für Wissenschaftsgeschichte, 2003.

Wallen, Martin. *City of Health, Fields of Disease: Revolutions in the Poetry, Medicine, and Philosophy of Romanticism*. Aldershot: Ashgate, 2004.

Nineteenth Century

Bailin, Miriam. *The Sickroom in Victorian Fiction: The Art of Being Ill*. Cambridge: Cambridge UP, 1995.

Bashford, Alison. *Purity and Pollution: Gender, Embodiment and Victorian Medicine*. Basingstoke: Macmillan, 2000.

Blair, Kirstie. *Victorian Poetry and the Culture of the Heart*. New York: Oxford UP, 2006.

Byrne, Katherine. *Tuberculosis and the Victorian Literary Imagination*. Cambridge: Cambridge UP, 2011.

Caldwell, Janis McLarren. *Literature and Medicine in Nineteenth-Century Britain: From Mary Shelley to George Eliot*. Cambridge: Cambridge UP, 2006.

Christensen, Allan Conrad. *Nineteenth-Century Narratives of Contagion: Our Feverish Contact*. London: Routledge, 2005.

Constable, Liz. "Fin-de-siècle Yellow Fevers: Women Writers, Decadence and Discourses of Degeneracy." *Esprit Créateur* 37.3 (1997): 25-37.

Gilbert, Pamela K. *Disease, Desire and the Body in Victorian Women's Popular Novels*. Cambridge: Cambridge UP, 1997.

Miller, Ian. *A Modern History of the Stomach: Gastric Illness, Medicine and British Society, 1800-1950*. London: Pickering and Chatto, 2011.

Pedlar, Valerie. *'The most dreadful visitation': Male Madness in Victorian Fiction*. Liverpool: Liverpool UP, 2006.

Penner, Louise. *Victorian Medicine and Social Reform: Florence Nightingale among the Novelists*. New York: Palgrave Macmillan, 2010.

Sigsworth, E.M. and T.J. Wyke. "A Study of Victorian Prostitution and Venereal Disease." *Suffer and Be Still: Women in the Victorian Age*. Ed. Martha Vicinus. Bloomington: Indiana UP, 1972. 77-99.

Smith, Andrew. *Victorian Demons: Medicine, Masculinity and the Gothic at the Fin-de-Siècle*. Manchester: Manchester UP, 2004.

Stern, Rebecca. "'Personation' and 'Good Marking Ink': Sanity, Performativity, and Biology in Victorian Sensation Fiction." *Nineteenth Century Studies* 14 (2000): 35-62.

Vrettos, Athena. *Somatic Fictions: Imagining Illness in Victorian Culture*. Stanford: Stanford UP, 1995.

Wood, Jane. *Passion and Pathology in Victorian Fiction*. Oxford: Oxford UP, 2001.

Twentieth and Twenty-First Centuries

Cooke, Jennifer. *Legacies of Plague in Literature: Theory and Film*. Basingstoke: Palgrave Macmillan, 2009.

Cosslett, Tess. *Women Writing Childbirth: Modern Discourses of Motherhood*. Manchester: Manchester UP, 1994.

Fahy, Thomas and Kimball King. *Peering Behind the Curtain: Disability, Illness, and the Extraordinary Body in Contemporary Theater*. New York: Routledge, 2002.

Goc, Nicola. "Mothers and Madness: The Media Representations of Postpartum Psychosis." *Interdisciplinary Perspectives on Health, Illness and Disease*. Ed. Peter L. Twohig and Vera Kalitzkus. Amsterdam: Rodopi, 2004. 53-66.

Goodman, Lizbeth, Helen Small, and Mary Jacobus. "Madwomen and Attics: Themes and Issues in Women's Fiction." *Literature and Gender*. Ed. Lizbeth Goodman. London: Routledge, with the Open University, 1996. 109-44.

Govan, Emma. "Entertaining Illness". *Making Sense of Health, Illness and Disease*. Ed. Peter L. Twohig and Vera Kalitzkus. Amsterdam: Rodopi, 2004. 125-40.

Keith, Lois. *'Take up thy bed and walk': Death, Disability and Cure in Classic Fiction for Girls*. New York: Routledge, 2001.

Pitt, Susan. "Midwifery and Medicine: Gendered Knowledge in the Practice of Delivery." *Midwives, Society and Childbirth: Debates and Controversies in the Modern Period*. Ed. Hilary Marland and Anne Marie Rafferty. London: Routledge, 1997. 218-31.

Raoul, Valerie, Connie Canam, Angela Henderson, and Carla Paterson. *Unfitting Stories: Narrative Approaches to Disease, Disability, and Trauma*. Waterloo: Wilfred Laurier UP, 2007.

Shannonhouse, Rebecca. *Out of her Mind: Women Writing on Madness*. Expanded ed. New York: The Modern Library, 2003.

Soricelli, Rhonda L. and David H. Flood. "(Un)Professional Relationships in the Gendered Maze of Medicine." *Teaching Literature and Medicine*. Ed. Anne Hunsaker Hawkins and Marilyn Chandler McEntyre. New York: MLA, 2000. 344-52.

Wald, Christina. *Hysteria, Trauma and Melancholia: Performative Maladies in Contemporary Anglophone Drama*. Basingstoke: Palgrave Macmillan, 2007.

Westfahl, Gary and George Edgar Slusser. *No Cure for the Future: Disease and Medicine in Science Fiction and Fantasy*. Westport: Greenwood Press, 2002.

Julika Loss, Miriam Banas, Andrea Baessler,
Edith Reuschel, Marina Kreutz,
Sven Schmalfuß and Iris M. Heid

Some Aspects of Medical Research on Sex and Gender Differences: Risky Lifestyle or Risky Genes?

For a long time, it has been acknowledged that biological processes differ between men and women, but only recently have these observations been drawn together to form a specific field of medical research: gender in medicine. In most instances, dosages of pharmaceutical products have been computed using patients' height and weight, but these computations did not take the sex of the patient into account. Since 2000, several countries have established gender-in-medicine centers, with Germany having started one at the Charité in Berlin (see Oertelt-Prigione and Regitz-Zagrosek 2012). These centers work towards comparisons of men and women in the medical field, while acknowledging that "women are not small men".

The lectures on 'Gender and Disease' delivered at the University of Regensburg by specialists from various medical areas highlighted aspects of sex differences in life style, genetics, body fat, immunology, and the health care system.

Risky Lifestyle

Differences in health status have been described for people from different social classes, but there are also health inequalities in gender. In 2005, life expectancy for women in the US was estimated at 80.8 years compared to 75.7 years for men (see Arias, Rostron and Tejada-Vera 2010). Men are more likely to die from myocardial infarction, suicide or accidents than women (see Statistisches Bundesamt 2012), and lung cancer is also more common among men.

From these estimated numbers the question arises whether these differences are socially or biologically determined. Studies investigating the life spans of nuns and monks show similar life expectancies for both sexes, approaching that of women in the population at large, and it therefore seems to follow that factors other than biology are causing the lower life expectancy among men. Several hazardous lifestyles have been identified that are known to cause the major common chronic diseases: heart disease, cancer, stroke, and respiratory disease in industrialized countries. Risky lifestyles are more frequently found among men: 98% of work-place accidents happen to men, as women are more likely to be employed in less risky occupations. Other lifestyle factors of common diseases are alcohol and tobacco consumption, low intake of fruit and vegetables, and lack of physical activity, which can lead to high blood levels of cholesterol, obesity, or high blood pressure.

But not only self-adopted lifestyles need to be considered: social norms can also produce gender-specific behavior that is detrimental to health. The roles and behavior of men and women in a given culture are dictated by that culture's gender norms and values. Pressures to conform to gender-stereotypes can encourage both women and men towards adopting a riskier lifestyle. More young women start smoking to underscore the new liberties they feel the need to demonstrate; women may not receive necessary health care if norms in their communities prevent them from travelling alone to a clinic; young men try to live up to the general expectations that men are bold risk-takers and subject themselves to risky adventures that may lead to accidents.

One factor attracting global attention is obesity, which is defined as a body-mass-index (computed as weight in kilogram divided by the squared height in meters) above or equal 30 kg/m^2. There is a worldwide epidemic and the effects on most common diseases are well known. Some reasons for the obesity epidemic are increasingly sedentary lifestyles and an abundance of readily available high-caloric food. Causes for obesity appear to differ according to gender as girls tend to be less engaged in physical activities, while boys frequently adopt unhealthier diets. Girls have a higher awareness of nutritional aspects and body size that are governed by female beauty ideals, whereas boys see muscularity and strength as the predominant feature of masculinity. Not only obesity, but also cultural pressure towards thinness feed health problems: about 25% of girls practice unhealthy methods of weight control including fasting, skipping meals, excessive exercise, laxative abuse, and self-induced vomiting. Women's magazines include 10 times more advertising on weight loss than men's magazines. An unhappy result of advertisements, TV shows, and movies is that 70 to 90% of women and girls are unhappy with their appearance. Weight control is even becoming a subject for girls as young as five years of age.

Another dangerous lifestyle factor is smoking. It is the leading cause of lung cancer and many other diseases and considered to be the single greatest cause of preventable death globally. While smoking rates are going down among men, they are going up among women. This is explained by the growing proportion of women in employment, the increasingly similar lifestyle of men and women and the erosion of cultural norms preventing women from smoking. The advertisements of the tobacco industry frequently represent the elegance of smoking beauty icons, or allude to potential weight loss effects, a new sense of freedom and independence, and heightened self-confidence. The downside of this lifestyle change can be observed in the high level of lung cancer with a time lapse of several decades. While smoking rates decreased among men from over 80% in the 1950s to 36% in 2000, and among women from 50% in the 1970s to 28% in the year 2000, lung cancer rates plummeted by 50% for men (from an annual death rate of 446 in the UK in 1970 to 254 in 2000) and doubled among women (annual death rate of 50 in 1970 to 120 in 2000, see Peto et al. 2000). Thus while lung cancer used to be mainly a male disease, lung cancer death rates have now equalized for men and women – due to women's lifestyle changes.

Generally, gender can influence health in terms of behavioral differences as well as access to health care. Gender differences regarding health are particularly apparent in countries where pregnancy and childbirth still pose a significant health risk to women due to health care structures and social or cultural aspects. The numbers of women dying during childbirth vary as much as from seven in 100,000 births in Germany to 1,400 in 100,000 births in Afghanistan.

Risky Genes

The genetic code of a person is like a book with four billion letters. In 1% of these letters, the genetic code varies between individuals making up the individual genetic profile. It is known that such genetic variation is linked to common diseases like myocardial infarction or type 2 diabetes, but also to obesity and smoking behavior.

Particularly for obesity it is interesting to note that the same genetic profiles that have produced lean persons during past centuries can now, in the affluent modern world, prove dangerous in the sense that it makes a person susceptible to obesity. It seems as if some genetic profiles make it difficult for the person to cope with the amount of food available everywhere and at all times. The genetics of body fat seem to modify the appetite signaling in the brain, while the genetics of whether the fat is deposited more around the abdomen or around the hips are connected to metabolic mechanisms. Interestingly, the genetic effects controlling where the fat is deposited are much stronger in women, and it is not completely surprising that women's waists are subjected to different biological control mechanisms than men's, although the concrete cause of this effect is not yet understood.

But what are the apparent sex differences? Women are smaller, lighter, have less muscle mass, more body fat, and thinner bones. Men are fertile throughout their adult lives, while women's fertility is restricted to the time around 15 to 50 years of age. Certainly, the sex chromosomes play a pivotal role, with men being distinguished by one Y chromosome inherited from the father and one X from the mother while women have two X chromosomes. Before birth, these sex chromosomes determine which primary sex organs are developed. The secondary sex organs mature during puberty mostly due to stimulation by the sex hormones. Puberty and the associated hormonal changes are accompanied by a growth spurt that is later in life for boys, but much stronger than for girls, which is the reason why men are taller. The different numbers of X chromosomes, however, cease to play an important role after birth as the second X of the women is then silenced and does not function in any biologically meaningful way. The Y chromosome carries almost no genes at all. So what makes the difference after birth? Could it be due to the sex hormones? Both men and women have the same hormones, albeit in different quantities. While men produce about 7000 micrograms testosterone (the "male" sex hormone) per day, women produce only about 300 microgram per day. Furthermore, what is produced from testosterone differs: women convert 50% of testosterone into estradiol (the "female" sex hormone), while men convert only 0.25%.

Recent research has also described sex differences in gene expression and regulation of genes on the autosomal chromosomes (all chromosomes except the sex chromosomes). This opens up a multitude of possibilities as to how genetics can trigger sex differences (see Ober et al. 2008). To make it even more complicated, the genetic function is modulated by effects from the environment called "epigenetic effects": If the person smokes or experiences famine, it has been observed that certain gene regions are silenced. The extent to which these epigenetic effects affect diseases or habits has not yet been fully understood, but, clearly, it mixes the mechanisms of genes with those of lifestyles. There is, therefore, no definite answer to the question whether health depends more on the effects of risky lifestyles or risky genes.

From the Abdomen to the Heart

Naturally, women show a body fat content 10 % higher than men for a given body mass index (see Romero-Coral et al. 2008). In addition, marked differences in body fat distribution, specifically in waist and hip circumference, are known between genders. Generally, women have smaller waists than men. This makes particularly younger women appear pear-shaped (round hips, small waist) and men apple-shaped (large waist, slim hips). However, it can also be noted that this difference diminishes with age, particularly after the female menopause when the shape of women and men approach each other. This is not only an aesthetic burden for both men and women, but the thickening of the waist can also lead to health problems increasing the risk for cardiometabolic diseases, if the change is substantial (see Bays et al. 2008 and Bays 2009). Fat around the waist is mostly located within or around the organs and is active in producing hormones that negatively influence the metabolic system, which can lead to high blood pressure, blood glucose and blood cholesterol – all components of the metabolic syndrome and all risk factors for cardiovascular disease and diabetes (see Lakka et al. 2002; see Wilson et al. 2005).

Cardiovascular disease or more specifically myocardial infarction is also a worthwhile area of gender research. Myocardial infarction is considered a disease of men, but it kills almost as many women as men. How can that be? Although women experience myocardial infarctions about 10 to15 years later than men, the longer life period of women leads to the fact that they experience a very similar absolute number of myocardial infarctions compared with men. Moreover, men are more likely to survive it. Early mortality of myocardial infarction is greater in women than in men and this is particularly pronounced in young women (see Vaccarino et al. 1999).

Recent analysis of hospitalization data and descriptions of symptoms by patients have shown that women experience a myocardial infarction with a greater diversity of symptoms like nausea, stomach ache, general weakness and sweating, while the typical chest pain is more often described by men. It appears that men describing the typical chest pain are more likely to be rapidly diagnosed as suffering from myocardial infarction – by themselves or the emergency doctor – and therefore seek help in the emergency room earlier. By contrast, women, and their doctors, attribute chest pain more frequently to an extracardiac origin and adequate treatment is delayed. In summary, diagnosis is more difficult in women, which means that women are often underdiagnosed and much time is lost before life-saving measures can start in hospital (see Daly 2006). This becomes clear when we examine data corroborating that the proportion of severe myocardial infarction is higher for hospitalized women than for men. The non-diagnosis of female myocardial infarction is thus a probable cause for women being more likely to die from this severe cardiac disease (see Jneid et al. 2008). Similar differences concerning other diseases might still continue to be underestimated.

The Gendered Immune System

Another important trigger or suppressor of diseases is the immune system. The task of the immune system is to protect the body against infection with microbes like bacteria or tumor cells. It discriminates between "self" and "other" and fights 'foreign intruders'. It also has a life-long memory.

Are there sex differences in the strength of the immune system? It appears so. On the one hand, men suffer more frequently from infection diseases and women get well more quickly and more completely after infections and even sepses and injuries. On the other hand, women are more prone to suffer from auto-immune diseases, which are diseases where the immune system works too well and starts fighting the "self" instead of the "other". One well-known auto-immune disease is rheumatoid arthritis, which affects and destroys the joints. Rheumatoid arthritis is three times as frequent among women than among men. It has been outlined above where these sex differences might originate: X chromosomes or sex hormones. Female hormones affect the activity of the immune cells, and many of the auto-immune diseases are X-linked, which means they are controlled by genes on the X chromosome. Despite the silencing of the second X, there remain differences in terms of the gene expression between men and women, some of which lead to auto-immune disease.

The immune system also plays a role in many types of cancer. Colorectal and liver cancer affects more men than women. Increased tumor growth can be found in men and the protective effect of the female sex hormone, estradiol, is evident.

A Woman's Kidney

The role of the immune system is particularly important where transplantation is concerned. Here, the 'foreign intrusion' needs to be protected. For example, if a kidney is not functioning properly, the blood is no longer purified, the regulation of the water content in the body is disturbed, and blood pressure control is lost. A dysfunctional kidney requires dialysis and eventually a replacement organ. Transplantation of the kidney or the liver is often the only option for a patient to survive, but depends heavily on people's inclination to donate their organs. Women are more often the donor and less often the recipient of an organ. Substantially more men are on the waiting list for an organ, for example in Regensburg on 31 December 2013, there were 97 women and 239 men on the transplantation lists. Data from Eurotransplant, the European organisation for transplant waiting lists and transplant distribution, from the year 2000 shows that 71% of non-biologically related donors for kidneys were wives and 64% of biologically related donors were women. This underscores a role of gender differences not only in disease development, but also in social aspects.

Obstetrics and Gynecology

Finally, obstetrics and gynecology in third-world countries are another preeminent example of the link between health risks and sex and gender difference. Women's biological role in reproduction, especially in third-world countries, puts them at risk for childbed death and for HIV infection. An HIV seroprevalence study was performed among pregnant women in Uganda in order to determine the prevalence of HIV infection (see Reuschel et al. 2013). In 2001 (n=466) and in 2007 (n=486), two groups of clinically healthy pregnant women aged 14 to 50 years were enrolled from a local prenatal care department. The seroprevalence of HIV-1 infection did not decrease significantly, dropping from 28.3% to 25.1% between 2001 and 2007. In the same period of time the prevalence of syphilis antibodies decreased from 27.9% to 11.1%. Thus, the HIV seroprevalence among pregnant women in Uganda is still critically high but – as other sexually transmitted diseases like syphilis demonstrate – will hopefully further decrease in the future. Nevertheless the proportion of HIV infections in Africa is much higher in women than in men due to higher female viral susceptibility (see Quinn and Overbaugh 2005). Additionally via vertical transmission the virus passes the placenta, which leads to children already born HIV-positive. The most effective strategy up to now to fight AIDS in Uganda remains prevention by education especially of girls but also boys before puberty in order to avoid further spread of the HI-virus.

Summary and Outlook

This article has dealt with some aspects of sex difference from diverse medical fields. Different reasons for sex and gender difference have been highlighted from a medical point of view, including lifestyle, sex chromosome variation, sex hormones as well as health care access and utilization. More research is necessary to fully understand the differences and similarities in order to work towards a more individualized medicine, starting with the differences between men and women.

List of Works Cited

Arias, Elizabeth, Brian L. Rostron and Betzaida Tejada-Vera. "United States Life Tables, 2005." *National Vital Statistics Reports* 58.10 (2010).

Bays, H. E. "'Sick Fat,' Metabolic Disease, and Atherosclerosis." *American Journal of Medicine* 122.1 (2009): S26-S29.

Bays, H. E., J. M. González-Campoy, R. R. Henry, D. A. Bergman, A. E. Kitabchi, A. B. Schorr and H. W. Rodbard. "Is Adiposopathy (Sick Fat) an Endocrine Disease?" *International Journal of Clinical Practice* 62.10 (2008): 1474-83.

Daly, C., F. Clemens, J. L. Lopez Sendon, L. Tavazzi, E. Boersma, N. Danchin, F. Delahaye, A. Gitt, D. Julian, D. Mulcahy, W. Ruzyllo, K. Thygesen, F. Verheugt and K. M. Fox. "Cardiovascular Disease in Women: Gender Differences in the Management and Clinical Outcome of Stable Angina." *Circulation* 113 (2006): 490-98.

Jneid H., G. C. Fonarow, C. P. Cannon, A. F. Hernandez, I. F. Palacios, A. O. Maree, Q. Wells, B. Bozkurt, K. A. Labresh, L. Liang, Y. Hong, L. K. Newby, G. Fletcher, E. Peterson, L. Wexler. "Sex Differences in Medical Care and Early Death after Acute Myocardial Infarction." *Circulation* 118.25 (2008): 2803-10.

Lakka, H.M., D. E. Laaksonen, T. A. Lakka, L. K. Niskanen, E. Kumpusalo, J. Tuomilehto and J. T. Salonen. "The Metabolic Syndrome and Total and Cardiovascular Disease

Mortality in Middle-Aged Men." *JAMA: The Journal of the American Medical Association* 288.21 (2002): 2709-16.

Ober, Carole, Dagan A. Loisel and Yoav Gilad. "Sex-Specific Genetic Architecture of Human Disease." *Nature Reviews Genetics* 9 (2008): 911-22.

Oertelt-Prigione, Sabine and Vera Regitz-Zagrosek (eds.). *Sex and Gender Aspects in Clinical Medicine.* London: Springer, 2012.

Peto, Richard, Sarah Darby, Harz Deo, Paul Silcocks, Elise Whitley and Richard Doll. "Smoking, Smoking Cessation, and Lung Cancer in the UK Since 1950: Combination of National Statistics with Two Case-Control Studies." *British Medical Journal* 321 (2000): 323-29.

Quinn, Thomas C. and Julie Overbaugh. "HIV/AIDS in Women: An Expanding Epidemic." *Science* 308.5728 (2005): 1582-83.

Reuschel, E., S. Tibananuka and B. Seelbach-Goebel. "HIV-1 Seroprevalence among Pregnant Women in Rural Uganda: A Longitudinal Study over Fifteen Years." *Gynecologic and Obstetric Investigation* 75 (2013): 169-74.

Romero-Coral, A., V. K. Somers, J. Sierra-Johnson, R. J. Thomas, M. L. Collazo-Clavell, J. Korinek, T. G. Allison, J. A. Batsis, F. H. Sert-Kuniyoshi and F. Lopez-Jimenez. "Accuracy of Body Mass Index in Diagnosing Obesity in the Adult General Population." *International Journal of Obesity* 32.6 (2008): 959-66.

Statistisches Bundesamt. *Gesundheit: Todesursachen in Deutschland 2012.* Wiesbaden: Statistisches Bundesamt, 2012.

Vaccarino, Viola, Lori Parsons, Nathan R. Every, Hal V. Barron and Harlan M. Krumholz. "Sex-Based Differences in Early Mortality after Myocardial Infarction." *The New England Journal of Medicine* 341 (1999): 217-25.

Wilson, P. W., R. B. D'Agostino, H. Parise, L. Sullivan, J. B. Meigs. "Metabolic Syndrome as a Precursor of Cardiovascular Disease and Type 2 Diabetes Mellitus." *Circulation* 112.20 (2005): 3066-72.

Edith Feistner

Krankheit als Heil?
Genderperspektiven auf das Opfer der Gesundheit in der Literatur des Mittelalters

Medizin und Geschlecht im Mittelalter – Hinführung zum Thema

Krankheit verband sich selbstverständlich auch im Mittelalter mit dem Wunsch nach Heilung. Die für mittelalterliche Heilkunde und Medizin geltende Grundannahme, wonach die Durchführung therapeutischer Maßnahmen nur dann zur Genesung der Kranken führe, wenn dies im Einklang mit dem göttlichen Willen stehe (vgl. Jankrift 2003: 29), änderte daran nichts. In ihrer (auch für alle anderen Bereiche des Lebens relevanten und wohl auch nicht nur auf das Mittelalter beschränkten) Allgemeinheit ließ diese Kautele genügend Freiraum für die Entfaltung medizinischer Aktivitäten. Freilich unterstanden diese einer Logik, die in ihrer Andersartigkeit aus heutiger Sicht als solche zunächst gar nicht erkennbar sein mag, jedenfalls aber zumindest befremdet. Drei Beispiele dafür, die aus Texten des 12. und 13. Jahrhunderts stammen, seien genannt und kurz betrachtet:

> 1. In dem zur frühesten deutschen Medizinliteratur zählenden, weitverbreiteten Bartholomäus wird als Mittel für die Einschätzung der Überlebenschance eines Kranken empfohlen, dessen Harn mit der Muttermilch einer Frau zu mischen, die von einem männlichen Säugling entbunden worden ist; wenn beide Flüssigkeiten ineinanderfließen, ist der Kranke heilbar, wenn sie getrennt bleiben, ist er unheilbar (vgl. Wegera 2011: 132).

> 2. Als Arznei gegen Lepra wird, so bei Hildegard von Bingen (Causae et curae) zu lesen, u.a. eine Salbe mit getrocknetem Schwalbenkot und Schwefel empfohlen (vgl. Jankrift 2003: 29f.).

> 3. Nach medizinischer Vorstellung der Zeit konnte eine Frau, die sexuellen Umgang mit einem Leprakranken gehabt hatte, diese Krankheit, ohne selbst zu erkranken, auf weitere Sexualpartner übertragen; diese Vorstellung wurde an der Wende zum 13. Jahrhundert (Livre au Roi) denn auch in Rechtsform umgesetzt: Die gesunde Ehefrau eines lehensfähigen Man-

nes, der an Lepra erkrankte, musste ihrerseits den Rest des Lebens „in der
Zurückgezogenheit eines Klosters verbringen"; man sah darin ein „proba-
tes Mittel zur Vorbeugung gegen eine mögliche Ausbreitung der Krankheit" (Jankrift 2003: 117).

Hinter diesen scheinbar disparaten Beispielen steht sehr wohl eine eigene,
durchaus rationale Logik: Die im ersten Beispiel genannte Harnschau verbindet
sich mit der Vorstellung vom höheren prognostischen Erkenntniswert der Mut-
termilch für einen männlichen Säugling. Sie verbindet sich auch mit der Vorstellung, wonach eine Frau, die mit einem männlichen Fötus schwanger geht, körperlich und geistig-moralisch in besonders guter, ja in besserer Verfassung ist
als sonst, weil sich die dem Körper der Frau zugewiesene kalte und feuchte ‚Natur' durch die dem Körper des Mannes zugewiesene heiße und trockene ‚Natur'
ausgleiche (vgl. Konrad von Megenberg 2003: I. 47). Die im zweiten Beispiel
genannte Lepra-Therapie gründet auf der Vorstellung, dass Lepra als Krankheit
mit den Qualitätsmerkmalen kalt und trocken durch den als heiß geltenden
Schwalbenkot und Schwefel zu temperieren sei (vgl. Jankrift 2003: 29). Die im
dritten Beispiel genannte Vorstellung, eine Frau könne die kalte und trockene
Krankheit auf einen Mann übertragen, ohne selbst zu erkranken, gründet ebenfalls auf der Logik der unterschiedlichen ‚Natur' des Körpers der Frau
(kalt/feucht) und des Mannes (heiß/trocken) (vgl. Jankrift 2003: 117).
      Die Logik, die hinter diesen Beispielen steht, ist die der Säftelehre, die für die
mittelalterliche Medizin maßgeblich ist, ihre Wurzeln aber bekanntlich schon in
der Antike hat und auf den berühmten Namen des Hippokrates (460/459 bis ca.
360 v. Chr.) zurückgeführt wird. Claudius Galenus hat im zweiten nachchristli-
chen Jahrhundert aus ihr sein im Mittelalter und noch darüber hinaus wirkmäch-
tiges Schema der Humoralpathologie entwickelt.[1] Demnach seien alle Dinge aus
den vier Elementen zusammengesetzt, denen ihrerseits die vier Qualitäten kalt,
trocken, heiß und feucht sowie die vier Kardinalflüssigkeiten des Körpers –
schwarze Galle (melancholia), Schleim (phlegma), gelbe Galle (cholera) und
Blut (sanguis) – zugeordnet werden. Da im Rahmen dieses ganzheitlichen
Schemas Krankheit als Störung des Gleichgewichts im Säfteverhältnis (Dyskra-
sie) definiert ist, besteht die Aufgabe des Arztes in der Wiederherstellung des
Gleichgewichts. Ähnlich wie die Krankheitsausprägungen selbst sind dabei die
zu verabreichenden Heilmittel wiederum in die vier Qualitäten kalt, trocken,
heiß und feucht eingeteilt.[2] Dass diese Qualitätsmerkmale auch dazu dienen, die
körperliche Grundkonstitution des Mannes von der der Frau zu unterscheiden,
haben meine Beispiele 1.) und 3.) bereits verdeutlicht.

---

[1] Abb. bei Wegera 2011: 143.
[2] Vgl. zusammenfassend Wegera 2011: 142f.; Jankrift 2003.

Im Mittelalter ist das galenische Schema der Humoralpathologie nicht nur übernommen, sondern noch zusätzlich durch eine ‚interpretatio christiana‘ untermauert worden. In Hildegards von Bingen *Causae et curae* etwa heißt es:

> Der Grund dafür, daß manche Menschen an […] Krankheiten leiden, liegt am Phlegma, das sie im Übermaß in sich haben. Wäre nämlich der Mensch im Paradiese geblieben, so würde er die Phlegmen […] nicht in seinem Körper haben, sondern sein Fleisch würde ganz gesund sein und frei von Schleim. Weil er aber dem Schlechten sich zugewandt und das Gute im Stich gelassen hat, wurde er der Erde ähnlich […]. Denn nach dem Genusse des Apfels wurde das Blut der Söhne Adams in das Gift des Samens verwandelt, aus dem die Nachkommen der Menschen entstehen. Daher ist auch ihr Fleisch geschwürig und durchlöchert. Diese Geschwüre und Löcher erzeugen in den Menschen sozusagen Sturm und einen feuchten Rauch, woraus dann die Phlegmen entstehen und zusammengerinnen […].
>
> (zitiert nach Wegera 2011: 143)

Im Gegensatz zu anderen Autoren, in der Regel Männern, leitet die heilkundige Äbtissin zwar ihrerseits die Norm des menschlichen Körpers vom Mann ab, macht aber zumindest an dieser Stelle erstaunlich wenig Aufhebens um die Verführung Adams durch Eva.[3] Doch man sieht immer: Mittelalterliche Medizin ist wie schon die antike ganz selbstverständlich kulturell kontextualisiert und unterscheidet dabei – die ‚interpretatio christiana‘ tut das Ihre dazu – auch ganz selbstverständlich zwischen der Disposition des Körpers von Mann und Frau. Anstelle der heute geläufigen Differenzierung zwischen ‚sex‘ und ‚gender‘ führt sie die (auch) medizinisch relevante Unterschiedlichkeit des Körpers von Mann und Frau auf eine unterschiedliche ‚Natur’ der Geschlechter zurück, die allerdings als Erbe Adams und Evas vom Menschen wie selbstverschuldet, also ihrerseits religiös-kulturell konditioniert erscheint. Der Topos, wonach Jesus Christus, der Erlöser, zugleich auch der beste aller Ärzte sei, und zwar nicht bloß im metaphorischen Sinn (vgl. Jankrift 2003: 30), steht in engem, gleichsam psychosomatischen Zusammenhang damit. Das Mittelalter bietet folglich, so befremdend andersartig die Logik der Bilder von Körper und Krankheit und der daraus resultierenden medizinischen Konzepte war, gerade wegen deren symbolisierungsträchtiger Ganzheitlichkeit ein besonders reiches Untersuchungsfeld für die Fragestellung dieses Bandes, der das Thema „Gender and Disease" im Kontext heutiger, laborgestützter Medizin mit mikroskopisch-parzellierender Untersuchungsmethodik und gleichzeitig aus kulturhistorischer Perspektive wieder bzw. neu zu entdecken sucht.[4]

---

[3] Vgl. im Einzelnen hier auch Moshövel 2005: 52-68.

[4] Die jüngst erschienene Publikation *Sex and Gender Aspects in Clinical Medicine* (2012) von Sabine Prigione-Oertelt etwa wird mit dem Schlagwort „Gender in der Medizin als Entdeckung der letzten zehn Jahre" beworben.

Aus dem weiten mediävistischen Untersuchungsfeld zum Thema greife ich als Nicht-Medizinerin und Nicht-Medizinhistorikerin, sondern Literaturwissenschaftlerin ein Problemfeld heraus, für das der Textbereich der Literatur auch einen ganz eigenen Erkenntniswert besitzt: Es geht mir in der Folge – jenseits von medizinischen Fragen der je spezifischen Diagnose, Therapie oder Prävention bestimmter einzelner Krankheiten – um die grundsätzliche Frage nach der Erfahrung von Krankheit und den Umgang mit Krankheit. Der Fokus liegt damit auf einer ‚patientenzentrierten' Perspektive und einer gesellschaftlichen Perspektive. Für beide Perspektiven liefern gerade ‚Krankengeschichten', wie sie in literarischen Texten des Mittelalters begegnen, ein wichtiges Anschauungsmaterial. Medizinische Sach- und Fachtexte waren dagegen weitgehend rezepthaft-theoretisch und, damit zusammenhängend, wesentlich arztzentriert (vgl. Riha 2009: 99-101), so dass sie für die Frage nach dem ‚Sitz im Leben', den Krankheit für den Betroffenen selbst und für seine soziale Umgebung hatte, wenig Aufschluss geben. Wenigstens zum Teil gilt das auch für den quantitativ wohl bedeutendsten Bereich der literarischen Thematisierung von Krankheit: den der Heilungswunder in der Hagiographie. Hier liegt der Akzent eo ipso auf dem Umschlag von der Krankheit in die spontane, wunderbare Genesung der Patienten durch die Fürsprache des jeweiligen Heiligen bei Gott anstatt auf dem Erleben der Krankheit selbst. Als gattungstypische Bestandteile der Vita von Heiligen sind diese katalogartig aufgezählten Heilungswunder ohnehin denn auch keine eigenständigen ‚Krankengeschichten'.

Die Geschichten von kranken Protagonisten beiderlei Geschlechts, die ich in der Folge aufgreife und im Blick auf die Gender-Thematik untersuche, bewegen sich in einem Spannungsfeld von unterschiedlich gestufter Historizität und Literarizität, ‚Biographik' und Fiktion. Der literarische Filter ist also bei der Bewertung der Geschichten zu berücksichtigen. Denn dieser ‚entobjektiviert' einerseits zwar den Einblick in die historische Lebenswirklichkeit von Kranken, setzt andererseits aber durchaus auch einen in ‚objektiven' Krankheitsprotokollen fehlenden Raum der Artikulation von Vorstellungen, Wünschen und Ängsten frei, der selbst wieder einen historischen Erkenntniswert besitzen kann. Das gilt umso mehr, wenn man bedenkt, dass im Mittelalter medizinisches Wissen und Laienwissen über körperliche Abläufe noch kaum auseinanderklafften, da die Grundzüge der Humoralpathologie allgemein bekannt waren und auch keine „hermetische Fachsprache" (Riha 2009: 100) existierte. Bei meinen Beispielen handelt es sich – angesichts der Absenz von Autorinnen entsprechender Werke notgedrungen – um Texte, deren Autoren allesamt Männer waren. Der literarische Filter ist zugleich also auch bereits ‚gegendert'. Es handelt sich um geistliche und höfisch-weltliche Autoren, aber durchweg nicht um Mediziner. Die Textbeispiele kreisen um zwei Krankheiten bzw. Symptomkomplexe:

1. die der Lepra und

2. die einer von Geburt an vorliegenden Lähmung.

Beide kommen meiner literatur- und kulturgeschichtlichen Frage nach Genderperspektiven auf die Erfahrung von und den Umgang mit Krankheit insofern besonders entgegen, als sie keine unmittelbare, akute Todesfolge nach sich ziehen, sondern mit einer chronisch andauernden Prozesshaftigkeit verbunden waren, deren spezifische Auswirkungen zudem noch über die in die kranken Protagonisten selbst projizierte Innenperspektive hinaus auch die Frage nach der gesellschaftlichen Isolation oder Integration der Kranken beleuchten.

1. Mittelalterliche Erzählungen von Leprakranken: Genderperspektiven auf Hartmanns von Aue *Der Arme Heinrich* im motivgeschichtlichen Kontext

1.1 Lepra ('Aussatz') im Mittelalter

Nachdem man im Mittelalter noch nichts von einem bakteriologischen Paradigma oder dem „Abgleich zwischen klinischer Symptomatik und pathologisch-anatomischem Substrat" (Riha 2009: 99) wusste, war unbekannt, dass Lepra von dem *mycobacterium leprae* verursacht ist. Die Übertragungswege sind bis heute noch nicht restlos geklärt, auch wenn Tröpfcheninfektion als wahrscheinlich gilt (vgl. Riha 2006: 17). Man wusste lediglich um die mit Lepra verbundene Ansteckungsgefahr als solche, die Krankheit selbst galt aber als unheilbar. Die förmlich-offizielle Feststellung der Indikation Lepra im Zuge der Lepraschau zog als Rechtsfolge die lebenslange Separierung der Kranken nach sich.

Lepröse vagabundierten als Bettler oder waren, vermehrt seit dem 13. Jahrhundert, in Leprosorien meist an Ausfallstraßen oder Wegkreuzungen außerhalb von Ansiedlungen und Städten untergebracht. Die Separierung der Kranken von den Gesunden verband sich „mit sehr drastischen Ausschlussriten". Diese konnten bis hin zur Teilnahme der Kranken an ihrer eigenen Totenmesse und symbolischer ‚Beerdigung' reichen, die zur Ausstattung der Kranken mit spezieller Kleidung (Umhang, Hut/Kapuze) und dem Segregationsgebot des Tragens dieser Kleidung sowie der zugehörigen Attribute (Handschuhe, Bettelsack, Klapper/Glocke/Horn) oft noch hinzukam (vgl. Jankrift 2003: 124; Uhrmacher 2005: 100f.).

Die Lepraschau selbst orientierte sich anders als in der naturwissenschaftlich begründeten Medizin an den sichtbaren (Körper-)Zeichen; es handelte sich deshalb eher um Semiotik als um Diagnostik im modernen Sinn (vgl. Jankrift 2003: 124). Bei aller damit verbundenen Gefahr von Missinterpretation konnten die

Zeichen der Lepra in der Tat als äußerlich gut sichtbar gelten (vgl. Jankrift 2003: ˙120),[5] großenteils schon im Gesicht des Kranken,[6] und daher als allgemein bekannt vorausgesetzt werden. Sie gingen denn auch in die Dichtung ein, wo das Erzählmotiv der Lepra als das exemplarische Paradigma schlechthin für das Phänomen des Ausgesetztseins einer Krankheit und zugleich des Ausgesetztseins aus der Gemeinschaft der Gesunden diente (vgl. Oswald 2008: 23-44)[7]: Die Beschreibung der Leprasymptomatik etwa aus dem ca. 1280 entstandenen *Arzneibuch* des in Würzburg tätigen, viel rezipierten Wundarztes Ortolf von Baierlant unterscheidet sich substanziell kaum von der Beschreibung des aussätzigen Dieterich aus der ebenfalls im 13. Jahrhundert entstandenen Versdichtung *Engelhard* des Konrad von Würzburg. So heißt es bei Ortolf von Baierlant:

> Man sal eynen außeczigen also erkennen: Jm vallen dy wintpran vß den augen vnd dy augen werden schiblot [= kreisrund] in dem hawbt. Er wirt heyszer in der kelen vnd hat pfinnen in dem münde vnter der zungen vnd an der zungen. Vnd der pal zwischen dem dawmen vnd den vingeren swindet im.

(zitiert nach Riha 2009: 103)

Und bei Konrad von Würzburg:

> Im [= dem kranken Dieterich] wurden hâr und bart
> dünn unde seltsæne.
> sîn ougen, als ich wæne,
> begunden sich dô gilwen.
> als ob si æzen milwen,
> sô vielen ûz die brâwen drobe.
> sîn varwe, die dâ vor zu lobe
> liutsælich was unde guot,
> diu wart noch rœter danne ein bluot
> und gap vil egebæren schîn.
> diu lûtersüeze stimme sîn
> wart ûnmâzen heiser.
> im schuof des himels kaiser
> grôz leit an allen enden.

---

[5] Lepraschauen konnten auch Nicht-Mediziner vornehmen (vgl. Meyer 2007: 145-52; Uhrmacher 2005: 102f.).

[6] Vgl. vier der sechs *signa univoca* von Lepra im Gesicht (*facies leonina*), z.B. nach Guy de Chauliac: „Augen und Ohren runden sich, die Augenbrauen schwellen an und verlieren die Haare, die Nase treibt auf […] und die Lippen nehmen eine Missgestalt an" (Meier 2007: 126).

[7] Vgl. auch die hier enthaltene ausführliche Verzeichnung neuerer Forschung zu Lepra im Mittelalter unter Einschluss der medizinischen, sozialen und religiösen Dimensionen der Thematik.

an füezen unde an henden
wâren im die ballen
sô genzlich în gevallen
daz mich sîn immer wundert.

(vv. 5150-5168)

Die äußerlichen Zeichen der Krankheit, wie sie in der Dichtung für die anderen Protagonisten wahrnehmbar werden, sind sogar detaillierter beschrieben als im *Arzneibuch* und zugleich – im Blick auf die Reaktion der Beteiligten – vom Erzähler emotionalisierend ausgestaltet.[8] Umgekehrt fehlt hier, wiederum ganz im Sinne der Funktion dieser *descriptio* innerhalb der erzählten Geschichte, der erst bei näherer Untersuchung zu erkennende Befund im Mund- und Rachenraum, wie ihn Ortolf beschreibt. Bereits an der Gegenüberstellung dieser beiden Beispiele wird also auch der unterschiedliche Erkenntniswert von Dichtung gegenüber Fachliteratur deutlich.

1.2 Silvesterlegende vs. *Armer Heinrich*:
Der Kranke und das Geschlecht des therapeutischen Blutes

Das Aussatzmotiv begegnet in der mittelhochdeutschen Literatur häufig. Schon vor Hartmann von Aue wird es mehrfach in der *Kaiserchronik* thematisiert und dient dort zur Figurenzeichnung heidnischer Herrscher.[9] Auch die im Mittelalter bekannteste Geschichte einer Aussatzheilung, diejenige aus der Silvesterlegende, begegnet unter anderem hier (vv. 7806-7948): Der von Gott wegen seiner Christenverfolgung mit Aussatz geschlagene Kaiser Konstantin d. Gr. erfährt

---

[8] Ausgabe: Konrad von Würzburg, *Engelhard*, 1963; vgl. dazu auch die Einleitungs- und Abschlussverse der *descriptio*: „Sîn lîp der wol gehandelte/wart vil schiere dort geslagen/mit dem vil armen siechtagen/den man dâ heizet miselsuht./diu viel ûf in mit der genuht/daz er mitalle ûzsetzic wart" (vv. 5144-5149) bzw. „sîn lîp der wart gesundert/vil gar von schœnen sachen/und wart mit ungemachen jæmerlichen überladen" (vv. 5169-5171).

[9] Ausgabe: Hartmann von Aue, *Der arme Heinrich*, 1993; Ausgabe: Schröder, *Deutsche Kaiserchronik*, 1964. In der Chronik dient insbesondere der heidnische Kaiser Domitian neben dem berüchtigten Nero als Negativbeispiel für das Verhalten des Aussätzigen (*Kaiserchronik* vv. 5662-5674): „Si swuoren alle gemainlîchen,/daz si in ze tôde sluogen/oder alsô lebendic in di erde begruoben./Alsô der kunic Domîcîânus vernam,/daz in Rômære wolten reslahen,/dô muos er in entrinnen./er hiez im ain ros gewinnen,/er kêrte ingegen der brucke./alsô er kom in almitten, –/daz liet saget uns ân zwîvel: – /daz ros sluog in in die Tîver./in gesah nie niemen mêre./die tievel wîzent sîn sêle." Ein positives und theologisch ‚korrektes' Gegenbeispiel stellt der zur Zeit des Pontius Pilatus amtierende Kaisers Tiberius dar, den die *Kaiserchronik* zugleich als Gründer Regensburgs herausstellt (vv. 671-852): Er wird vom Aussatz durch seine Meditation über dem Schweißtuch gereinigt, in das Jesus auf dem Weg nach Golgatha, wo er sein Blut zur Erlösung der Menschheit hingab, sein Gesicht abgedrückt hat. (Vgl. zum Schweißtuch der Veronika im Kontext der Lepra: Meier 2007: 132).

von einem weisen Mann, dass ihn Blut von bis zu zwei Jahre alten Säuglingen heilen kann. Er zwingt alle Mütter dazu, ihre *kindelîn* nach Rom zu bringen, um deren Blut in einem großen Bad zu sammeln. Als Konstantin die verzweifelten Klagen der Mütter vom Kapitol aus wahrnimmt, wird er nachdenklich. Die Apostel Petrus und Paulus erscheinen ihm im Traum und verweisen ihn auf Papst Silvester. Konstantin wird von diesem zum Christentum bekehrt. Im Taufwasser fällt der Aussatz von ihm ab, und das Christentum wird fortan zur Staatsreligion: soweit die Ursprungserzählung von der christlichen Verfasstheit der europäischen Politik und Kultur. Dass derartiger therapeutischer Einsatz von Blut ein Erzählmotiv, aber keine historische Realität war – weder in der Antike noch im Mittelalter (vgl. Eis 1973: 135-51) –, braucht kaum betont zu werden, wenngleich sich christlicherseits die Vorstellung vom Blut auch mit dem Erlösungswerk Jesu am Kreuz verbinden konnte[10] und medizinischerseits bei der Lepradiagnostik die sog. Seihprobe, wonach durch Erhitzung von Aderlassblut des Aussätzigen erdige Bestandteile zu Tage träten, mit Blut in Verbindung stand (vgl. Jankrift 2003: 30; Riha 2009: 103).

Die Geschichte vom Armen Heinrich kennt anders als die in der Silvesterlegende keinen epochalen Umschlag vom Heidentum zum Christentum, wie er in der Figur von Aussatzerkrankung und -heilung des Kaisers abgebildet wird. Sie profiliert auch nicht die damit verbundene geschichtsphilosophische Demonstrationslogik. Hartmanns Figur des Armen Heinrich ist vielmehr ein für die hochmittelalterliche deutsche Dichtung typischer höfisch-christlicher Protagonist, weder ein Heiliger noch ein Übeltäter, sondern tatsächlich ein ‚Patient': Durch den Aussatz wird der kranke Adlige aus seinem Leben in der Gesellschaft gerissen und zieht sich, nachdem er die besten Ärzte vergeblich konsultiert hat, von Hoffnungslosigkeit erfüllt auf einen Meierhof zurück, den einer seiner Dienstleute bewirtschaftet. Das einzige Heilmittel, das er von einem Arzt in Salerno erfahren hat, steht ihm nicht zur Verfügung: ein Bad im Blut einer Jungfrau, die ihr Leben freiwillig für seine Genesung opfert. Verzweifelt bringt er seine Tage damit zu, mit Gott und mit sich selbst zu hadern. Als sich ihm wider Erwarten in Ge-stalt der zum Opfer bereiten Tochter seines Bediensteten die Heilungsmöglichkeit anbietet, ergreift er die Gelegenheit und reist mit dem Mädchen nach Salerno. Im letzten Moment, unmittelbar bevor der Arzt das Operationsmesser ansetzt, besinnt sich Heinrich und verzichtet auf den Tod des Mädchens, obwohl dieses wütend darauf besteht, für ihn sterben zu wollen. Auf wunderbare Weise wird er wegen seines Verzichts auf das Opfer geheilt und heiratet schließlich das Mädchen.

An die Stelle einer Symbolik der Bekehrung zum christlichen Glauben, wie sie in der Silvesterlegende mit der Ersetzung des Kinderblutes durch Taufwasser

---

[10] Theologisch ‚korrekt' ist diese Vorstellung freilich nicht (vgl. Dieckmann 2011: 183).

vorliegt, rückt in Hartmanns Erzählung die Programmatik einer Krankenge-schichte, genauer: einer Geschichte des Kranken und einer Geschichte der Men-schen in seiner Umgebung, insbesondere des opferbereiten Mädchens. Bemer-kenswert ist hier schon der Befund, dass parallel zur nunmehr vorausgesetzten Freiwilligkeit des Opfers (im Unterschied zu dessen gewaltsamer Anordnung in der Silvesterlegende) auch die Spezifikation einhergeht, wonach das Opfer weiblichen Geschlechts und jungfräulich-rein zu sein hat. Man wird darin durch-aus eine Art Gender-Automatismus sehen können, der eher soziale als medizini-sche Perspektiven aufweist.

1.2.1 Das Selbstverhältnis des kranken Heinrich

Der Kranke braucht die ‚weibliche' Opferbereitschaft, um in einem langen inne-ren Prozess an den Punkt zu gelangen, seine Krankheit nicht nur als Gegensatz zu einem allein mit Gesundheit verbundenen Begriff von Leben wahrzunehmen, gleichsam als Weder-Leben-noch-Sterben. Seine Absolutsetzung des Heilungs-wunsches kann der Kranke erst dann reflektieren, als er das ersehnte, einzige Heilmittel wirklich vor Augen hat, um es zu erproben: Die literarische Inszenie-rung führt vor, wie der Protagonist an diesem Punkt endlich seine Krankheit an-nimmt, weil er erkennt, dass auch er ein neues, würdiges Leben gewinnt, wenn er das Leben der aufopferungsvollen (Jung-)Frau bewahrt. Eine *niuwe güete* tritt an die Stelle seiner bisherigen Haltung (vv. 1238-1240). Das Annehmen der Krankheit ist Voraussetzung für die Heilung und damit zugleich conditio sine qua non für das wunderbare Eingreifen Gottes. Die Opferbereitschaft der (Jung-) Frau ist für die literarische Inszenierung von Heinrichs innerem Prozess also nö-tig, gleichzeitig aber am Ende entbehrlich, ja suspekt.

1.2.2 Das Selbstverhältnis des opferbereiten Mädchens

Die Innenperspektive, die der opferbereiten (Jung-)Frau zugeschrieben wird, ist denn auch genau passförmig mit dem inneren Prozess des Kranken verzahnt: Die ‚weibliche' Opferbereitschaft erfüllt das Kriterium der Freiwilligkeit, ist da-rum aber keineswegs schon uneigennützig. Das zeigt die handfeste Argumenta-tion des Mädchens, als es im Gespräch mit seinen Eltern die Entscheidung für das Opfer legitimiert: Neben religiösen Argumenten dominiert hier der Aspekt lebenspraktischer und sozialer Vorteilhaftigkeit für das Mädchen selbst und für seine vom Wohlergehen wie von der Geneigtheit des Dienstherren abhängigen Familie. Nur ein kleiner Auszug aus der Rede sei hier als Beispiel zitiert:

> wir hân niht gewisses mê
> wan hiute wol und morgen wê

und ie ze jungest der tôt:
daz ist ein jæmerlîchiu nôt.
[...]
belîbe ich âne man bî iu
zwei jâr ode driu,
sô ist mîn herre lîhte tôt,
und komen in sô grôze nôt
vil lîhte von armuot,
daz ir mir selhez guot
zeinem man niht muget geben,
ich enmüeze alsô swache leben,
daz ich iu lieber wære tôt.
[...]
mîn gert ein vrîer bûman, dem ich wol mînes lîbes gan.
zewâre, dem sult ir mich geben,
sô ist geschaffen wol mîn leben.
im gât sîn phluoc harte wol,
sîn hof ist alles râtes vol.
da enstirbet ros noch daz rint,
da enmüent diu weinenden kint,
da enist ze heiz noch ze kalt,
da enwirt von jâren niemen alt
(der alte wirt junger),
da enist vrost noch hunger,
da enist deheiner slahte leit,
da ist ganziu vreude âne arbeit.
ze dem wil ich mich ziehen
und selhen bû vliehen,
den der schûr und der hagel sleht
und der wâc abe tweht,
mit dem man ringet unde ie ranc.

(vv. 712-715, 747-755, 775-793)

Die heftige, geradezu hysterische Abwehrreaktion des Mädchens auf die Ver-
schonung vor dem Blutopfer ist entsprechend, sieht es doch die Erfüllung seines
Wunsches dahinschwinden, aus dem beengten, mühseligen Leben in die para-
diesische ,Hofhaltung' beim himmlischen Bräutigam zu gelangen. Am Ende
heißt es nur:

Swie vil sî vlüeche unde bete
unde ouch scheltens getete,
daz enmohte ir niht vrum wesen:
sî muose iedoch genesen.

(vv. 1333-1336)

1.2.3 Sucht nach Heilung – Sucht nach Heil:
Gegenderte literarische Rolleninszenierung als Funktion gegenderter
sozialer Handlungsspielräume?

Trotz aller genderspezifischer Variation bei der Besetzung der Opferrolle nimmt
in den Erzählungen von Aussatzheilungen durch Blutopfer stets ein Mann die
Figur des Kranken ein. Liegt das nur daran, dass Männer die Autoren dieser Erzählungen waren, oder besaß im Kontext patriarchalischer Geschlechterlogik die
Auseinandersetzung mit (eigener) Krankheit und Ohnmacht bei Männern nicht
doch womöglich auch eine spezifische Relevanz? In Hartmanns Erzählung will
der Kranke nur als Gesunder leben. Als Gesunder hatte er eigene Handlungsspielräume und als Geheilter gewinnt er diese auch wieder zurück. Das Mädchen
hingegen will aus seinem beengten Leben ins Paradies entfliehen. Es hatte selbst
als gesundes Mitglied der Gesellschaft keine Handlungsspielräume und gewinnt
diese am Ende auch nur vermittelt durch den/ihren Mann. Der Körper ist ihr
hauptsächliches (bzw. einziges) Kapital. ‚Weibliche' Hingabe an den Mann und
Selbstdefinition über das Wohlergehen des Mannes werden damit ebenso bestätigt wie die Überlegenheit des Mannes. Wenn in der modernen Hartmann-Re-
zeption Dichter wie Wilhelm Grimm oder Gerhard Hauptmann die Opferbereitschaft des Mädchens als Ausdruck oder Entdeckung ‚reiner' Liebe zu neuen Eh-
ren gebracht haben, ändert sich daran übrigens wenig. Es ist dies bloß eine andere, ‚zeitgemäße' Form, das Gleiche zu legitimieren, die die Pille der Geschlech-
terhierarchie noch dazu mit einer verführerisch süßen Hülle umgibt.

1.3 (Kranker) Körper und Geschlecht: Körper haben – Körper sein

Mit gesellschaftlichen Rollenzuschreibungen korrespondiert im Mittelalter auch
der Stellenwert des Körpers bzw. der Körperhaftigkeit, der dem Mann und der
Frau zugeschrieben wird. Ausgehend von den Beobachtungen zu Hartmanns
Erzählung vom Armen Heinrich und dem opferbereiten Mädchen sei dies
zumindest kurz noch vertieft, um so auch einen Anschluss an den folgenden
Punkt meines Beitrags herzustellen. Gemäß einer langen Auslegungstradition
zur Genesiserzählung definierte man die Frau, Erbin Evas, als vom Körper des
Mannes (der Rippe Adams) abgeleitetes, also ganz und gar ‚körperliches' Ge-
schöpf, das nur in Vermittlung über Geist und Seele des Mannes seinen Anteil
an der Göttlichkeit des Schöpfers bezieht. Der spätantike Kirchenlehrer Au-
gustinus attestierte demzufolge, wirkmächtig für das Mittelalter, der Frau lediglich eine Hilfsfunktion für die Fortpflanzung des Mannes, bevor Thomas von
Aquin im 13. Jahrhundert mit seinem berühmten *dictum* von der Frau als miss-
glücktem Mann (*femina est mas occasionatus*) der Frau sogar den Status des

‚anderen' Geschlechts absprach.[11] Dass in den bildlichen Sündenfalldarstel-
lungen stets Eva die Hand zum Apfel führt, ist eines von vielen Beispielen für
die Auffassung von der auf Nahrung und leiblichen Genuss ausgerichteten
Körperverhaftetheit der Frau. In diesem Sinn geht die Frau im Körperlichen auf,
‚ist' sie Körper, während der Mann einen Körper ‚hat' und kraft seines Geistes
entscheidet, ob er diesem nachgibt (wie Adam) oder nicht. Es liegt nahe, den
hier zugrundeliegenden Gegensatz zwischen Mann und Frau zunächst einmal
wenigstens hypothetisch auch auf den Umgang von Mann und Frau mit dem
kranken Körper zu übertragen. Gilt also:

Körper haben (Mann) vs. Körper sein (Frau)

=

Krankheit haben (Mann) vs. Krankheit sein (Frau) ?

Für die gesellschaftlich konditionierte (Selbst-)Wahrnehmung eines kranken
Mannes und einer kranken Frau resultierte dann daraus, dass es als ‚männlich'
kodiert ist, genauso wie den gesunden Körper auch die körperliche Krankheit zu
beherrschen, d.h. wie einen Gegner zu bekämpfen, als ‚weiblich' hingegen, sich
mit ihr zu identifizieren. Um dem genauer nachzugehen, ist eine Fallanalyse
notwendig, die es ermöglicht, die Krankengeschichte eines Mannes auch direkt
mit der Krankengeschichte einer Frau zu vergleichen. Dies soll nun am Beispiel
von Hermannus contractus, dem ‚Lahmen', und von Margareta contracta, der
‚Krüppel', wenigstens noch skizziert werden.

2. Mittelalterliche Viten von Gelähmten:
Genderperspektiven auf Hermannus contractus und Margareta contracta

2.1 Lähmung im Mittelalter

Lähmung sei hier als Sammelbegriff verstanden, der sich im Sinn mittelalterlicher Medizin am sichtbaren Zeichen orientiert und deshalb auch auf eine Unter-
scheidung zwischen Krankheit als Ursache und Behinderung als symptomati-
scher Folge verzichtet. Das Spektrum dessen, was im Mittelalter unter ‚Lähmung' kursierte, reicht so von der Apoplexie- bis zur Unfallfolge. Heilungsmi-
rakel in Legenden erwähnen besonders häufig Gelähmte, und hier wiederum besonders gelähmte Kinder (vgl. Goetz 2009: 21-55; Wittmer-Butsch 2003). Ab-
gesehen von Unfallfolgen dürften sich hinter diesen Lähmungen vor allem die

---

[11] Vgl. zu diesem viel behandelten Thema u.a. Feistner 1999, Fritsch-Staar 1999, Haag 1999,
Spreitzer 1999.

ansteckende Virusinfektion der Poliomyelitis oder infantile Cerebralparese infolge von Komplikationen beim Geburtsvorgang verborgen haben. Meine Beispiele sind zumindest dadurch spezifiziert, dass in beiden Fällen eine Lähmung

1. (wohl) von Geburt an vorliegt, dass sie sich

2. nicht nur an den Extremitäten manifestiert, sondern am ganzen Körper bis hin zu erschwerter Artikulation und Nahrungsaufnahme, und dass sie

3. einen Schweregrad aufweist, der den Betroffenen ohne fremde Hilfe weder Fortbewegung noch Aufrechtstehen, z.T. nicht einmal Aufrechtsitzen oder Zurseitedrehen ermöglichte, sie also existentiell von Dauerpflege abhängig machte.

Gerade in Fällen derart gravierender körperlichen Beeinträchtigung aber besitzt Gender als soziales Geschlecht eine hohe Relevanz: Behinderte wurden zwar als Objekte der Fürsorge betrachtet, doch diese Fürsorge hatte durchaus ihre Grenzen (vgl. Goetz 2009: 21-55; Irsigler 2009: 165-81).[12] Umso entscheidender muss der jeweilige Sozialstatus gewesen sein, wenn es um die Frage ging, wie Behinderte gesellschaftlich integriert waren bzw. ob sie nicht innerhalb der Gesellschaft ähnlich isoliert waren wie Lepröse am Rande der Gesellschaft. Sicher nicht zufällig unterscheidet sich der Fall des Hermannus contractus so stark von dem der Margareta contracta, selbst wenn es sich nur um je einen Einzelfall handelt und schon die Tatsache als solche, dass für eine(n) Körperbehinderte(n) überhaupt eine eigene Vita vorliegt, als Ausnahme gelten kann.

2.2 Beschreibungshorizonte:
Zum Blick auf die Körperbehinderung eines Mannes und einer Frau

2.2.1 Hermannus contractus (Hermann von Reichenau)

Hermann von Reichenau, im Mittelalter unter dem Namen Hermannus contractus bekannt, ist u.a. urkundlich gut dokumentiert[13] und lebte vom 18. Juli 1013 bis zum 24. September 1054. Als Adeliger entstammte er dem Geschlecht der Grafen von Altshausen und fand dank der engen Beziehungen, die sein Vater zum Benediktinerklosters Reichenau als dessen Förderer hatte, dort mit sieben Jahren Aufnahme als Schüler, dann als Mönch, Wissenschaftler und Lehrer. Entgegen kirchenrechtlicher Vorschrift erhielt er sogar trotz seiner körperlichen Gebrechen die Priesterweihe. Aus seiner Vita, die Berthold von Reichenau, ehe-

---

[12] Hierzu auch Horn 2009: 303-16; Knackmuß 2009: 335-68.
[13] Die folgenden Angaben nach Berschin 2005: 15-32; vgl. auch Benz 2007.

maliger Schüler, Mitbruder und Freund Hermanns verfasste (vgl. Robinson 2003: 163-74), geht hervor, dass man dem Gelähmten eigens einen Tragstuhl gebaut und wohl auch Sekretäre gestellt hat, damit sein umfangreiches Werk aufgezeichnet werden konnte, da er selbst nur mit Einschränkungen in der Lage war zu schreiben.[14] Der Abt des Klosters, Bern von Reichenau, schätzte sein Potenzial und ermöglichte ihm großzügig gelehrte Buchkommunikation. Als Chronist und geistlicher Dichter, vor allem aber als Mathematiker und Astronom war Hermannus nicht nur bis in die frühe Neuzeit bekannt, sondern hat sich seit den Anfängen der Wissenschaftsgeschichte bis heute einen Namen gemacht. Als Behinderter ist er auch aktuelle Vorbild- und Identifikationsfigur – Peter Radtke hat seiner Person ein Theaterstück gewidmet –, eben deswegen, weil er nicht nur Behinderter war, sondern trotz Behinderung ein renommierter Gelehrter. Schon im Mittelalter wird er auf Abbildungen hoch aufgerichtet, z.T. sogar im Stehen, und meist überhaupt bloß mit äußerst diskreter, auf das Krückenattribut beschränkter Andeutung seiner Behinderung dargestellt.[15]

Eine solche Perspektive zeigt sich auch in Bertholds *Vita Herimanni*. Diese stellt sich als Produkt literarischer Stilisierung hinsichtlich Struktur und Diktion trotz Anklängen an die Hagiographie in die rhetorische Tradition des Personenlobs. Schon ihr Aufbau ist signifikant: Eingeteilt in fünf Kapitel, beginnt sie mit einer allgemeinen lobenden Würdigung Hermanns, auf die im II. Kapitel eine gerafft abstrahierende Skizze seiner Lebensweise, seiner Vorzüge und Eigenschaften folgt. Die beiden letzten Kapitel berichten über Hermanns letzte Lebensphase, darüber, wie sich sein Gesundheitszustand verschlechtert, er gewünscht habe, „aus dem beschwerlichen Gefängnis dieser Welt" (Berschin 2005: 11) endlich befreit zu werden (Kap. IV), und er wenig später auch tatsächlich starb (Kap. V). Genau im Zentrum aber, im III. Kapitel, stehen, in zwei der Überlieferungszeugen durch die Überschrift *Studium Her(i)manni* optisch noch eigens markiert (Berschin 2005: 8), seine literarischen und wissenschaftlichen Werke. Kern der Vita ist also das, was nicht den behinderten Körper tangiert. Dementsprechend wird bereits in den beiden ersten Kapiteln die körperliche Beeinträchtigung zwar zumindest insoweit, wie es der Diskretion des rhetorischen *aptum* entspricht, durchaus beschrieben, aber konsequent durch Adversativpartikel von Hermanns geistiger Leistungsfähigkeit abgegrenzt, so dass diese in ein umso helleres Licht rückt.

---

[14] Vgl. Kapitel I und II der *Vita Herimanni* (Berthold von der Reichenau 2005: 6, 8).
[15] Vgl. Benz 2007, mit reichem Anschauungsmaterial vom Mittelalter bis zur Gegenwart.

2.2.2 Margareta contracta (Margareta von Magdeburg)

Als Verfasser der Vita Margaretas von Magdeburg nennt sich der Dominikaner Johannes von Magdeburg, Beichtvater der Gelähmten.[16] Weder über ihn noch über Margareta selbst weiß man außerhalb dieser Vita irgendetwas. So wenig mithin die Historizität des dort Berichteten als solches überprüfbar ist, so sicher ist dennoch die Historizität der Vita als Dokument eines literarischen Interesses am Blick auf das Leben einer körperlich schwer behinderten Frau. Die volkssprachlichen Bearbeitungen der lateinischen Vita des Johannes von Magdeburg sind bis heute freilich nicht einmal ediert.[17] Das wissenschaftliche Interesse liegt, wenn überhaupt, innerhalb der Mystikforschung. Vielfach stand dabei bislang jedoch der ‚höhere' Zweck von Margaretas körperlichem Leid im Fokus, ihr Zwiegespräch mit Gott, während der Blick auf die Art, wie der Text ihr körperliches Leid selbst beschreibt, dahinter zurücktrat.[18]

   Die Vita wird auf ca. 1260/70 datiert. Nachdem sie Margaretas Geburtsdatum nicht nennt und auch nicht bis zu deren Tod reicht, sind keine exakten Angaben möglich; ob Margareta, wie ihr von Johannes als prophetisches Vorwissen zugeschrieben wird, im „Alter Jesu Christi", also mit 32 Jahren, gestorben ist, muss offen bleiben (vgl. Schmidt 1992: 85 [Kap. 63]). Laut Vita entstammt sie (dies eine Parallele zu dem Mädchen in Hartmanns Erzählung) einem inferioren sozialen Kontext, wo körperliche Leistungsfähigkeit überlebenswichtig ist. Dass Margareta, so lange sie als Kind noch klein und leicht genug dafür ist, auf dem Arm einer blinden Arbeitskraft bzw. ihrer eigenen blinden Mutter die Aufgabe einer Seh-Hilfe übernimmt,[19] setzt ins Bild: Nur in dem Maß, wie ihr Körper als ‚Krücke' für andere funktioniert, kommt sie selbst voran. Nachdem man Margareta mit den Jahren spüren lässt, dass sie für den Dienstbetrieb im Haushalt hinderlich ist (Schmidt 1992: 4 [Kap. 3]),[20] schließt sie sich mit 12 Jahren der seinerzeit institutionalisierten Lebensform des Reklusentums an, d.h. sie bezieht eine ‚Klause' in der Stadt, lebt dort von Almosen der Bewohner und übernimmt

---

[16] Zitiergrundlage ist die Ausgabe von Paul Gerhard Schmidt (Schmidt 1992).

[17] Ruh (*Verfasserlexikon* 1978ff., Sp. 788) erwähnt eine unedierte niederländische Übertragung aus dem 17. Jh. (Antwerpen, Kapuzinerarchiv, cod. V 149). Ich beziehe mich in der Folge auf die deutsche Abbreviatur in der Handschrift mgq 191 (Staatsbibliothek zu Berlin, Preußischer Kulturbesitz), fol. 244r-256r.

[18] Vgl. Ruh 1993: 125-29; besonders deutlich Weiß 1995. Ganz anders als bei Hermannus contractus hat man bei Margareta contracta bezeichnenderweise auch kein Interesse an einer medizinischen Krankheitsdiagnostik gezeigt (vgl. die Diskussion des Mediziners Christoph Brunhölzl: Brunhölzl 1999: 239-43).

[19] Ersteres in der lateinischen Vita (Schmidt 1992: 3 [Kap. 2]), Letzteres in der deutschen Bearbeitung (mgq 191, fol. 244r).

[20] In der genannten deutschen Version ist zumindest die grausame Rücksichtslosigkeit der eigenen Mutter abgemildert.

dafür die Dienstleistung des Gebets und des religiösen Zuspruchs. Bedingt durch ihren schlechten Gesundheitszustand und durch das teils unliebsame Aufsehen, das sie erregt, wird sie aber schließlich in ein Frauenkloster verbracht (vgl. Schmidt 1992: 88 [Kap. 64] bzw. 51 [Kap. 47]). Dort sorgt man, freilich ohne sie als reguläre Nonne aufzunehmen, für ihr Überleben, und gelegentlich wird sie von dem Dominikaner Johannes besucht, der sie schon als Rekluse seelsorgerlich betreut hat. Seine *Vita Margarete contracte* wirkt streckenweise auch tatsächlich wie eine Aneinanderreihung von Gesprächseindrücken.

Diese konzeptionelle Perspektive führt zusammen mit der gender- bzw. hierarchiebedingten Verfügbarkeit des Beschreibungsobjekts dazu, dass Krankheit und Behinderung hier ungleich detaillierter beschrieben sind als in Bertholds *Vita Herimanni*. Schon deshalb, weil Johannes die Leiden der Margareta im Zusammenhang mit jedem seiner Besuche stets aufs Neue thematisiert, zieht sich der Blick auf den Körper wie ein roter Faden durch den gesamten Text: Man erfährt, wie sie hinfällt und hilflos liegen bleibt, wie sich ihre Gesichtszüge infolge spasmischer Kontraktionen verzerren und sie Probleme bei der Nahrungsaufnahme oder mit unkontrollierbarem Schluckauf hat, wie Tränenflüssigkeit aus ihren Augen und Schleim aus Nase und Mund herausläuft, wie ihr Hemd nach Schweißausbrüchen durchnässt ist, wie sie an unerträglichen Kopfschmerzen leidet.[21] Und da der leidende Körper zugleich Dreh- und Angelpunkt für die religiösen Gespräche der Margareta mit ihrem Beichtvater ist, stellt er überhaupt das beherrschende Thema dieser Vita dar. Noch mehr als für den lateinischen Text gilt dies für die bisher unerforschte deutsche Bearbeitung in der Berliner Handschrift mgq 191, denn die dogmatisch verallgemeinernden Lehrkapitel, die Johannes in die ‚Krankengeschichte' inseriert,[22] sind dort systematisch getilgt. Als auch wirkungsgeschichtlich besonders relevant erweist sich damit vor allem zweierlei: der durchaus indiskrete Blick auf den kranken Körper der Frau und das bewundernde Interesse daran, wie sie diesen Körper nicht nur hinnimmt, sondern mit aller Konsequenz bejaht. Denn sie betrachtet ihn als Liebesgabe Jesu Christi und sieht sich durch ihr Leiden nicht nur gezeichnet, sondern ausgezeichnet. Das Leiden bedarf, derart zur *raison d'être* nobiliert, keiner Linderung. Nur so erlangt Margareta immerhin auch innere Unabhängigkeit von menschlicher Zuwendung und Hilfe. Johannes von Magdeburg erlebt dies selbst, als sein Versuch scheitert, die Kranke durch Besuchsverweigerung zu strafen, um sie dahin zu bringen, ihrem Körper nicht auch noch durch Askese zuzusetzen.

---

[21] Zusammenfassend auch in der Einleitung zur Ausgabe von Schmidt 1992: XI; vgl. als kleine Auswahl von Beispielen ebenda: 18, 22f., 51, 53, 84, 88.
[22] Vgl. in der Ausgabe von Schmidt 1992: XIIIf.

2.3 Deutungshorizonte:
Behinderung und Geschlecht im Paradigma von Geist und Körper

Das unterschiedliche Maß der Körperlichkeit, das bei der Definition von Mann und Frau im Mittelalter als gleichsam ‚genetisch' bedingtes Differenzierungskriterium ausschlaggebend war und beide Geschlechter unterschiedlichen Verhaltensmaßstäben unterwarf, manifestiert sich auch in den Viten der beiden Gelähmten: Die *Vita Herimanni* zeichnet das Bild eines am Körper behinderten Mannes, dessen Geist – als das definitorisch ‚Bessere' und ‚Höhere'[23] – in einen Gegensatz zum Körper tritt. Der Geist bricht die Herrschaft des Körpers und erobert sich den Freiraum einer Beschäftigung mit Inhalten, die über den Körperbezug wesentlich hinausgehen, bis der (allen Menschen gemeinsame) endliche Körper den Geist ohnehin loslässt. Die Abgrenzung des Geistes von der Erfahrung des Körpers, die dem Mann zugeschrieben und von ihm gefordert wird, tritt der Vita gemäß bei Hermann gerade wegen seiner lebenslangen Körperbehinderung besonders zu Tage: Hermann verwirklicht das Potenzial des Mannes diszipliniert, lotet die *conditio humana* bis an die Grenzen aus und erfährt dabei von seiner sozialen Umgebung, wiederum Männern, alle erdenkliche Unterstützung.

Demgegenüber entwirft die *Vita Margarete contracte* ein invertiertes Verhältnis von Geist und Körper. An die Stelle des geistig-geistlichen Heraustretens aus dem Körper, das diesen in seine Schranken zu weisen sucht, tritt, ganz im Sinn der als ‚weiblich' interpretierten Identifikation mit dem Körper, bei der behinderten Frau (oder ist dies den Augen des Beobachters/Autors ihrer Vita zuzuschreiben?) ein meditatives Umkreisen der Körpererfahrung. Die Vita zeichnet das Bild einer Frau, deren Geist eine zuallererst auf den Körper bezogene Reflexionsinstanz darstellt und darauf ausgerichtet ist, den Körper in seiner als gottgewollt verstandenen kreatürlichen ‚Gegebenheit' anzunehmen, jeden Widerstand dagegen aber konsequent zu brechen. So entsteht buchstäblich aus der Not eine Tugend: aus dem Leiden am behinderten und kranken Körper und an der Verachtung durch die anderen wird ein göttliches Gnadengeschenk, aus der „Hölle" des Körpers wird eine „Hölle der Erlösung", die noch in der religiösen Übertragung auf das Jenseits den gleichen Status eines Erlösungsortes hat wie das Paradies (vgl. Ruh, 1993). Angesichts des krankheitsbedingten und sozial immer weiter eingeschränkten Handlungsspielraums bleibt Margareta allerdings wenig anderes zu tun übrig, als den Körper selbst zum ‚Buch des Lebens' und das Lesen in diesem ‚Buch' zum Lebensinhalt zu machen. Als *contracta* verkörpert sie ganz konkret die ihrem Geschlecht symbolisch zugeschriebene defizitäre

---

[23] In der ebenfalls um Hermann kreisenden Bärenlegende (vgl. Handschin 1935: 1-8) wird dementsprechend auch eigens erzählt, wie sich dieser schon als Kleinkind bewusst für den Geist und gegen den Körper entschieden habe.

‚Natur'[24] ebenso wie die Defizienz der *conditio humana* überhaupt, an der bei aller genderspezifischen Abstufung auch der Mann Anteil hat. Insofern wirkt Margareta auch aus dem Blickwinkel des Erzählers interessant und in ihrer machtvollen Selbstaufgabe so befremdlich wie beeindruckend.

Vergleicht man die beiden Viten insgesamt miteinander, so wird deutlich: Die Vita der behinderten Frau setzt in permanenter Nahaufnahme genau das ins Bild, was die Vita des behinderten Mannes zwar nicht verbirgt, aber doch so weit wie möglich an den Rand zu schieben sucht: den Körper. Die ‚männliche' Metapher vom Gefängnis des Körpers impliziert die Logik, dass der Mensch die ihn einschränkenden Mauern zu durchbrechen oder zu versetzen strebt, um seinen Lebensspielraum zu erweitern. In der auf Margareta contracta projizierten (bzw. von ihr verinnerlichten) ‚weiblichen' Wendung dieser Metapher erscheint das Gefängnis des Körpers ganz im Gegenteil wie ein Rückzugsort, dessen Ummauerung allein einen Schutzraum für die Seele garantiert, und sei dieser auch so eng, dass er Paradies und Hölle zugleich ist.[25]

Entsprechend unterschiedlich sind beide Viten im Gattungs- und Diskursfächer mittelalterlicher Vitentypen eingeordnet. Diese Einordnung schafft, vom Einzelfall abstrahierend und unabhängig von der Frage nach der historisch-biographischen Authentizität des Beschriebenen, genderrelevante Fakten, selbst dort, wo sich diese ‚nur' als literarische artikulieren.[26] Gerade der aus heutiger Sicht so befremdliche Fall der Margareta contracta ist durchaus kein Einzelfall: Alix von Schaerbeek, die, wohl nur wenig älter, ebenfalls im 13. Jh. lebte und Zisterzienserin im Kloster Mariä Kammeren (La Cambre) bei Brüssel war, erkrankte laut der ihr gewidmeten Vita eines anonymen (geistlichen) Verfassers[27] im Alter von 22 Jahren an Lepra. Sie wurde infolgedessen aus der Klostergemeinschaft isoliert, musste während der drei Jahre bis zu ihrem Tod in einer Behausung außerhalb des Klostergebäudes leben und konnte nicht mehr vollständig an der Eucharistie teilnehmen. Auch hier wird der Verfasser nicht müde zu unterstreichen, dass das (über Erblindung und Lähmung als sukzessive Auflösung ihres Körpers beschriebene) Leid dieser Leprösen als Zeichen ihrer Erwählung durch Gott aufzufassen sei. Alix selbst sei über ihre Erblindung regelrecht

---

[24] Vgl. in diesem Sinn auch die Hinweise zur ‚Normalität' der Krankheit bzw. des Wunsches nach Krankheit in den Nonnenviten u.a. bei Knackmuß 2009: 335-68.

[25] Vgl. Schmidt 1992: 99 (Kap. 69): „Tantum habuit securitatem, quod certa fuit, quod a Deo numquam debuit separari. Sed magis propter hanc eandem certitudinem se contempsit, quia cogitavit: ‚Deus ligat te sua gratia et ista magna securitate, quam tu habes. […] Ipse facit tibi sicut malefactori, qui in carcerem proicitur et ligatur. Quamdiu iacet in carcere, et ligatus, non perpetrat mala.'"

[26] Vgl. dazu besonders Ursula Peters (Peters 1988) und Susanne Bürkle (Bürkle 1999).

[27] Acta Sanctorum. Iunii tomus secundus (Henschen 1969); vgl. den Hinweis bei Oswald 2008: 30.

beglückt gewesen, weil sie sich so auch von der letzten Ablenkung auf dem Weg zur *unio mystica* mit Jesus Christus befreit gefühlt habe (vgl. Henschen 1969: 473, I/3; 475, II/23; 476, III/27).

Und noch ein letztes Beispiel: In der von Fra Arnaldo da Foligno verfassten Vita der Franziskaner-Tertiarin Angela da Foligno heißt es, diese Frau habe sich nicht nur für die Pflege Aussätziger aufgeopfert, sondern sogar gezielt die Absicht verfolgt, sich bei der Pflege der Kranken selbst anzustecken, um das Martyrium in der Nachfolge Christi zu erleiden (vgl. Oswald 2008: 38). Damit hat sich auch der Kreis zu Hartmanns von Aue Dichtung über den an Aussatz erkrankten Armen Heinrich und das zum Blutopfer bereite Mädchen geschlossen. Was über Angela da Foligno geschrieben wird, ist nur eine im Vergleich zu Hartmanns Erzählung medizinisch ‚rationalisiertere' Spielart des Opfers von Gesundheit und Leben. Die Bereitschaft zu diesem Opfer beim Umgang mit Kranken wird Frauen zugeschrieben – Frauen, die mit dem ‚Kapital' ihres Körpers Heilung anderer und auf diesem Weg auch das eigene Heil bewirken wollten.

3. Schlussfolgerungen: Krankheit und Gesundheit, Heilung und Heil

Blickt man von heute aus auf die mittelalterlichen Fallbeispiele zurück, so dürfte vor allem auffallen, welch große Differenz den Geschlechtern zugeschrieben ist – auch und gerade im Umgang mit Krankheit. Ich habe als Grund dafür in erster Linie den Aspekt der sozialen Handlungsspielräume geltend zu machen versucht, auf dem auch das aus der Genesiserzählung abgeleitete Legitimierungsmodell letztlich aufruht. Kulturgeschichtlich bedingte Veränderungen von Handlungsspielräumen können ebenfalls erklären, warum sich gender-Konstruktionen zur Gegenwart hin mehr oder weniger stark gegeneinander verschoben haben. Mehr noch als der Befund als solcher, dass Krankheit, zumal eine lebensbedrohliche und/oder eine unheilbare, eine gravierende Erfahrung darstellt, hat sich die Art und Weise geändert, wie Krankheit erlebt wird.

Die Fallbeispiele aus dem Mittelalter legen den Befund nahe, dass parallel zur klaren Differenzlinie, die zwischen den Geschlechtern gezogen und mit einer ebenso klaren Bewertungshierarchie verbunden wurde, auch die Grenzen zwischen ‚gesund' und ‚krank' unterschiedlich verliefen: Beim Mann, verstanden als Verkörperung des ‚voll' ausgeprägten Menschen, rücken Gesundheit und Krankheit weit auseinander. Krankheit erscheint daher wie ein Einbruch in die Männlichkeitskonstruktion, ein Kontrollverlust, gegen den es sich so weit nur irgend möglich zu stemmen gilt. Anders als die Verbindung von Krankheit und Heilung liegt die Vorstellung, dass Krankheit selbst mit Heil verbunden sei, hier ungleich ferner, als sie im Blick auf die Frau bzw. als Projektion auf die Frau erscheint: Frauen ist ohnehin eine schon konstitutionelle Affinität zur Krankheit zugeschrieben und Raum, diese Zuschreibung ebenso wie das durch sie abgebildete Wertgefälle nicht auch tatsächlich zu internalisieren, bleibt ihnen oft wenig. Dieser Logik entsprechend hat sich der Mann, konkret oder im übertragenen Sinn, im Kampf – Mann gegen Mann – zu opfern, die Frau aber hat sich der Krankheit zu opfern – ihrer eigenen, ‚konstitutionellen‘, und derjenigen von anderen, nicht zuletzt von Männern. Sie hat ganz buchstäblich das Heil in der Krankheit zu suchen. In der Theorie wird, wenn man an die spätmittelalterliche Exegese zum Buch Hiob denkt, der himmlische Lohn für krankheitsbedingtes Leiden allen Menschen in Aussicht gestellt, die ihre Krankheit, je nachdem, als Strafe oder Prüfung gottergeben ertragen, umso mehr aber jenen, die Krankheit als Auszeichnung durch Gott anzunehmen verstehen (vgl. Johanek 1992: 43f.). Konkret vorgeführt wird das aber dann doch weniger von Männern als von Frauen, die – das ist die Kehrseite der dahinter stehenden Gender-Logik – es auch leichter damit haben, sich im ‚Gefängnis‘ eines kranken Körpers einzurichten, wenn wirklich kein Entrinnen möglich ist.

Genesis, Buch Hiob oder Hoffnung auf himmlischen Lohn sind aus unserer Kultur ausgezogen. Heute hofft man auf Labordiagnostik, medizinische Apparaturen oder Technologien, und Medizin ist (auch) ‚weiblich‘ (geworden). Und doch markiert, so denke ich, das an mittelalterlichen Beispielen Beschriebene nicht nur eine Etappe auf dem Weg, der über viele weitere Etappen zur Gegenwart geführt hat. Es zieht vielmehr, wenngleich die Ursachen meist nicht mehr bekannt sind, zumindest auf der Ebene der Symptomatik seine Spuren auch in die Gegenwart hinein. Diesen Spuren nachzugehen, wäre ein anderes Thema.

Literaturverzeichnis

Benz, Wolfram, et al. *„Hermann der Lahme" – Graf von Altshausen*. Lindenberg: Fink, 2007.

Berschin, Walter. „Hermann der Lahme. Leben und Werk in Übersicht." *Hermann der Lahme. Gelehrter und Dichter (1013-1054)*. Hrsg. Walter Berschin und Martin Hellmann. Heidelberg: Mattes 2005. 15-32.

Berthold von der Reichenau. „'Vita Herimanni'. Lateinisch und deutsch, übersetzt von Walter Berschin." *Hermann der Lahme. Gelehrter und Dichter (1013-1054)*. Hrsg. Walter Berschin und Martin Hellmann. Heidelberg: Mattes 2005. 6-13.

Brunhölzl, Christoph. „Gedanken zur Krankheit Hermanns von Reichenau". *Sudhoffs Archiv – Zeitschrift für Wissenschaftsgeschichte* 83 (1999): 239-43.

Bürkle, Susanne. *Literatur im Kloster. Historische Funktion und rhetorische Legitimation frauenmystischer Texte des 14. Jahrhunderts*. Tübingen: Francke, 1999.

Dieckmann, Bernhard. „Von Blutmagie zum Sühnopfer. Der Arme Heinrich zwischen Hartmann von Aue und Gerhart Hauptmann." *Im Drama des Lebens Gott begegnen. Einblicke in die Theologie Józef Niewiadomskis*. Hrsg. Nikolaus Wandinger, und Petra Steinmair-Pösel. Wien, Berlin: LitVerlag, 2011. 175-91.

Eis, Gerhard. „Salernitanisches und Unsalernitanisches im 'Armen Heinrich' des Hartmann von Aue." *Hartmann von Aue*. Hrsg. Hugo Kuhn und Christoph Cormeau. Darmstadt: Wissenschaftliche Buchgesellschaft, 1973. 135-51.

Feistner, Edith. „Der Körper als Fluchtpunkt: Identifikationsprobleme in geistlichen Texten des Mittelalters." *Manlîchiu wîp, wîplîch man. Zur Konstruktion der Kategorien 'Körper' und 'Geschlecht' in der deutschen Literatur des Mittelalters*. Hrsg. Ingrid Bennewitz und Helmut Tervooren. Berlin: Erich Schmidt Verlag, 1999, 131-42.

Fritsch-Staar, Susanne. „*Uterus virgineus thronus est eburneus*. Zur Ästhetisierung, Dämonisierung und Metaphorisierung des Uterus in mhd. Lyrik." *Manlîchiu wîp, wîplîch man. Zur Konstruktion der Kategorien 'Körper' und 'Geschlecht' in der deutschen Literatur des Mittelalters*. Hrsg. Ingrid Bennewitz und Helmut Tervooren. Berlin: Erich Schmidt Verlag, 1999, 182-203.

Goetz, Hans-Werner. „'Debilis'. Vorstellungen von menschlicher Gebrechlichkeit im frühen Mittelalter." *Homo debilis. Behinderte – Kranke – Versehrte in der Gesellschaft des Mittelalters*. Hrsg. Cordula Nolte. Korb: Didymos, 2009. 21-55.

Haag, Christine. „Das Ideal der männlichen Frau in der Literatur des Mittelalters und seine theoretischen Grundlagen." *Manlîchiu wîp, wîplîch man. Zur Konstruktion der Kategorien 'Körper' und 'Geschlecht' in der deutschen Literatur des Mittelalters*. Hrsg. Ingrid Bennewitz und Helmut Tervooren. Berlin: Erich Schmidt Verlag, 1999, 228-48.

Handschin, Jacques. „Hermannus contractus-Legenden – nur Legenden?" *Zeitschrift für deutsches Altertum und deutsche Literatur* 72 (1935): 1-8.

Hartmann von Aue. *Der arme Heinrich*. Übers. Siegfried Grosse. Hrsg. Ursula Rautenberg. Stuttgart: Reclam, 1993.

Henschen, Gottfried. *Acta Sanctorum. Iunii tomus secundus*. Antwerpen, 1698. Nachdruck, Brüssel, 1969.

Horn, Klaus-Peter. „Überleben in der Familie – Heilung durch Gott. Körperlich beeinträchtigte Menschen in den Mirakelberichten des 9. und 10. Jahrhunderts." *Homo debilis. Behinderte – Kranke – Versehrte in der Gesellschaft des Mittelalters*. Hrsg. Cordula Nolte. Korb: Didymos, 2009. 303-16.

Irsigler, Franz. „Mitleid und seine Grenzen. Zum Umgang der mittelalterlichen Gesellschaft mit armen und kranken Menschen." *Homo debilis. Behinderte – Kranke – Versehrte in der Gesellschaft des Mittelalters*. Hrsg. Cordula Nolte. Korb: Didymos, 2009. 165-81.

Jankrift, Kay Peter. *Krankheit und Heilkunde im Mittelalter*. Darmstadt: Wissenschaftliche Buchgesellschaft, 2003.

Johanek, Peter. „Stadt und Lepra." *Lepra – Gestern und Heute. 15 wissenschaftliche Essays zur Geschichte und Gegenwart einer Menschheitsseuche. Gedenkschrift zum 650-jährigen Bestehen des Rektorats Münster-Kinderhaus*. Hrsg. Richard Toellner. Münster: Regensberg, 1992. 42-47.

Knackmuß, Susanne: „'Moniales debiles' oder behinderte Bräute Christi. (Chronische) Krankheit, Behinderung und Familienbande im Frauenkloster um 1500." *Homo debilis. Behinderte – Kranke – Versehrte in der Gesellschaft des Mittelalters*. Hrsg. Cordula Nolte. Korb: Didymos, 2009. 335-68.

Konrad von Megenberg. *Das „Buch der Natur". Kritische Edition nach den Handschriften, Band I*. Hrsg. Robert Luff, und Georg Steer. Tübingen: Niemeyer, 2003.

Konrad von Würzburg. *Engelhard*. Hrsg. Paul Gereke. Tübingen: o.V., 1963. 192-249.

Meier, Esther. „Die heilende Kraft des Angesichts Christi. Leprakranke und das Schweißtuch der Veronika." *Gesund und krank im Mittelalter*. Hrsg. Andreas Meyer, und Jürgen Schulz-Grobert. Leipzig: Eudora, 2007. 125-43.

Meyer, Andreas. „Lepra und Lepragutachten aus dem Lucca des 13. Jahrhunderts." *Gesund und krank im Mittelalter.* Hrsg. Andreas Meyer und Jürgen Schulz-Grobert. Leipzig: Eudora, 2007. 145-210.

Moshövel, Andrea. „Der hât ainen weibischen muot. Männlichkeitskonstruktionen bei Konrad von Megenberg und Hildegard von Bingen." *Männer – Macht – Körper. Hegemoniale Männlichkeit vom Mittelalter bis heute.* Hrsg. Martin Dinges. Frankfurt am Main/New York: o.V., 2005, 52-68.

Oertelt-Prigione, Sabine und Vera Regitz-Zagrosek. *Sex and Gender Aspects in Clinical Medicine.* London: Springer, 2012.

Oswald, Marion. „Aussatz und Erwählung. Beobachtungen zu Konstitution und Kodierung sozialer Räume in mittelalterlichen Aussatzgeschichten." *Innenräume in der Literatur des deutschen Mittelalters.* Hrsg. Burkhard Hasebrink et.al.. Tübingen: Niemeyer, 2008. 23-44.

Peters, Ursula. *Religiöse Erfahrung als literarisches Faktum. Zur Vorgeschichte und Genese frauenmystischer Texte des 13. und 14. Jahrhunderts.* Tübingen: Niemeyer, 1988.

Riha, Ortrun. „Aussatz. Geschichte und Gegenwart einer sozialen Krankheit." *Sitzungsberichte der Sächsischen Akademie der Wissenschaften zu Leipzig, Mathematisch-naturwissenschaftliche Klasse 129/5.* 2004. Stuttgart/Leipzig: S. Hirzel, 2006. 5-31.

---. „Chronisch Kranke in der medizinischen Fachliteratur des Mittelalters. Eine Suche nach der Patientenperspektive." *Homo debilis. Behinderte – Kranke – Versehrte in der Gesellschaft des Mittelalters.* Hrsg. Cordula Nolte. Korb: Didymos, 2009. 99-120.

Robinson, Ian S. „Die Chroniken Bertholds von Reichenau und Bernolds von Konstanz 1054-1100." *MGH: Scriptores rerum Germanicarum Nova Series 14.* Hannover: Hahn, 2003. 163-74.

Ruh, Kurt. *Geschichte der abendländischen Mystik. Bd. 2: Frauenmystik und Franziskanische Mystik der Frühzeit.* München: Beck, 1993.

Schmidt, Paul Gerhard. *Johannes von Magdeburg O.P., Die Vita der Margareta contracta, einer Magdeburger Rekluse des 13. Jahrhunderts.* Leipzig: o. V., 1992.

Schröder, Edward. „Deutsche Kaiserchronik: die Kaiserchronik eines Regensburger Geistlichen." *MGH: Deutsche Chroniken I.1.* Hannover, 1895. Nachdruck, Berlin: Weidmann, 1964. 216-77.

Spreitzer, Brigitte. „Störfälle. Zur Konstruktion, Destruktion und Rekonstruktion von Geschlechterdifferenz(en) im Mittelalter." *Manlîchiu wîp, wîplîch man. Zur Konstruktion der Kategorien 'Körper' und 'Geschlecht' in der deutschen Literatur des Mittelalters.* Hrsg. Ingrid Bennewitz, und Helmut Tervooren. Berlin: Erich Schmidt Verlag, 1999, 249-63.

Uhrmacher, Martin. „Die Lepra in Köln vom 12. bis 18. Jahrhundert." *Krank – gesund. 2000 Jahre Krankheit und Gesundheit in Köln.* Hrsg. Thomas Deres. Köln: Kölnisches Stadtmuseum, 2005. 98-113.

Verfasserlexikon – Die deutsche Literatur des Mittelalters. Johannes von Magdeburg OP. Nachtragsband. Hrsg. Kurt Ruh, und Burghart Wachinger. Berlin/New York: de Gruyter. 1978ff.

Wegera, Klaus-Peter, Simone Schuetz-Balluff, und Nina Bartsch. *Mittelhochdeutsch als fremde Sprache: Eine Einführung für das Studium der germanistischen Mediävistik.* Berlin: Schmidt, 2011.

Weiß, Bardo. *Margareta von Magdeburg. Eine gelähmte Mystikerin des 13. Jahrhunderts.* Paderborn: Schöningh, 1995.

Wittmer-Butsch, Maria und Constanze Rendtel. *Miracula – Wunderheilungen im Mittelalter. Eine historische-psychologische Annäherung.* Wien: Böhlau, 2003.

Dorothea Heitsch

Soulless Animals?
Some Renaissance Discussions
Concerning Women's Immaterial Parts

> l'animal sensuel et faux chez qui l'âme n'est point, chez qui la pensée ne circule jamais comme un air libre et vivifiant, elle est la bête humaine
>
> (Maupassant 1902: 136)

Within this volume's inquiry into the relationship between ideas of gender and disease from a socio-historical, medico-historical, and narratological perspective the question I ask is whether early modern women have souls. Whether the female human being is endowed with a soul, since according to a tendentious reading of *Genesis* 2: 21-24 God breathed the soul into Adam exclusively before he created Eve from Adam's rib, might not actually be a question worth pursuing, because women are baptized, they must go to confession and they can have kindred souls with men or may even be considered as the soul of a man.[1] Yet Renaissance authors did ask this question and a host of related ones, often influenced by theological debates, such as whether woman was a human being, whether she was made in the image of God, in what form she would be resurrected, how she related to man in matters of sin and malediction, what disqualifications she suffered in the life of the Church, and in what ways she was the equal or the superior of man (Maclean 1980: 7, 1977: 2).[2] The fact that the issue of soulless women has been raised at some intervals from the Mâcon case of the Middle Ages (Nolan 1998: 13f., Nolan 1993: 501-9, Blamires 1992), through the Reformation and Counter-Reformation[3] to, more recently, funda-

---

[1] A literary example of female confession can be found in Hélisenne de Crenne's *Les angoysses douloureuses qui procèdent d'amours* (1538); a case of male-female soul mates is the friendship between Marie de Gournay and Michel de Montaigne (see below).

[2] See similarly also Mujica 2003: 11. Mujica's introduction gives a useful survey of the general situation of women in early modern Europe.

[3] The case of a pamphlet published in 1595 whose anonymous author denied women the status of human beings, its rebuttals, translations, and seventeenth-century reactions up to Archangela Tarabotti's *Che le donne siano della spetie degli huomini* (1651, *Women are of the Human Race*) seems to be more of an exception, even though it came to be taken quite seriously in the course of sixty years. See, for example, Fleischer 1981.

mentalist debates in France[4] may prove that it either poses a genuine
Reformation to, more recently, fundamentalist debates in France may prove that
it either poses a genuine problem in the eyes of certain beholders, both historical
and contemporary, or that it reflects particular tendencies within a developing
public discourse.

So why would Renaissance readers, and we with them, be interested in
whether early modern women have souls? Whether animals and plants can have
a soul is certainly a question discussed during that time, and not by Michel de
Montaigne alone in his "Apologie de Raymond de Sebond."[5] Indeed, not merely
animal souls, but those of stones or worms are equally analyzed with great
interest,[6] which has given rise to a new direction of research in our days.[7] It
should therefore be logical, both then and now, to grant souls to women (and all
human beings that are perceived as different).[8] The other reason for Renaissance
readers' and our curiosity would be that one way, if not the only one, to
approach gender equality before Descartes is through the equivalence of the
male and female soul (Hassauer 2008: 18).[9] Yet can those early modern women
who, according to Aristotle and his followers, are created as imperfect males and
who, according to Galen, are severely hampered by their supposed cold physicality actually have a soul? The short answer is that women, in keeping with the
(mostly male) authorities, seem to have a soul but that this organ is more
wedded to their bodies and it is more fraught with passion than guided by
reason. General discussions concerning the early modern soul in literary and
medical texts are only beginning to be undertaken, often in connection with the
question of immortality, and they remain mere sketches.[10] In the following pages

[4] In particular a discussion between Marcel Bernos (Bernos 2003) and Pierre Darmon who
answers him and sees the renewed interest in the question as part of an attempt to defend the
Catholic church against those who are said to accuse it of having denied women a soul, that is,
a fictitious accusation used by fundamentalist Catholics to build scapegoats since the 1980s.
The question of soulless women therefore seems to reappear in moments of crisis (Darmon
2012: 27-38).

[5] See, for example, Brancher 2008. Paracelsus discovers female forces in stones and plants
(Pagel 1962).

[6] See, for example, Cohen 2013.

[7] See Steel and McCracken 2011. Karen Raber's study of animals follows this trend into the
Renaissance (Raber 2013).

[8] Fundamental texts that touch on this problem are Huet 1993 and Schiebinger 1993.

[9] Hassauer rightly asserts that until the separation of "res cogitans" from "res extensa,"
equality can only be argued through the equality of souls. Her claim – until Poulain de la
Barre makes his Cartesian statement "l'esprit n'a point de sexe" it is the affirmation by Maria
de Zayas ("las almas ni son hombres ni mujeres") that sets the tone for equality – needs some
nuancing, which I propose to offer in this essay.

[10] See Heitsch 2010, Hirai 2011 and Solomon 2012. For some basic notions on the early
modern soul, see the section on psychology in Schmidt 1996: 453-534.

I therefore discuss the etymological dimension of the problem, the theological one, the medico-anatomical aspect, and literary examples. I will consult texts by men and women, antifeminist and proto-feminist writings. My examples will be tipped toward the French tradition, though I will endeavor to diversify.

In asking whether early modern women have souls I build on much feminist scholarship[11] and analyses of corporeality,[12] but first and foremost I am indebted to the studies by Ian Maclean.[13] Thus, I take up and refine a series of issues this scholar presented in his ground-breaking work. Obviously, the question concerning women's souls touches on several disciplines, in the same way that Maclean pointed it out for the notion of woman in general; and though it would be possible to divide my deliberations into neat categories, such as medicine, theology, law, and ethics, for example,[14] many of the texts I analyze are hybrids, neither entirely medical nor entirely theological, but rather medico-ethical or ethico-legal, and the boundaries between them are always fluid. In this respect, the question of soulless women is similar to the "Querelle des femmes" of which it is a part: the battle involving physical, metaphysical, theological, philosophical, literary, rhetorical, legal, medical, political, and economical facts about the physical equipment of the female body, the moral equipment of the female soul, the intellectual equipment of the female mind, and the cognitive equipment of the female brain; and as a result a battle about the rank of the sexes and the order of the world.[15] Accordingly, the textual genres used by the participants in this battle are amorphous and their content often is cross-disciplinary, just as this is the case with writings about the early modern female soul.

---

[11] For a very concise survey of early modern women's situation in general see the introductions by Margaret L. King and Albert Rabil to each volume of the series *The Other Voice in Early Modern Europe* as well as, for example, Jordan 1990.

[12] In particular Evelyne Berriot-Salvadore's monumental work in which, however, she hardly discusses the soul (Berriot-Salvadore 1993).

[13] "As will be seen, the notion of woman is, as it were, molecular in structure, consisting of an interdependent network of assumptions taken from different intellectual spheres; for the sake of clarity, woman's status in theology, in anatomy and medicine, in law, and finally in moral philosophy and politics will be considered in turn" (Maclean 1977: 1).

[14] "In one sense at least, theology in Christian Europe precedes ethics, law and medicine. In another sense, the organon in which Aristotelian method is established precedes these disciplines. Medicine can be said to precede ethics, as it provides natural justifications for moral and political precepts; both medicine and ethics underlie law. The relationship between disciplines is not, however, uniquely hierarchical; it is also molecular, for different disciplines reflect different aspects of human existence" (Maclean 1980: 83).

[15] For definitions of the Querelle, see Hassauer 2008: 15, Wunder and Engel 1998, Maihofer 1998 and Kelly 1984. More recent surveys of Querelle studies are given by Warner 2011 and Campbell 2013.

Etymology

Etymologically, "anima" in Latin means something breathing or blowing in the sense of wind or breath (from the Greek "anemos"–wind) and, metaphorically, may signify the breath of life, the vital principle, and the soul (Simpson 1968). The Greek term is "psyche" and in Christian contexts "anima" becomes the soul, but can also mean the spirit. In old French texts we find both the noun "animal," in the sense of "being" or "beast" in the twelfth century, and the adjective "animal" in the thirteenth century derived from the Latin "animalis," animated. In the fourteenth century, the verb "animer" means "to give life" or, rather, "to give movement" and "to render more lively" (Dauzat 1938). From the feminine noun "alme," "arme," or, in the *Chanson de Roland*, "anme," and "aneme" in the *Vie de Saint Alexis* the term develops by the thirteenth century into "âme" (Gamillscheg 1969). In Christian terms, "âme" is the spiritual principle of divine creation tied to the human being whose body it leaves after death. It becomes regenerated by baptism and is saved through Christ's death, therefore surviving after the death of each believer, including women's, according to commentators.

Robert Estienne's *Dictionnaire français-latin* of 1539 adds a moral aspect to the definitions: it renders "cultus animi" as the jewel of the soul, like virtue and similar things;[16] "vitiositas" as a quality of the soul discordant with itself and in perpetual dissension with all that it does;[17] and "umbrae infernae" as the souls in the underworld.[18] "Ame," in sixteenth-century France, is also used in the sense of "person," in the combination "âme moutonnière" by François Rabelais (Rabelais 1994: 706), and by Estienne Pasquier in the expression "rendre l'âme en l'autre monde" (Huguet 1925-73).[19] This short overview reminds us of the multiple connotations of the word. And, for the purpose of this essay, it is useful to point to the closeness of "anima" and "animal," of soul and a living principle and of the fact that descriptions of the soul, though often made through notions of immortality, are, of course, also achieved through analysis of the passions, emotions, and affect. Moreover, early modern arguments in favor of women's subordinate role are often based on pseudo-etymologies, such as in the case of Heinrich Kramer (known as Henricus Institoris) and Jacob Sprenger's *Malleus Maleficarum* (Speyer, 1487). In this authoritative and detailed manual for the witch hunt women are etymologically defined as weak in faith because "the word 'femina' is spoken as 'fe' and 'minus,' because she has and keeps less

---

[16] "[O]rnement de l'ame comme vertu & semblables" (Estienne 1539).

[17] "[U]ne qualité de l'ame qui est discordante de soymesme & en perpetuelle dissension en tout ce qu'elle fait" (Estienne 1539).

[18] "[L]es ames estans es enfers." (Estienne 1539)

[19] For a condensed version of the etymological information, see Rey 1998.

faith."[20] And Johann Weyer, who did attempt a medical explanation of dia-
bolism as what he perceived to be melancholia, still defines woman, "mulier," as
seemingly derived from "mollis," soft (Weyer 1991: 181f.).[21]

Spiritual Matters

It is the Bible, its exegesis, and religious institutions that determine much of the
early modern woman's subordination to her husband,[22] though "all commentators stress that she will share equally in the joys of paradise. In theological
terms, woman is, therefore, the inferior of the male by nature, his equal by
grace" (Mclean 1980: 27). One exception is Tertullian (160-220 AD) who imagined a fusion of body and soul and their joint resurrection as sexed bodies in
the afterlife, in a concrete "imitatio Christi" (Elliott 2013: 91). Even though this
position was eventually rejected, it influenced some Western theologians' view
of an embodied and sexed afterlife (ibid.). With regard to the soul's faculties,
not all parts of the tripartite soul were considered to be equal and the rational
soul was thought to be given to the human being only, yet it was itself divided.
This division between the lower rational soul, which negotiated the outer world
via the senses and the imagination, and the higher rational soul, which alone
bore the image of God, was mainly due to Augustine. Woman and her weaker
body was said to be subject to her inferior physical condition to the extent that it
influenced the lower part of the rational soul. The only way she could separate
herself from her body would be in mystical rapture (Elliott 2013: 94f.).

One striking example of male mysticism has recently been analyzed in its
cognitive and religious aspects by Jessica Boon (Boon 2012), but there also is a
considerable number of early modern women mystics, such as Saint Catherine
of Genoa (1447-1510) who wrote a treatise on Purgatory (see Nugent 1987) and
Saint Theresa of Jesus (1515-1582) who in the first chapter of her autobiography
describes how the Lord began to awaken her soul to virtue in her childhood (see
Morón-Arroyo 1987: 402-31). Mystical rapture is then carried into depictions of
female friendship in Spanish convent life (see Bilinkoff 2008) and into the
practical tasks a nun needs to carry out in her daily routine (see Diefendorf

---

[20] "Dicitur enim femina 'fe' et 'minus,' quia semper minorem habet et servat fidem"
(Institoris and Sprenger 2006: 42C).

[21] Rebecca Wilkin mentions this in the context of her study on female imagination (Wilkin
2008: 13f.)

[22] See a compilation of the Biblical texts that Renaissance writers refer to most frequently in
Aughterson 1995: 9-40.

2008).[23] Katherine Phillips in England (1632-1664) (see Hageman 1987) and Marie de Gournay in France (1565-1645) (see Heitsch 2010) will take spiritual ecstasy to different heights in their lay friendships. So will, in a way, the metaphysical poets in their descriptions of love and friendship. To a certain extent the so-called "honnête amour" inspired by Neoplatonism, outlined by Castiglione's interlocutors in book three of the *Cortegiano* (Venice, 1528), and celebrated by Tullia d'Aragona in parts of her dialogue on the infinity of love (Venice, 1547) is also a transcending experience.[24]

Mystical yearnings also foster women's confidence to undertake theological and metaphysical writing. Two hurdles are to overcome in this pursuit, that is, women's limited access to learning in general and, in particular, the prohibition imposed on them that they interpret Scripture.[25] Margaret Roper (1505-1544),[26] Marie Dentière (1495-1561) (see Head 1987), and Marguerite de Navarre (1492-1549) (see Tétel 1987) are examples of women who endeavor to prove that humanistic and theological erudition is good for the female soul, yet they do not always do it to the acclaim of their male contemporaries. Of course, there is the influence of Juan Luis Vives' *Education of a Christian Woman* (1524) in which he accepts female intellectual abilities and Sir Thomas Elyot in *Defence of Good Women* (1540) proposes similarly that women should participate in civic life and military pursuits. Such ideas will be taken up by Olympia Morata (1526-1555) who refers back to a frequent Renaissance source:

> I could mention others of this and preceding ages, but there exist entire volumes on famous women and they prove what Plato taught in the fifth book of the Republic and in the seventh book of the Laws is true: that there should be the same training for women and for men both in arts and letters as well as in gymnastics and military science. He sets them in charge of the protection of the city, and assigns commands to them. And while he concedes that they are weaker in body than men, he makes them equals in soul.

(Morata 2003: 72)

A century later, Anna Maria van Schurman will prove this point in her friendly dispute *Amica dissertatio inter Annam Mariam Schurmanniam et Andr. Rivetum de capacitate ingenii muliebris ad scientias* (Paris, 1638). And María de Zayas

---

[23] Diefendorf describes the case of Carmelite Barbe Acarie (1566-1618), who practices and teaches that one can be united in the highest part of one's soul with God while pursuing acts of charity or routine tasks of daily life.

[24] For a definition, see Villemur 1999: 242.

[25] See Kelso 1956, King 1991 and Timmermans 1993.

[26] Margaret Roper, the eldest daughter of Sir Thomas More, translated Erasmus's commentary on the Lord's Prayer into English. See McCutcheon 1987.

(1590-1661) will confirm the spiritual equivalence of the male and female mental apparatus, before it is proposed in Marguerite Buffet's *Nouvelles Observations sur la langue française* (Paris, 1668) and before it is laid out in the first male treatise on gender equality by François Poulain de la Barre, *De l'Egalité des deux sexes* (Paris, 1673).[27]

Woman's Body Plan and the Soul

The theological and moral problem of woman's souls was reinforced by much contemporary medical discourse. Within the Western cultural tradition women had historically been seen as incomplete and as more defined by their bodies and bodily functions. With regard to the first point Aristotle stipulated that the female is a deviation from the norm and that whatever is not perfect is monstrous.[28] A frequently cited collection of Arabic, Greek, Medieval, and Renaissance treatises entitled *Gynacea* (1566) circulates until the end of the sixteenth century,[29] and the interrelationship of commonplaces about woman will be maintained in interdisciplinary studies, such as Franciscus Vallesius's *De iis quae scripta sunt physicè in libris sacris* (Lyon, 1588), in which Aristotle's "imperfect male" theory is reinforced and justified by an exegesis of Genesis, by Simon Majolus's *Colloquia physica* (Mainz, 1615), where a theologian, a doctor, a philosopher, and a soldier discuss the nature of women, and Sebastian Meyer's *Augustae laudes Divinae Majestatis e Galeni de usu partium libris xvii selectae* (Freiburg, 1627).[30]

What did the soul consist of anatomically? Both Juan Luis Vives in *De anima* (Basel, 1538) and Thomas Vicary in *The anatomie of mans bodie* (1548) do not go beyond medieval knowledge, that is, Aristotle and Galen before his 1525 Aldine edition. Andreas Vesalius refuses to address the organ entirely in the 1543 and 1555 editions of *De humani corporis fabrica* (Brussels, 1543):

---

[27] See more on equality below.

[28] "The first beginning of this deviation is when a female is formed instead of a male, though this indeed is a necessity required by Nature, since the race of creatures which are separated into male and female has got to be kept in being" (Aristotle 1963: IV.iii, 401-3); "The female is as it were a deformed male" (Aristotle 1963: II, iii, 175); "The female is passive, the male is active" (Aristotle 1963: I.xxi, 113). In the *Metaphysics*, this polarity is outlined as male-female, limited-unlimited, odd-even, one-plurality, right-left, square-oblong, at rest-moving, straight-curved, light-darkness, good-evil (Maclean 1980: 2). See a summary of these views in Cadden 1993, ch. 1.

[29] See some excerpts in Aughterson 1995: 48-54.

[30] See Maclean 1977: 23, who also points out the parallels between Judaeo-Christian and Classical commonplaces.

To avoid running afoul of some "idle talker" here, or some critic of doctrine, I shall completely avoid this dispute concerning the types of soul and their location. For, today, you will find many judges of our most truthful and sacred religion, especially among the natives of my country, and if they heard anyone muttering about the opinions of Plato, Aristotle, Galen, or their interpreters, about the soul, even when the subject is Anatomy (when these subjects are especially likely to be discussed), they leap to the conclusion that such a person is in doubt about the faith or has some uncertainty about the immortality of Souls, without taking into consideration that physicians (provided they do not come rashly into their art or wish to apply inappropriate remedies to a sickened member) must think about the faculties that govern us, how many kinds there are, how each is marked, in what member of a living thing each is established, and besides these (if we can grasp it with the mind) chiefly what the substance and essence of the soul is.

(Vesalius 2014: 2.6.15, 1202)

Vesalius stipulates that the head is formed for the sake of the eyes by nature,[31] and not as the temple of the soul by God as some poets of the time would have it, and he also determines that the heads of men do not always differ from those of women, that is, they each may have the same anatomical flaws.[32] In book seven on the brain he gives an account of "the source of sensation, arbitrary motion, and the ruling spirit[33] (by means of which we form mental pictures, reason, and remember), [...] and will describe the brain and all its parts as well as the sense organs."[34] Here he rejects the three ventricle theory and in doing so refuses the authority of Aristotle – and that of the theologians on women's psychology with it:

But I do not have a satisfactory grasp of how the brain performs its functions in imagination, reasoning, thought, or memory (or however else you might like to subdivide or enumerate the powers of the chief spirit in accordance with anyone's theories). If, however, by meticulous and untiring examination of the parts of the brain – and then by observation of other parts of the body whose use is readily known to one trained in dissection – I can grasp something that is even likely by discovering a similarity, that would surely not be accomplished without staining the most sacred

[31] In that he follows Galen and Avicenna; see Vicary 1888: ch. 3.

[32] "The head is formed for the sake of the eyes by nature;" "The Heads of Men do not always differ from those of Women;" the example illustrating the latter point is the continuation of the sagittal suture as metopic suture which, according to the anatomist, "occurs very rarely in men, and still more rarely or hardly ever in women" (Vesalius 2014: 1.1.6, 58). According to current medicine, this suture persists in about 8% of adult skulls, whereas in all other skulls it fuses about the fifth year (Vesalius 2014: 1.1.6, 58 and note 53).

[33] Princeps anima: most highly refined of the spirits in the body sent out through the nerves to govern bodily movement.

[34] "The Brain is Constructed for the Sake of the Primary Spirit, and for sensation and voluntary movement" (Vesalius 2014: 2.7.1, 1256).

faith. […] For who, immortal God, will not be astonished at the crows of the philosophers of this age – and, I might add, of theologians – who make such fools of themselves by disparaging the divine and supremely admirable machine of the human brain in their impious dreams against the Maker of the human fabric no differently than if they were Prometheuses. They invent the most witless falsehoods about some structure of the brain […].

(Vesalius 2014: 2.7.1, 1258)

By acknowledging, on the basis of his trademark parallel dissections, that the only difference between human and animal brains is that their size is proportionally smaller, he implicitly also grants equal brain power to women.[35]

Charles Estienne, Vesalius's rival and the loser in the mid sixteenth-century race for a modern anatomical manual, merely indicates the soul in his *Dissection of the Parts of the Human Body* (Paris, 1545 in Latin and 1546 in French). He speaks about the soul in the context of the anatomy of the eye, where he mentions that which Plato named the soul by which he says we see and discern all things that are represented to us.[36] This seems to be the only mention Estienne makes of the organ in question. In contrast, Philipp Melanchthon dedicates the entire *Commentarius de anima* (Wittenberg, 1540) to the soul which he wants to understand by first analyzing the body, later changing and revising his findings into *Liber de anima* (Wittenberg, 1553) under the influence of Vesalius's anatomy; interestingly he entirely avoids the tricky issue of the imagination.[37] Jean Fernel devotes the fifth book of his *Physiologie* (1554) to the soul, yet he does not go into female and male souls and avoids discussions of immortality. Instead, he minutely analyzes all the faculties and also returns, like Melanchthon, to early Galen and Aristotle.[38] Ambroise Paré, in his *Anatomie universelle du corps humain* (Paris, 1561), attempts a definition of the soul as an incorporeal, invisible, and intellectual substance that is alive itself and gives life and movement to the body when it is joined to it. It is the receptacle of divine

---

[35] "The Construction of the Brain of animals does not differ from that of man." And he adds in 1555: "I do not think anything more can be learned from anatomy, given that theologians deny all power of reason and every faculty of what we call the pre-eminent spirit to brute animals, even though the ape, dog, horse, cat, and every other quadruped I have ever seen, all birds, and many species of fish, resemble man almost everywhere in the construction of their brain" (Vesalius 2014: 2.7.1, 1260).

[36] "[…] quem solum esse animum, eaque nos cernere Plato ait" (Estienne 1545: 304). "qui est ce que Platon a nommé l'Ame: par laquelle dit que nous voyons et discernons toutes choses qui nous sont representées" (Estienne 1546: 332.9).

[37] Gantet 2010: 96. See also Nutton 1990.

[38] "il faut entierement destruire et renverser l'opinion absurde et ridicule de presque tous les plus jeunes et modernes, qui met en place la memoire au derriere du cerveau, et la phantaisie, c'est à dire la faculté de penser, mediter et de feindre au devant, cette opinion est premierement venuë des Arabes" (Fernel 2001: 392-3).

illumination created from nothing to enliven the human body and is called "anima" because it animates and vivifies the body.[39] Yet in *De hominis generatione* (Paris, 1573) Paré determines that female souls are infused precisely five days later into the embryo than male souls, a fact which confirms once more woman's subordinate status.[40] Conrad Gesner composes a *Liber de anima* (Zurich, 1563) in which he maintains Aristotelian psychology. Paracelsus, who discusses women throughout his work, has some interesting passages in his *Philosophia sagax* (1537/38) and *Opus paramirum* (1531). He admits a differing male and female physiology but stresses that women are comparable as human beings, that is, equivalent. Women's bodies are different from men's and therefore require different treatments, in the same way that their psychological sufferings are of a different nature. Though he considers the matrix as the center of woman, he does not mean by it the uterus or sex organs, but a (somewhat occult) central image and an essence that cannot be determined. And though he discusses the importance of the female imagination for the development of the fetus, he thinks that both men and women's imagination can run wild and should be kept in check by physical activity (see Wiesner-Hanks and Scholz-Williams 1998).

As a result we can say that the anatomists and medical practitioners either avoid discussing the soul entirely or they resort to the authority of Aristotle, Plato, and the pre- (and post-)Aldine Galen. They also do not usually define women's souls in particular. It is female imagination that early modern physicians tend to discuss. In their opinion it is particularly active and leads, according to the authority Jacques Ferrand and his *Traicté de l'essence et guerison de l'amour ou de la melancholie érotique* (Toulouse, 1610), to more frequent cases of love melancholy in women than in men.[41] Moreover the disorder of the maternal imagination during conception or pregnancy may produce monstrous progeny. This thesis seems to be due to a lost text attributed to Empedocles who credits the mother's imagination with the shape of her progeny (Huet 1993: 4).[42] Gregor Reisch, together with medico-ethical litera-

---

[39] "C'est le receptacle d'illumination divine, immortelle et perpetuele, creée par la puissance de Dieu, faite de rien pour vivifier le corps humain. [...] Elle est appellee Ame, pour ce qu'elle anime & vivifie le corps. Ell'est dite esprit, pour ce qu'elle aspire au corps, & qu'elle est comme un rayon de la divinité [...]" (Paré 1561).

[40] In this he apparently follows Augustine (Nutton 1990: 141).

[41] Much scholarship has been devoted to love-melancholy, see Ciavolella 1976, Wack 1990, Wells 2007, Dawson 2008 and Folger 2009.

[42] Ambroise Paré in *Des monstres et prodiges* (1573) quotes the "ancients" (Aristotle, Hippocrates, Empedocles) for blaming the mother's ardent and obstinate imagination at the moment of conception, but he can also draw on Pierre Boaistuau and Claude de Tesserand's *Histoires prodigieuses*, Loys Lavater's, *Les Trois Livres des apparitions des esprits*, Johan Weyer's *Cinq livres de l'imposture et tromperie des diables* (1563). There seem to be two

ture, may enlighten us on why women's imagination is said to be the way it is. In Reisch's *Margarita philosophica* (Freiburg, 1503) we find a depiction of the soul and its faculties typical of the time: the precise localization of physical processes happens in the three ventricles of the brain (according to Galen), which was later criticized by Vesalius.[43] According to Galen, it was perception that collected data of the five senses, whereas for Augustine it was the imagination that influenced data (Gantet 2010: 17-22, 93-97). This accepted opinion is complemented by the theory of the humors which is basically a theory of heat and which stipulates that women's colder humors result in a different physiognomy with narrower shoulders and fatter hips as well as insufficient energy to drive matter up towards the head (Maclean 1980: 31).

One important sixteenth-century compiler on this issue is Juan Huarte de San Juan who in *Examen de ingenious para las sciencias* (Baeza, 1575) makes it clear that women are, as was generally accepted, naturally inferior to man (their sex is cold and moist) and therefore not endowed with any profound judgment. Yet their defect in wit qualifies them all the better for childbearing. In the medical discussion surrounding the nature of women he clearly falls on the side of those who regard the female as the imperfect copy of the male whose lack of heat prevented her from pushing out the sexual organs and who would, if she could, turn herself into a male.[44] Still he does acknowledge that there are certain exceptional women who have been endowed with exceptional gifts. One female author who turned Huarte's presentation of the Galenic temperaments to her advantage is Marie de Gournay. According to the former's manual, she has a temperament that is perfect for studying, for writing, and for intellectual pursuits in general.[45]

Martin Akakia, physician to François I, and the Portuguese medical practitioner Rodrigo de Castro maintain that women are equal to men in the "operationes animi," just as they are the equal of men in the perfection of their

strands, one describing the imagination as playing a role in exiting the emotions, such as in Thomas Fienus, *De Viribus Imaginationis* (Leuven, 1609), Pietro Pomponazzi, *De Naturalium Effectuum Admirandorum Causis, sive De Incantationibus* (Basel, 1556) and Fortunio Liceti, *De monstrorum causis* (Padua, 1616). Second, the role of images during conception as in Konrad Lycosthenes *Prodigiorum Liber*, Jacob Rueff's *De Conceptu et Generatione Hominis*, Pierre Boaistuau's *Histoires Prodigieuses*, Ambroise Paré's *Des monstres et prodiges*, Fortunio Liceti *De Monstrorum Causis, Natura et Differentiis*, and Ulysses Aldrovandi's *Monstrorum Historia* (see Céard 1971, Park and Daston 1981). This second strand may become especially dangerous for women, because it plays into the discussion of sorcery that is fuelled by the *Malleus Maleficarum* at the end of the fifteenth century and taken up by Weyer and Bodin (see Wilkin 2008).

[43] In this context, see also Green 2003.

[44] For a discussion of this position, see Berriot-Salvadore 1997.

[45] I show this in a chapter on my manuscript on *Writer-Physicians in Early Modern France*.

sex (Maclean 1977: 43). André Du Laurens, physician to Henri IV, even accords them superior powers of the mind (ibid.). In this they seem to approach a position acknowledging that the mind has no sex and they may be indebted to Jerome who asserts that sex is not of the mind and to Aquinas' similar though not identical argument that sex is not of the soul (ibid.). Another suggestion is made by Theodore Collado, a French physician, who puts forward the theory of a random distribution of mental strengths and weaknesses in both sexes (ibid.). In 1555, the writer François de Billon declares women and men equally intelligent in his *Le Fort inexpugnable de l'honneur du sexe Femenin* (Billon 1970: 152). He will be influenced by Agrippa von Nettesheim.

Defense of Woman's Soul

Neoplatonism combined with "dignitas homini" or "dignitas feminae" literature like Giovanni Boccacio's *De mulieribus claris* (1374) and Christine de Pisan's *Cité des dames* (1405)[46] counters the view of women as imperfect males. Symphorien Champier, who is said to have introduced Neoplatonism to France,[47] stipulates in his *Nef des dames vertueuses* (Lyon, 1503) not that women are less or better than men but that they are equal to some extent.[48] Yet it is Heinrich Cornelius Agrippa von Nettesheim who starts his *Declamatio de nobilitate et praecellentia foeminei sexus* (Antwerp, 1529) with a passage on the equality of souls:

> Sexual distinction consists only in the different location of the parts of the body for which procreation required diversity. But he [God] has attributed to both man and woman an identical soul, which sexual difference does not at all affect.[49] Woman has been allotted the same intelligence, reason, and power of speech as man and tends to the same end as he does, that is, [eternal] happiness, where there will be no restriction by sex. For according to the truth of the gospel, although all will return to life in their own sex, they will no longer carry out the functions of their sex, but it has been

---

[46] Lyndan Warner explores this connection between the Querelle des femmes on the nature of woman and the Renaissance debate on the dignity and misery of man, see Warner 2011. Jean Céard gives a useful survey of "Listes de femmes savantes au XVIe siècle", see Céard 1999.

[47] James Wadsworth considers the fourth book as the first French expression of Ficinian Neoplatonism in his edition of *Le Livre de vraye amour de Symphorien Champier* (Champier 1962: 13). Roland Antonioli compares Champier and Agrippa's *Declamatio* and thinks that they present a new image of woman purer to man, closer to God, and able to see the future and interpret divinity (Antonioli 1990: 61).

[48] "Et la femme aulcunement et en aulcune chose est esgalle à son mari" (Champier 2007: 134). Champier's *Nef* may be a direct response to Josse Bade's *Nef des folles* (ca. 1500) and he invites men to treat women like "compagnes et égales," but without granting them complete equality.

[49] See Luke. 20, Matth. 22, Mark. 12B7.

promised to them that they will be similar to angels. Thus there is no preeminence of nobility of one sex over the other by reason of the nature of the soul, rather, inwardly free, each is equal in dignity.

(Agrippa von Nettesheim 1996: 43)

Agrippa goes on to say that woman as the last creation is the perfection of the universe and therefore the most noble creature; that God gave his benediction to man thanks to woman; that man was the cause of original sin having eaten of the apple and having closed for us the doors of Paradise; and that man's tyranny deprives woman from the freedom she receives at birth.[50] Agrippa's treatise on women is fundamental because it takes up and answers a series of previous writings and will inspire many others.[51] Yet this author, like Michel de Montaigne after him, also made fun of his contemporaries' attempts to locate and define the human soul in *De incertitudine et vanitate scientiarum atque artium declamatio invectiva* (Cologne, 1527) (Agrippa von Nettesheim 1993:101).

One reader of Agrippa's treatise on women was without doubt Marguerite Briet alias Hélisenne de Crenne who in a three-volume romance entitled *Les Angoysses douloureuses qui procèdent d'amours* (Paris, 1538) shows us a heroine (and an author) claiming independence and equality by inverting literary topoi, such as the "innamoramento" which is here described from a female point of view, female love melancholy, the quest of a lovesick knight and his companion, and the composition of a therapeutic text, among others.[52] Hélisenne has been called a champion of women's rights for her proto-feminist literary writings (see delle Robbins-Herring 1987), and in the context of this essay, I would like to mention her use of confession, because it seems to me to illustrate some issues concerning moral and spiritual equality both on the textual and personal level.[53] At one point of the married heroine's infatuation with a young man, her husband, at the recommendation of a servant, has her speak to a monk so that she can confess what he perceives as an illicit love affair: "I began to premeditate my confession to this monk, and I said to myself: 'Oh lord, how tiresome

---

[50] In that he may be inspired by a passage in Mario Equicola's *On Women* (*De mulieribus*, 1501). See Albert Rabil's introduction to the *Declamation* (Rabil 1996: 24).

[51] Ian Maclean sees Agrippa as a seminal work (Mclean 1977: 26). Anita Traninger analyzes the literary tradition in which Agrippa writes and points to one direct female imitator, see Traninger 2008. Precursors are many, in Spain for example we have Juan Rodríguez de la Cámara, *El triunfo de la donas* (1443), Álvaro de Luna, *El libro de la virtuosas e claras mujeres* (1446), Mosén Diego de Valera, *Tratado en defense de mujeres* (1440), Fray Martín Alonso de Córdoba, *Jardín de las nobles doncellas* (1500), see Mujica 2003: 4; for France, see Swift 2008. For followers in England, see Woodbridge 1984.

[52] I have described this elsewhere, see Heitsch 2009.

[53] For some general ideas on confession in this work, see Krause 2004.

and painful it is to feign and dissimulate! I say this because I have no will or desire to communicate the secret of my love through confession, for I am neither contrite nor repentant.'" (Crenne 1996: 43). She will go into the arranged meeting fully intending to lie. In chapter fourteen of the novel, the monk is striving to gain her soul and make her return to God, but in vain, because Hélisenne obstinately cleaves to her infatuation and remains faithful only to love. As a result, she is not admitted to a Christian heaven at the end of her quest, but to a Virgilian one instead: "[…] the souls of Guenelic and Hélisenne were being carefully examined. When Minos had heard everything, he judged them, and determined that without delay they should be taken to the Elysian Fields, where souls repose in sweetness and felicity. Then Mercury took us to the lake called Lethe, and had the two blessed souls drink the water of oblivion" (Crenne 1996: 196). The paradox that many scholars have seen is that the confession does not take place in the privacy of a conversation with a monk, but it is performed with rhetorical skill and much pleasure in the public sphere of a book written by a female author who is subverting literary commonplaces and questioning spiritual authority.[54]

A number of women writers play expressly with the topos of souls' equality. One of them is Marie de Romieu (ca. 1545-1590) who in her witty poem *Discours que l'excellence de la femme surpasse celle de l'homme* (1581) mocks traditional male stereotypes regarding women, doubts that men have reason, and states that women, equipped with nicer and more delicate bodies, have corresponding minds and reason (Romieu 1972: 16, 18). Similarly, Lucrezia Marinella (ca. 1571-1653) maintains "I would say that women's souls were created nobler than men's, as can be seen from the effect they have and from the beauty of their bodies." This is what she proceeds to prove in the third chapter of her treatise on the basis of textual sources (Marinella 1999: 55). Veronica Franco (1546-1591) claims that equality with men is only a matter of proof, which can be undertaken once women have the same opportunities of training: "When we women, too, have weapons and training, we will be able to prove to all men that we have hands and feet and hearts like yours" (Franco 1998: 163). An analogous argument will be offered by Moderata Fonte (1555-1592) in *Il merito delle donne* (1600) which will inspire Maria de Zayas (1590-1661) who states outright: "Why, vain legislators of the world, do you tie our hands so that we cannot take vengeance. Because of your mistaken ideas about us you render us

---

[54] "D'un côté on entend une exhortation à éviter ou à délaisser 'l'amour sensuel,' en raison des conséquences fâcheuses de celui-ci; de l'autre, ce que l'on nous montre est une expérience amoureuse qui, tout en étant une source de difficultés et d''angoisses,' s'impose de telle façon que l'individu est voué à y succomber, en goûtant les satisfactions (ou les promesses de satisfaction) qui font le contrepoids de la morale sociale" (Crenne 2005: 24). This has lead to questioning the existence of the female author (Reach-Ngo 2013).

powerless and deny us access to pen and sword. Isn't our soul the same as a man's soul?" (Zayas y Sotomayor 1948: 21). But it is Marie de Gournay (1565-1645) who in her treatise *Equality of Men and Women* (first version 1622, final version 1644) states:

> Further, the human animal, taken rightly, is neither man nor woman, the sexes having been made double, not so as to constitute a difference in species, but for the sake of propagation alone. The unique form and distinction of that animal consists only in its rational soul. And if it is permitted to laugh in the course of our journey, the jest would not be out of season that teaches us that there is nothing more like a cat on a windowsill than a female cat. Man and woman are so thoroughly one that if man is more than woman, woman is more than man. Man was created [male] and female – so says scripture, not reckoning the two except as one; and Jesus Christ is called Son of Man, although he is that only of woman – the whole and consummate perfection of the proof of this unity of the two sexes.
>
> (Gournay 2002: 86f.)

Whether Marie de Gournay builds on an androgynous view of human equality, as attempted in Louys Le Bermen's *Le Bouclier des dames* (Rouen, 1621),[55] or whether she writes in a pre- and post-Cartesian spirit may be decided by the reader. She definitely is part of a group of writers in France who contribute to a peak of publications on the woman question in the middle of the seventeenth century.[56] She not only develops her self-portrait as temperamentally, that is, physically or constitutionally, suited to writing, according to Juan Huarte, but, together with her comrades-in-arms, moves the discussion of gender equality away from proving the existence of female souls and their equivalence with male souls, away from a definition of the soul as tied to gender differences, and toward an egalitarian argument based on natural philosophy.

Conclusion

Does the early modern woman have a soul? The polemical doubt that she may not be human is treated more or less as a joke, even at the time and in spite of the attack launched in a satirical treatise at the end of the sixteenth century which provokes a series of written replies and is pursued into the Schurman circle and, by Arcangela Tarabotti, far into mid-seventeenth-century Italy.[57] For

---

[55] See Constance Jordan's chapter on "Equality" in *Renaissance Feminism*, where she criticizes Le Bermen's androgyne for being male-centered (Jordan: 271-2).

[56] Jeannette Geffriaud Rosso, *Etudes sur la féminité aux XVIIe et XVIII siècles*, Pisa: Libreria Goliardica, 1984, 189-211.

[57] Gisbertus Voetius dismisses it in the two first sentences of his treatise *Concerning Women* (van Schurman 1998: 97). At stake here is the *Disputatio nova contra mulieres, qua probatur*

as long as the three ventricle theory reigns, woman is granted a soul that is tainted by its unruly imagination and whose rational faculty is frailer than man's. This is why she is barred from learning in general and from pursuing the study of theology. Erudite women and women mystics counter these restrictions in practice as well as in theory. Some anatomists and medical practitioners avoid the topic of the soul entirely (Vesalius), but those who decide to dissect this organ and its faculties either confirm the theories and findings of Plato, Aristotle, and Galen (Estienne) or they reassess them (Paré, Fernel, Melanchthon). Paracelsus and Huarte who distinguish between male and female souls resort to proto-psychoanalysis. Literary and ethical writers seem to be most unencumbered by the weight of authority; they emphasize the identical nature of male and female souls (Agrippa, Gournay), fight for women's opportunity to prove their souls' equivalence to that of men (Marinella, Franco, Fonte, Zayas), and some furnish that proof in their work (Hélisenne de Crenne). In conclusion, we can say that when it comes to seventeenth-century egalitarian treatises in Europe that evolve from comparing men's and women's souls Louis Le Bermen, Marie de Gournay and François Poulain de la Barre are an avant-garde.[58]

List of Works Cited

Agrippa von Nettesheim, Heinrich Cornelius. *Über die Fragwürdigkeit, ja Nichtigkeit der Wissenschaften, Künste und Gewerbe*. Berlin: Akademie Verlag, 1993.

---. *Declamation on the Nobility and Preeminence of the Female Sex*. Trans. and ed. Albert Rabil. Chicago: U of Chicago P, 1996.

Antonioli, Roland. "Songes prophétiques et dames vertueuses." *Le songe à la Renaissance, actes du Colloque international de Cannes, 29-31 mai 1987*. Saint-Etienne: Institut d'Etudes de la Renaissance et de l'Age Classique, 1990. 61-69.

Aristotle. *Generation of Animals*. Trans. A. L. Peck. Cambridge: Harvard UP, 1963.

Aughterson, Kate (ed.). *Renaissance Woman: A Sourcebook. Constructions of Femininity in England*. London: Routledge, 1995.

Bernos, Marcel. *Femmes et gens d'Église dans la France classique (XVIIe-XVIIIe siècle)*. Paris: Cerf, 2003.

Berriot-Salvadore, Evelyne. *Un corps, un destin. La femme dans la médecine de la Renaissance*. Paris: Champion, 1993.

---. "Le discours médical sur la nature féminine à la Renaissance." *Littérarture et medicine*. Ed. Jean-Louis Cabanès. Bordeaux: Université Michel de Montaigne, 1997. 57-68.

eas homines non esse (1595), allegedly by Valens Acidalius. For an evaluation, see Maclean 1980: 12 f. The entire quarrel is traced in Kenney 1998.

[58] See Sturman 1998. For an interesting analysis of how Marie de Gournay and François Poulain de la Barre negotiate authority in different ways, see Longino Farrell 1988.

Bilinkoff, Jodi. "Soul Mates: Spiritual Friendship and Life-Writing in Early Modern Spain (and Beyond)." *Female Monasticism in Early Modern Europe: An Interdisciplinary View*. Ed. Cordula van Wyhe. Aldershot: Ashgate, 2008. 143-53.

Billon, François de. *Le Fort inexpugnable de l'honneur du sexe Femenin*. Ed. Michael A. Screech. East Ardsley: S. R. Publishers. New York: Johnson Reprint Corp, 1970.

Blamires, Alcuin. *Woman Defamed and Woman Defended. An Anthology of Medieval Texts*. Oxford: Clarendon Press, 1992.

Boon, Jessica. *The Mystical Science of the Soul: Medieval Cognition in Bernardino de Laredo's Recollection Method*. Toronto: U of Toronto P, 2012.

Brancher, Dominique. "L'anthropocentrisme à l'épreuve du végétal: botanique sensible et subversion libertine." *La Renaissance décentrée*. Ed. Frédéric Tinguely. Geneva: Droz, 2008. 193-214.

Cadden, Joan. *The Meanings of Sex Difference in the Middle Ages: Medicine, Science, and Culture*. Cambridge: Cambridge UP, 1993.

Campbell, Julie. "The Querelle des femmes." *The Ashgate Research Companion to Women and Gender in Early Modern Europe*. Ed. Allyson M. Poska, Jane Couchman and Katherine A. McIver. Farnham: Ashgate, 2013. 361-79.

Céard, Jean. "Listes de femmes savantes au XVIe siècle." *Femmes savantes, savoir des femmes*. Ed. Colette Nativel. Geneva: Droz, 1999. 85-94.

Champier, Symphorien. *Le Livre de vraye amour de Symphorien Champier*. Ed. James B. Wadsworth. S'-Gravenhage: Mouton, 1962.

---. *La Nef des dames vertueuses*. Ed. Judy Kem, Paris: Champion, 2007.

Ciavolella, Massimo. *La malattia d'amore dall'antichità al Medioevo*. Roma: Bulzoni, 1976.

Cohen, Jeffrey J. "The Sex Life of Stone." *From Beasts to Souls. Gender and Embodiment in Medieval Europe*. Ed. E. Jane Burns and Peggy McCracken. Notre Dame: U of Notre Dame P, 2013. 17-38.

Crenne, Hélisenne de. *The Torments of Love*. Trans. Lisa Neal and Steven Rendall. Minneapolis: U of Minnesota P, 1996.

---. *Les angoisses douloureuses qui procèdent d'amour*. Saint-Etienne: Publications de l'Université de Saint-Etienne, 2005.

Darmon, Pierre. *Femme, repaire de tous les vices. Misogynes et féministes en France (XVIe-XIXe siècles)*. Bruxelles: André Versaille, 2012.

Dauzat, Albert. *Dictionnaire étymologique de la langue française*. Paris: Larousse, 1938.

Dawson, Lesel. *Lovesickness and Gender in Early Modern English Literature*. Oxford: Oxford UP, 2008.

Diefendorf, Barbara. "Barbe Acarie and her Spiritual Daughters: Women's Spiritual Authority in Seventeenth-Century France." *Female Monasticism in Early Modern Europe: An Interdisciplinary View*. Ed. Cordula van Wyhe. Aldershot: Ashgate, 2008. 155-71.

Elliott, Dyan. "Rubber Soul. Theology, Hagiography, and the Spirit World of the High Middle Ages." *From Beasts to Souls. Gender and Embodiment in Medieval Europe*. Ed. E. Jane Burns and Peggy McCracken. Notre Dame: U of Notre Dame P, 2013. 89-120.

Estienne, Charles. *De dissectione partium corporis humani libri tres*. Paris: S. de Colines, 1545.

---. *La dissection des parties du corps humain divisee en trois livres*, Paris: S. de Colines, 1546.

Estienne, Robert. *Dictionaire Francois-latin. Contenant les motz & manieres de parler Francois, tournez en Latin*. Paris: 1539.

Fernel, Jean. *La Physiologie*. 1554. Paris: Fayard, 2001.

Fleischer, Manfred. "Are Women Human? The Debate of 1595 Between Valens Acidalius and Simon Gedik." *The Sixteenth Century Journal* 12.2 (1981): 107-20.

Folger, Robert. *Escape from the Prison of Love: Caloric Identities and Writing Subjects in Fifteenth-Century Spain.* Chapel Hill: U of North Carolina P, 2009.

Franco, Veronica. *Poems and Selected Letters.* Trans. and ed. Ann Rosalind Jones and Margaret F. Rosenthal. Chicago: U of Chicago P, 1998.

Gamillscheg, Ernst. *Etymologisches Wörterbuch der französischen Sprache.* Heidelberg: Winter, 1969.

Gantet, Claire. *Der Traum in der Frühen Neuzeit.* Berlin: de Gruyter, 2010.

Geffriaud Rosso, Jeanette. *Etudes sur la féminité aux XVIIe et XVIII siècles.* Pisa: Libreria Goliardica, 1984.

Gournay, Marie de. *Apology for the Woman Writing.* Trans. Richard Hillman and Colette Quesnel. Chicago: Chicago UP, 2002.

Green, Christopher D. "Where Did the Ventricular Localization of Mental Faculties Come From?" *Journal of History of the Behavioral Sciences* 39.2 (2003): 131-42.

Hageman, Elizabeth H. "Katherine Philips: The Matchless Orinda." *Women Writers of the Renaissance and Reformation.* Ed. Katharina M. Wilson. Athens: U of Georgia P, 1987. 566-608.

Hassauer, Friederike. "Die Seele ist nicht Mann nicht Weib. Stationen der Querelle des femmes in Spanien und Lateinamerika vom 16. zum 18. Jahrhundert." *Querelles-Jahrbuch für Frauenforschung 1997.* Ed. Gisela Bock und Margarete Zimmermann. Stuttgart: Metzler, 1997. 203-38.

---. "Der Streit um die Frauen." *Geschlechterperspektiven. Forschungen zur frühen Neuzeit.* Ed. Heide Wunder and Gisela Engel. Königstein: Ulrike Helmer Verlag, 1998. 255-61.

---. "Sexus der Seele, Geschlecht des Geistes. Zwei Kapitel aus der Geschichte der Konstruktion des Zusammenhangs von Körper und Bewusstsein." *Inszenierung und Geltungsdrang.* Ed. Jörg Huber and Martin Heller. Zürich: Museum für Gestaltung, 1998. 77-95.

---. "Seelen ohne Körper, Geist ohne Geschlecht. Zur Theoriegeschichte der Konstruktion weiblichen Intellekts in Spanien." *Sosein – und anders. Geschlecht, Sprache und Identität.* Ed. Johanna Hofbauer et al. Frankfurt: Lang, 1999. 125-40.

--- (ed.). *Heisser Streit und kalte Ordnung. Epochen der Querelle des femmes zwischen Mittelalter und Gegenwart.* Wallstein: Göttingen, 2008.

Head, Thomas. "A Propagandist for the Reform: Marie Dentière." *Women Writers of the Renaissance and Reformation.* Ed. Katharina M. Wilson. Athens: U of Georgia P, 1987. 260-83.

Heitsch, Dorothea. "Female Love-Melancholy in Hélisenne de Crenne's *Les Angoysses douloureuses qui procedent d'amours* (1538)." *Renaissance Studies* 23.3 (2009). 335-353.

---. "Cats on a Windowsill: An Alchemical Study of Marie de Gournay." *Gender and Scientific Discourse in Early Modern Culture.* Ed. Kathleen P. Long. Farnham: Ashgate, 2010. 217-38.

---. "Renaissance Soul-Searching (1555-1584): Maurice Scève, Jacques Peletier du Mans, Pierre de Ronsard, Guillaume Du Bartas, René Bretonnayau." *Appositions: Studies in Renaissance / Early Modern Literature & Culture* 3 (2010). http://appositions.blogspot.com.

Hirai, Hiro. *Medical Humanism and Natural Philosophy: Renaissance Debates on Matter, Life, and the Soul.* Leiden: Brill, 2011.

Huet, Marie-Hélène. *Monstrous Imagination.* Cambridge: Harvard UP, 1993.

Huguet, Edmond. *Dictionnaire de la langue française du seizième siècle*. Paris: Champion, 1925-1973.

Institoris, Henricus and Jacobus Sprenger. *Malleus Maleficarum*. Ed. and trans. Christopher S. Mackay. Cambridge: Cambridge UP, 2006.

Jordan, Constance. *Renaissance Feminism. Literary Texts and Political Models*. Ithaca Cornell UP, 1990.

Jung, Ursula. "Ingenium und Tradition. Moderata Fontes *Il merito delle donne* (1600) und María de Zayas' *Desengaños amorosos* (1647)." *Heisser Streit und kalte Ordnung. Epochen der Querelle des femmes zwischen Mittelalter und Gegenwart*. Ed. Friedericke Hassauer. Wallstein: Göttingen, 2008. 230-55.

Kelly, Joan. "Early Feminist Theory and the *Querelle des femmes*." *Women, History, and Theory*. Chicago: U of Chicago P, 1984. 65-109.

Kelso, Ruth. *Doctrine for the Lady of the Renaissance*. Urbana: U of Illinois P, 1956.

Kenney, Theresa M. *Women Are Not Human. An Anonymous Treatise and Responses*, New York: Crossroads, 1998.

King, Margaret L. *Women of the Renaissance*. Chicago: U of Chicago P, 1991.

---. and Albert Rabil (eds.). *The Other Voice in Early Modern Europe*. 60 vols. Chicago: U of Chicago P, 1996-2010.

Krause, Virginia. "Confessions d'une heroïne romanesque: *Les Angoysses douloureuses qui procedent d'amours*." *Hélisenne de Crenne. L'écriture et ses doubles*. Ed. Jean-Philippe Beaulieu and Diane Desrosiers-Bonin. Paris: Champion, 2004. 19-34.

Longino Farrell, Michèle. "Theorizing on Equality: Marie de Gournay and Poullain de la Barre." *Cahiers du dix-septième: An Interdisciplinary Journal* 2.1 (1988): 67-79.

Maclean, Ian. *Woman Triumphant. Feminism in French Literature 1610-1652*. Oxford: Clarendon Press, 1977.

---. *The Renaissance Notion of Woman*. Cambridge: Cambridge UP, 1980.

Maihofer, Andrea. "Die Querelle des femmes: Lediglich literarisches Genre oder spezifische From der gesellschaftlichen Auseinandersetzung um Wesen und Status der Geschlechter?" *Geschlechterperspektiven. Forschungen zur frühen Neuzeit*. Ed. Heide Wunder and Gisela Engel. Königstein: Ulrike Helmer Verlag, 1998. 262-72.

Marinella, Lucrezia. *La Nobilta et l'eccellenza delle donne, co' difetti et mancamenti degli uomoni / The Nobility and Excellence of Women and the Defects and Vices of Men*. 1600. Trans. and ed. Anne Dunhill. Chicago: U of Chicago P, 1999.

Maupassant, Guy de. "Fou?" *Mademoiselle Fifi*. Paris: Société d'éditions littéraires et artistiques, 1902. 135-44.

McCutcheon, Elizabeth. "The Learned Woman in Tudor England. Margaret More Roper." *Women Writers of the Renaissance and Reformation*. Ed. Katharina M. Wilson. Athens: U of Georgia P, 1987. 449-80.

Morata, Olympia. *The Complete Writings of an Italian Heretic*. Trans. and ed. Holt N. Parker. Chicago: U of Chicago P, 2003.

Morón-Arroyo, Ciriaco. "The Human Value of the Divine. Saint Theresa of Jesus." *Women Writers of the Renaissance and Reformation*. Ed. Katharina M. Wilson. Athens: U of Georgia P, 1987. 402-431.

Mujica, Bárbara (ed.). *Women Writers of Early Modern Spain*. New Haven: Yale UP, 2003.

Nolan, Michael. "The Mysterious Affair at Mâcon: The Bishops and the Souls of Women." *New Blackfriars* 74 (1993): 501-9.

---. "The Myth of Soulless Women." *First Things* 72 (April 1998): 13-14.

Nugent, Donald Christopher. "Mystic of Pure Love. Saint Catherine of Genoa." *Women Writers of the Renaissance and Reformation*. Ed. Katharina M. Wilson. Athens: U of Georgia P, 1987. 67-95.

Nutton, Vivian. "The Anatomy of the Soul in Early Renaissance Medicine." *The Human Embryo. Aristotle and the Arabic and European Tradition*. Ed. G. R. Dunstan. Exeter: U of Exeter P, 1990. 136-157.

Pagel, Walter. *Das medizinische Weltbild des Paracelsus*, Wiesbaden: Steiner, 1962.

Paré, Ambroise. *Anatomie universelle du corps humain*. Paris: Jehan Le Royer, 1561.

---. *Des monstres et prodiges*. Ed. Jean Céard. Geneva: Droz, 1971.

Park, Katherine and Lorraine Daston. "Unnatural Conceptions: The Study of Monsters in Sixteenth- and Seventeenth Century France and England." *Past and Present* 92 (1981). 20-54.

Rabelais, François. *Oeuvres completes*. Ed. Mireille Huchon. Paris: Gallimard, 1994.

Raber, Karen. *Animal Bodies, Renaissance Culture*. Philadelphia: U of Pennsylvania P, 2013.

Rabil, Albert. "Agrippa and the Feminist Tradition." Heinrich Cornelius Agrippa von Nettesheim. *Declamation on the Nobility and Preeminence of the Female Sex*. Trans. and ed. Albert Rabil. Chicago: U of Chicago P, 1996. 3-32.

Reach-Ngo, Anne. *L'Écriture éditoriale à la Renaissance. Genèse et promotion du récit sentimental français (1530-1560)*. Geneva: Droz, 2013.

Reisch, Gregor. *Margharita philosophica nova*. Salzburg: Universität Salzburg, 2002.

Rey, Alain. *Dictionnaire historique de la langue française*. Paris: Le Robert, 1998.

Robbins-Herring, Kittye delle. "Champion of Women's Rights. Hélisenne de Crenne." *Women Writers of the Renaissance and Reformation*. Ed. Katharina M. Wilson. Athens: U of Georgia P, 1987. 177-218.

Romieu, Marie de. *Les premières oeuvres poétiques*. Geneva: Droz, 1972.

Schiebinger, Londa. *Nature's Bodies. Gender in the Making of Modern Science*. Boston: Beacon Press, 1993.

Schmidt, Charles B. et al. *The Cambridge History of Renaissance Philosophy*. Cambridge: Cambridge UP, 1996.

Simpson, D. P. *Cassell's Latin Dictionary*. New York: Macmillan, 1968.

Solomon, Julie. "You've Got to Have Soul: Understanding the Passions in Early Modern Culture." *Rhetoric and Medicine in Early Modern Europe*. Ed. Stephen Pender and Nancy S. Struever. Aldershot: Ashgate, 2012. 195-228.

Steel, Karl and Peggy McCracken. "The Animal Turn in Medieval Studies." *Postmedieval: A Journal of Medieval Cultural Studies* 2.1 (2011).

Sturman, Siep. "L'égalité des sexes qui ne se conteste plus en France. Feminism in the Seventeenth Century." *Perspectives on Feminist Political Thought in European History. From the Middle Ages to the Present*. Ed. Tjitske Akkerman and Siep Stuurman. London: Routledge, 1998. 67-84.

Swift, Helen J. *Gender, Writing, and Performance. Men Defending Women in Late Medieval France, 1440-1538*. Oxford: Clarendon Press, 2008.

Tétel, Marcel. "Marguerite of Navarre: The Heptameron, A Simulacrum of Love." *Women Writers of the Renaissance and Reformation*. Ed. Katharina M. Wilson. Athens: U of Georgia P, 1987. 99-131.

Timmermans, Linda. *L'Accès des femmes à la culture (1598-1715)*. Paris: Champion, 1993.

Traninger, Anita. "Wandelbare Orte. Zur Rhetorizität und 'Toposhaftigkeit' der Querelle des femmes bei Cornelius Agrippa (1486-1535) und Lucrezia Marinella (1571-1635)."

Heisser Streit und kalte Ordnung. Epochen der Querelle des femmes zwischen Mittelalter und Gegenwart. Ed. Friedericke Hassauer. Wallstein: Göttingen, 2008. 183-205.

van Schurman, Anna. *Whether a Christian Woman Should be Educated and Other Writings from Her Intellectual Circle.* Trans. and ed. Joyce L. Erwin. Chicago: U of Chicago P, 1998.

Vesalius, Andreas. *The Fabric of the Human Body: An Annotated Translation of the 1543 and 1555 Editions.* 2 vols. Basel: Karger, 2014.

Vicary, Thomas. *The Anatomie of the Bodie of Man.* 1548. London: EETS, 1888.

Villemur, Frédérique. "Éros et Androgyne: la femme comme un autre soy-mesme?" *Royaume de féminie. Pouvoirs, contraintes, espaces de liberté des femmes de la Renaissance à la Fronde.* Ed. Kathleen Wilson-Chevalier and Éliane Viennot. Paris: Champion, 1999. 237-60.

Wack, Mary. *Lovesickness in the Middle Ages. The Viaticum and Its Commentaries.* Philadelphia: U of Pennsylvania P, 1990.

Warner, Lyndan. *The Ideas of Man and Woman in Renaissance France. Print, Rhetoric, and Law.* Aldershot: Ashgate, 2011.

Wells, Marion. *The Secret Wound. Love-Melancholy and Early Modern Romance.* Stanford: Stanford UP, 2007.

Weyer, Johann. *Witches, Devils, and Doctors in the Renaissance: Johann Weyer, De praestigiis daemonum.* Trans. John Shea, ed. George Mora and Benjamin Kohl. Binghamton: MRTS, 1991.

Wiesner-Hanks, Mary and Gerhild Scholz-Williams. "Paracelsus über Geschlecht, Weisheit und die menschliche Natur." *Geschlechterperspektiven. Forschungen zur frühen Neuzeit.* Ed. Heide Wunder and Gisela Engel. Königstein: Ulrike Helmer Verlag, 1998. 301-12.

Wilkin, Rebecca. *Women, Imagination, and the Search for Truth in Early Modern France.* Aldershot: Ashgate, 2008.

Woodbridge, Linda. *Women and the English Renaissance. Literature and the Nature of Womankind, 1540-1620.* Urbana: U of Illinois P, 1984.

Zayas y Sotomayor, María de. *Novelas amorosas y ejemplares.* Ed. Augustín G. de Amezúa. Madrid: Aldus, 1948.

Clark Lawlor

Fashionable Disease and Gender in the Long Eighteenth Century

> Two handmaids wait the throne: alike in place,
> But diff'ring far in figure and in face.
> Here stood Ill Nature like an ancient maid,
> Her wrinkled form in black and white array'd;
> With store of pray'rs, for mornings, nights, and noons,
> Her hand is fill'd; her bosom with lampoons.
>
> There Affectation, with a sickly mien,
> Shows in her cheek the roses of eighteen,
> Practis'd to lisp, and hang the head aside,
> Faints into airs, and languishes with pride,
> On the rich quilt sinks with becoming woe,
> Wrapp'd in a gown, for sickness, and for show.
> The fair ones feel such maladies as these,
> When each new night-dress gives a new disease.

(Pope 2006: 92, ll. 25-38)

The eighteenth century was, notoriously, an age of fashionable disease. Much literary representation centred on the inauthenticity of claims to such fashionable conditions as the spleen and vapours, and often reeked of anti-feminist discourse. Pope's infamous lines from *The Rape of the Lock* (1714) in the melancholic Cave of Spleen depict the ladies of the fashionable world as paradoxically subject to the vagaries of their wombs ("Hail wayward Queen! / Who rule the sex to fifty from fifteen" (Pope 2006: 92, ll. 57-58)) and yet cunningly manipulating the symptoms of melancholy: "The fair ones feel such maladies as these, / When each new nightdress gives a new disease". Here the better-known world of female fashion combines with the fashionability of disease, even if negatively framed by Pope's profoundly ambiguous misogyny, both attracted and repelled as he was by the women of the upper ranks, and of whatever religious denomination.

This essay will map out some of the main issues concerning fashionable diseases in this period, although the subject is vast and requires a much more exhaustive treatment than can be provided in this essay. Here I will be considering how fashionable disease can be defined, how gender relates to fashionable diseases (with gout as a masculine disease and the key examples of consumption and melancholy being more complicated in their construction), the role of literature in fashionable disease and the importance of multiple discourses (gender, class, religion, medicine etc.). We need to examine the flexi-bility of symptomatology, the 'narrative' of symptoms for diseases such as me-lancholy and consumption and how they enable the insertion of these diseases into different discourses (such as consumption and the good death for Christians, and the relationship between melancholy, consumption and genius in both men and women).

We also acknowledge the role played by medical theory and its effect on lit-erary practice – changing medical models of the body did affect fashionable dis-ease. By the eighteenth century melancholy and nervous diseases became more acceptable across the whole of society, rather than certain groups, although there was a trickle-down effect in terms of class that increased as the century went on. Melancholy also became feminised (through sensibility and nervous models of the body, as did consumption). We track the turn from Sensibility to Roman-ticism, where we find that fashionable diseases like melancholy were the subject of a tussle between a remasculinised literary tradition (invoking Hamlet) versus a female appropriation by the likes of Charlotte Smith. We conclude that con-sumption's fashionability was gendered – via a masculine tradition of con-sumptive genius against female beauty and spirituality – and yet contested and unstable.

The Paradox of Fashionable Disease

Initially we face the large question of how a disease (physical or mental) can be perceived as a positive phenomenon in human experience. What factors can lead us to overcome the basic obstacle of disease as an unpleasant if not devastating facet of human life? How can gender feed into this equation? The answers are not simple, and we turn to the example of gout to get us started, as gout was a more clearly gendered condition than some others. Gout, as the late Roy Porter and G.S. Rousseau's book of the same title has shown, was 'The Patrician Malady'.[1] Portraits like that of William Pitt, 1st Earl of Chatham (1708-78) (after a painting by Brompton) depicted the subject as suffering from a disease brought about by an elite lifestyle, a malady to which only rich men, with their port and expensive French food, could cleave. It was a badge of honour, a sign of class distinction, a painfully double-edged sword that nevertheless confirmed a man's place in the social hierarchy.

On the other hand, gout was an object of satire – which was an index of an-other type of fashionability, but much less positive. One coloured engraving by Isaac Maddox after Henry W. Bunbury depicted a "A gouty man surrounded by

---

[1] See Porter and Rousseau 1998.

horse-riding accoutrements", or "Geoffrey Gambado Esq.".[2] This cartoon was again a display of the patrician in his element, but the artistic medium lent a degree of critique to the corpulent hunting type. Consumption and melancholy were a little more complicated in that they could be diseases of distinction for both male and female, as we will see shortly.

Another piece in the jigsaw for constructing fashionable diseases is the influence of creative literature in this period (before radio, television and the internet), which was a major vehicle for shaping responses to disease. Literature provided generic 'templates' through which people could understand or even experience their diseases. Narratives and representations were especially important, and different diseases suited different genres and different types of representation. The comic or tragic genres were significant elements in the fashionability of certain diseases (think of Romantic suicide, for example, with sentimental tragedy as its metier). We must also ask about the mesh of disease with cultural and social functions, such as the consumptive good death in which the disease had a 'fit' with the needs of the Christian to make peace with God. This is also a question of how diseases like melancholy and consumption work their way into the social and cultural nexus via their range of symptoms and narratives.

Biology and Culture

Arthur Kleinman has argued, and I agree with him, that the facts of biology are transformed by social and cultural factors, so that biology is constantly being reshaped (often radically) by our varying social environments (Kleinman 1988). This biological embedding can occur either synchronically between cultures in our own time, or diachronically between (for example) the depression/ tuberculosis of our day and the melancholy/consumption of previous centuries. Social discourses therefore become a crucial factor in generating the fashionability of a disease, discourses that include gender, religion and class – and medico-literary movements like sensibility in the eighteenth century. All these converge in the melancholic and consumptive character of Samuel Richardson's Clarissa Harlowe (from *Clarissa* 1747-8) – as we shall see later.

Gender is our chosen determinant of identity in this essay, but the weighting of gender's influence on fashionable disease is historically specific – it works in different ways in different periods and in different social groups. We do not find a straightforward narrative of patriarchal construction of 'inferior' diseases of women versus the 'superior' and 'fashionable' diseases of men.

[2] See this image at the *Wellcome Images* website:
http://images.wellcome.ac.uk/indexplus/result.html?*sform=wellcome-images&_IXACTION_=query&%24%3Dtoday=&_IXFIRST_=1&%3Did_ref=V0010867&_IXSPFX_=templates/t&_IXFPFX_=templates/t&_IXMAXHITS_=1

Defining Melancholy and Consumption – Flexible Disease Narratives

Melancholy works well as a case study for fashionable diseases in the period, and demonstrates how symptomatology can work with social requirements. Sadness varied in intensity – from crippling (Anne Finch – "Now a Dead Sea thou'lt represent, /A Calm of stupid Discontent" (Lawlor and Suzuki 2003: 69)) to mildly pleasant (Thomas Gray – "white melancholy, or rather Leucocholy for the most part [...] is a good easy sort of state" (Gray 1935: i.209)). As a condition often defined (although not always) by psychological symptoms that were internal rather than external physical marks, melancholy was amenable to appropriation by a wider range of people, in some ways like the usually mild external marks of consumption, a lung disease.

But – the early modern definition of melancholy was also irreducibly physical, having run through medical explanations from the original classical humoural one of malfunctioning black bile to the mechanical and then nervous of the late seventeenth and eighteenth centuries. Alistair Gowland's work on melancholy has demonstrated the cultural and discursive flexibility of an apparently 'soft' disease like melancholy in the early modern period (Gowland 2006: 86). Consumption was also flexible in its symptomatology and amenability to a variety of discourses, like the Christian 'good death' or secular love melancholy.

At the heart of this matter there is the basic issue of the condition's severity: we have 'Leucocholy' as Thomas Gray would later term it, where the melancholic individual can wallow in a relatively symptomless isolation from society. Gray defined a sort of "white melancholy, or rather Leucocholy for the most part [...] [which] is a good easy sort of state, and ca ne laisse que de s'amuser" (Gray 1935: i.209). This, to all intents, is a form of self-indulgence, a freeing oneself from social obligations in order to engage in a creative (or possibly entirely unproductive) use of the imagination. Sufferers from consumption often followed a similar disease process where, at first, they rather enjoyed the comparatively symptomless early stages of consumption and later, when symptoms of greater severity came forward, the realisation that they were condemned to suffering for the rest of their possibly brief existence brought on psychological depression, or at least a more negative view of their supposedly beneficial condition (Lawlor 2006: 30).

Melancholy (or melancholia, the two tended to be used interchangeably) was particularly flexible in its symptoms and outcomes. At one level, following Robert Burton's encyclopaedic *Anatomy of Melancholy*, symptoms (and causes) are often legion and include many physical manifestations. Burton's 'Contents' page states that the general symptoms of the body include: "ill digestion, crudity, wind, dry brains, hard belly, thick blood, much waking, heaviness, and palpitation of heart, leaping in many places, &c." (Burton 1989: 120). Psychological symptoms might be similarly various: Head Melancholy might mean "Continual fear, sorrow, suspicion, discontent, superfluous cares, solicitude, anxiety, perpetual cogitation of such toys they are possessed with, thoughts like dreams, &c." (ibid.). Hypochondriacal, or 'windy melancholy' deviated from the core features of fear and sadness: "Fearful, sad, suspicious, discontent, anxiety, &c. Lascivious by reason of much wind, troublesome dreams, affected by fits, &c." (ibid.). The thorny issue of gender also played itself out on the symptom-matology of melancholia: one part was entitled "Symptoms of nuns, maids, and widows melancholy, in body and mind, &c", in which Burton cited the classical yet ongoing concept of the womb's (*hystera*) role in deranging female physio-logy and psychology (ibid.).

But was melancholy primarily a mental state characterised by causeless fear and sadness and therefore capable of social functions above and beyond those of physical disease? Burton seeks to identify and explain the symptoms of "General Melancholy" that were "Common to all or most": "Fear and sorrow without a just cause, suspicion, jealousy, discontent, solitariness, irksomeness, continual cogitations, restless thoughts, vain imaginations" (ibid.). The positive representation of melancholy appears most related to this further stage of mental symptoms: the less severe the symptoms, the more positively a disease can be regarded and represented. This is partly why the consumption could be trans-formed into the exciting and poetic Romantic disease: because its progress and developing symptoms were relatively mild in comparison to other illnesses. Consumption was slow (good news for the devout Christian who wanted to be ready for death); there was no physical scarring; it was relatively painless be-cause of the low number of nerves in the lungs; there was no mental illness. Consumption had a number of symptomatological aspects that could be – and were – regarded positively: the bodily wasting might be seen as a pious rejection of the world and the flesh or a sign of refined nerves and female beauty; the alternating hectic rougeing and pallor of the cheeks could also be seen in terms of classical female beauty; because sufferers were often unaware of the severity of their condition the term 'spes phthisica' or 'hope of the consumptive' had been invented in classical times to describe the feverish creativity of the con-sumptive until the final moments of life (Lawlor 2006: 46-7).

Melancholy-depression, when compared in this manner, have much in com-mon. Historically the two were related, as consumption was a common result of love and religious melancholia, according to the doctors and popular narratives in literature and art. Romantic poets were almost encouraged to be both con-sumptive and melancholic, as the examples of minor poet Henry Kirke White and the more familiar John Keats amply prove. Melancholy could begin, like consumption, in a 'gentle' manner with mild symptoms; it could end, however, in disaster and death – like consumption. What was the symptom-complex of melancholy and consumption that could be positively construed? Some aspects we have already noted: melancholy could leave the body unmarked, unstigmatised, and free from pain, much like consumption.

The imagination is a key component in melancholy and in consumption. The imagination's effects in melancholia were initially explained by medical theory in terms of humoral disorder (vapours, arising from the indigestion and burning of black bile in the spleen and hypochondries, supposedly ascended to the brain). In the eighteenth century it was mechanical-hydraulic or chemical dysfunctions relating to the digestion that affected the supply of 'animal spirits' to the brain; and later in the period disordered nerves (again stemming from digestive malfunctions) wrought havoc with the physical operation of the brain and led to psychological problems. Further aspects of this theme might be elaborated, such as the astrological influence of Saturn on the humoural constitution, but the centrality of the imagination in the general understanding of melancholy was certain. Although the medical theory changed in its rationale, its implications for the imagination had a certain amount of continuity. The disrupted yet productive imagination might be beneficial for creative types, and not merely for the Romantics and their new valorisation of the concept of originality.

Melancholy and consumption were usually chronic. Some conditions, like smallpox, might strike swiftly, painfully and obviously. For the literary and studious person, a slow duration of disease had certain benefits: there was time for composition of creative literature. Chronic diseases favoured the development of thought and writing: dying of consumption or suffering from melancholy (including love melancholy) might inspire a poet or writer to put the experience into their work. Melancholy's chronicity and the tendency to introspection and imaginative inspiration were a paradoxically fortunate combination for the creative person. The time taken for melancholy and consumption to develop was a central feature in the connection between disease and creativity.

It is not a closed debate on the question of whether this story of melancholy's progress is a biological element in the manner of conditions with clear causes (at least to modern science) of consumption, cholera, smallpox or the Black Death (however those disease structures might vary in their outcomes in themselves).[3] The eighteenth century, despite elements of modernity, took its cue from the Classical writers in regarding mind and body as fundamentally interrelated, and such a view continued until the rise of positivist science in the nineteenth century.

Fashionable melancholy itself is necessarily a dilution of the illness: we reduce our focus towards the form of melancholy described by both Burton and Gray, in which the symptoms are chronic and the 'story' of the disease follows

---

[3] See Horwitz and Wakefield 2007 for a clear exposition of the problems involved in defining modern-day depression.

an arc that allows an initially pleasant form of melancholy. Burton suggests a tragic end, with the progressive worsening of the melancholy state, unless some intervention is forthcoming, and ultimately death through disease or suicide results. The suicide' option' itself became fashionable in the Romantic period, from Goethe's character of young Werther to the spectacular (alleged) suicide of Chatterton, the iconic poet of sensibility driven into suicidal depression by a cruel and negligent world (at least as represented by Victorian artists like Henry Wallis, who painted "The Death of Chatterton" (1856), a notoriously melodramatic rendition of the 'suicide'). The fate of the consumptive Keats – his disease allegedly brought on by a harsh review – echoes that of Chatterton in the connection of illness and biography. The discourse of the poet of sensibility being nervously maladapted to the harsh circumstances of literary production prevalent at the end of the eighteenth and start of the nineteenth centuries plugged straight into the symptoms and 'narratives' of consumption and melancholy, both of which suited a certain cultural construction of the role of a lower-class poet (Lawlor 2006: 146).

Melancholy also had the advantage that it could go into remission, thus allowing at least some lucid intervals necessary for creative activity, thus mitigating the worst debilitations of its fear and sadness as basic features. Nevertheless it was possible to write even when suffering more severe states of emotion, and, in certain cases, writers could be inspired by such extreme emotions to express and even contain melancholy's agonies. Also, melancholy was not usually thought to disengage the individual from reality completely, as in the 'raving' lunatic represented in Caius Cibber's statue on the gates of Bedlam. Imprisonment due to melancholy was not usually necessary because melancholics were perfectly capable of functioning in society most of the time: one cure for melancholy was to seek out company and occupation: "If you are idle, be not solitary; if you are solitary, be not idle" said Dr Johnson, via Robert Burton (Boswell 1934: 415). The doomed hero and poet in William Cowper's poem "The Castaway" (1803) actually fled society rather than causing disruption within it. It is the case that the hallucinatory element of the early-modern complex of melancholy does not sit well with this more 'friendly' discourse on the disease, but even these visions were largely benign, in the sense that they were not a permanent event: the individual might have a vision, but then usually returned to lucidity and reality. Hallucinations were part of the advantageous imaginative disorder – all contributed to the inspired melancholic individual artist.

These diseases, be they melancholy or consumption, detached one from society just enough to liberate the imagination, and indeed body, from social constraints that might be inconvenient to the creative process. Love-sick melancholy and/or consumptive poets, Renaissance or Romantic (and even a few

earlier eighteenth-century examples), could take advantage of such illness. The
women also could retire into a quiet grove of one's own (like an Anne Finch, as
we will see later in this essay) in order to nurse both their melancholy and their
poetic imagination, and with the added advantage of avoiding onerous domestic
duties. Due to melancholia's psychological core, due to its potential extremes of
severity (like consumption), due to the difficulty of diagnosing the exact
motivation and authenticity of the condition (also a problem with consumption),
it was a disease that allowed a higher degree of self-expression: a poetic and
creative disease indeed, and one ripe for fashionability.

Masculine Melancholy and Genius

Aristotle, or at least pseudo-Aristotle, put forward the contentious but highly
influential concept of the melancholic (male and upper-class) genius in the
Classical period. In the Renaissance this idea of disease as a vehicle for
intellectual prowess and creativity was seized upon by the melancholic scholar
Marsilio Ficino (1433-99) in Italy and thence disseminated across Europe, cul-
minating in the dramatic character of Shakespeare's Hamlet.[4] Robert Burton
summarised the view of the Aristotelian tradition succinctly: "Melancholy men
or all others are most witty, [and their melancholy] causeth many times divine
ravishment, and a kind of *enthusiasmus* […] which stirreth them up to be excellent Philosophers, poets, Prophets, etc." (Burton 1989: 461). This tinge of the
Platonic, the hint of a connection with the divine, chimed well with the Renaissance alchemy and astrology of Ficino and his peers, and the new version of
Renaissance melancholy spread like wildfire across Europe.

   Robert Burton may be the most famous actual melancholic of the Renaissance, but Hamlet is the template of the melancholic man of distinction for
future ages, just as Ophelia becomes the archetype of female lovesickness, a
blend of passionate sexual desire and virginal purity that ends in suicide. Much
has been written about Hamlet and his relationship to both traditions of melancholy, the more prosaic and gritty Galenic inheritance and the 'genial' melancholy of Ficino and Aristotle – Hamlet is a complex blend of the two. Shakespeare's spectacularly successful and influential portrait of Hamlet as a tortured
soul, an alienated intellectual, almost anti-hero, with great psychological depth,
set the seal on melancholy's glamorous reputation in literature and, to some
extent, life.

---

[4] See Ficino 1549.

Gendered Discourses of Melancholy

The fashionable vogue of melancholy as it emerged from the Renaissance was in the main masculine, but women did attempt to take advantage of the connection between literary genius and melancholy. Those higher up the ranks had better access to an education that could equip women to exploit the pose of the melancholic thinker, even if they were not suffering from the illness in reality. Margaret Cavendish (1661-1717) was the Duchess of Newcastle, and a prolific writer in all manner of genres, including natural philosophy. Samuel Pepys called her "mad, conceited, ridiculous", irritated as he was by her efforts to display the powers of her own intellect (Pepys 1976: 123).

One of these self-conscious poses adopted by Cavendish was that of the melancholic figure, shy, and a lover of books and isolation. Her frontispiece to *The Philosophical and Physical Opinions, written by her Excellency, the Lady Marchionesse of Newcastle* (1655) has a poetic caption that explains the meaning of the image:

> Studious She is and all Alone
> Most visitants, when She has none,
> Her Library on which She looks
> It is her Head her Thoughts her Books.
> Scorninge dead Ashes without fire
> For her owne Flames doe her Inspire.

(Cavendish 1655: frontispiece)[5]

It is well documented that female authors had genuine causes for depression, given the often aggressive opposition to their writings, even if there were supportive men in their circles who did encourage them in the life of the mind. Pepys's reaction is notable, but in this caption Cavendish draws upon a certain kind of 'madness' that actually validates her as an intellectual of distinction, and draws on the iconography of the melancholy scholar, posing alone with the tools of her trade: desk, pen, ink, books. The image is clearly a form of role-playing, but its goal is to indicate her authentic genius. The flames that inspire her have the Platonic spark of the divine that we saw in Burton's discussion of melancholy genius, and the caption boldly claims that innate inspiration for Cavendish, a mere woman. We will see that female intellectuals continue to tap into the possibilities for self-expression opened up by melancholy genius in the following centuries.

Many women were prevented from participating in an education sufficient to allow them to exploit scholarly melancholy in the manner of a Cavendish, but the fact that women were thought of as cold and dry in a humoural sense meant

---

[5] For further analysis of this image see Rippl 2011.

that they could be considered as melancholic. The renewal of Galenism in the earlier period also left an opportunity for women to argue that they too contained black bile, and that they too could be possessed by it for the forces of good and intellect rather than merely as deluded witches, although the theory of the humours could, as with other philosophies, be used in the service of patriarchy. It has been argued that the Aristotelian mode excluded women, but this ignores the importance of the humours and Galen in the construction of melancholy.[6] Medieval woodcuts depicted melancholy either as a despairing scholar or a (female) spinster. Cavendish's image was late enough to be present at the birth of the New Science, in which the concept of the four humours was shunted aside for a new mechanical/hydraulic idea of the body, but it took a long time for popular images and illness narratives to catch up with the new thinking on the function of the heart and so on, as indeed did many medical treatments. The humours were very persistent as an element of theory and practice in both medicine and wider culture.

Some critics state that any positive perception of female melancholy was reversed when a new form arose in the seventeenth century that was related to disorder of the female reproductive organs and was more akin to hysteria in the modern sense, but throughout the history of melancholy that sexual difference has been continuously reformulated according to developing notions of the body and deployed against the idea of female intellectual equality.[7] For the solitary male scholar, Robert Burton, melancholy was masculine, and he only discussed women in one chapter of the *Anatomy of Melancholy*, added in 1628, not the 1624 original: "Symptoms of Nuns, Maids and Widows Melancholy, in body and mind, &c.". The source of disruption that led to a specific form of melancholy was the underemployed womb in Burton's world. Despite this obstacle, women continued to claim fashionable disease for themselves.

Melancholic Female Self-Fashioning

This deployment of a feminised fashionability to melancholia continued further into the eighteenth century. Anne Finch's popular poem "A Pindaric Ode on the Spleen" (originally written around 1694) shows a female poet carefully delineating different types of authentic and inauthentic melancholy, and ultimately situating her own particular form of real suffering as a proof of her poetic iden-

---

[6] See for example Schiesari 1992.

[7] See Hodgkin 2005, chapter 4 "Melancholy: A Land of Darkness", 60-85. Hodgkin uses the work of Carol Thomas Neely to show that a new form of female melancholy arises where women's melancholy is not the genius type but one related to "disordered female wombs and genitals" (Neely, quoted in Hodgkin 2005: 83).

tity.[8] Finch attacks those fops and fools who pretend to the fashionable Spleen, but the female poet has a further strategy to pursue:

> The fool to imitate the wits
> Complains of thy pretended fits
> And dullness born with him would lay
> Upon thy accidental sway;
> Because sometime thou do'st presume
> Into the ablest heads to come.
>   That often men of thought refin'd,
>   Impatient of unequal sense,
> Such slow returns, where they so much dispense,
> Retiring from the croud, are to thy shades inclin'd.
>   O'er me, alas, thou do'st too much prevail,
>   I feel thy force, whilst I against thee rail.

> (Lawlor and Suzuki 2003: 70-71)

Finch portrays melancholy as a fashionable malady that attracts the pretentious and the stupid, but it is also a real illness that afflicts "men of thought" who flee from the fashionable city mob. The solitary person of true sense finds consolation in the "shades" of rural peace, reflecting the clear moral victory of the country over the city in Finch's pastoral of illness. She positions herself as a true melancholic person, shifting, in a clever move, from the "men of sense", who retire into the country shades, to her own painful experience ("O'er me, alas") and a similar flight away from the falsely fashionable urban environment:

> Whilst in the Muses paths I stray,
> Whilst in their groves and by their secret springs
> My hand delights to trace unusual things,
> And deviates from the known and common rules.

> (Lawlor and Suzuki 2003: 71)

Longinus and, in Finch's period, Alexander Pope had promoted the idea of the poet as being able to break the rules of poetry; Finch latches onto this individualist turn and relates it to her own poetic wanderings in the pastoral retreat of traditionally male genius. The diseased woman becomes a genuine melancholic poet via Finch's cunning manoeuvre, and the "secret springs" of genius are now those of Finch too. Her melancholy is fashionable but also real. She uses the winding and even digressive Pindaric form of the ode to reflect the protean nature of her splenetic condition, a smart use of poetic form that further proves

---

[8] In an intriguing combination of science and literature not uncommon in the eighteenth century, Finch's poem was published within William Stukeley's *Of the Spleen*, 'Diseases', Sect. XVII, 64-69 [1723]; including Ann[e] Finch, 'A Pindaric Ode on the Spleen', 6-9; reprinted in facsimile in Lawlor and Suzuki 2003: 69-72.

her point: Finch is a true poet. By spurning false melancholy, she depicts her own as genuine, and ironically conveys an image of herself as authentically suffering for her art in a sophisticated set-piece of a poem.

Diseases of Gender and Rank

We turn to Burton (again) to remind us that gender was not separate from rank in the seventeenth or eighteenth centuries:

> For seldom should you see a hired servant, a poor handmaid, though ancient, that is kept hard to her work and bodily labour, a coarse country wench, troubled in this kind, but noble virgins, nice gentlewomen, such as are solitary and idle, live at ease, lead a life out of action and employment, that fare well, in great houses and jovial companies, ill-disposed peradventure of themselves, and not willing to make any resistance, discontented otherwise, of weak judgment, able bodies, and subject to passions [...] such for the most part are misaffected, and prone to this disease.
>
> (Burton 1989: 417)

These sentiments were echoed by George Cheyne in his influential *English Malady* in the eighteenth century. The explanations of melancholy might have shifted into the spleen and vapours via the new mechanistic model of the body (now not sign of a sick soul but blocked pipes, although it could be caused by psychological factors as part of the six 'non-naturals'), but the divisions of class continued. Importantly, Cheyne's and other popular definitions of the English Malady in the eighteenth century avoided the stigma of lunacy and paved the way for the development of melancholy as 'polite' disease.[9] Melancholy became a disease of civilisation: a sign of refined nerves and taste.

Sensibility and Melancholy

The displacement of the 'man-machine' by advances in nerve theory after mid-century blended melancholy with sensibility, and these medical discourses coincided in an exemplary fashion with others in the literary case of Samuel Richardson's character Clarissa Harlowe, who suffers from love melancholy which then transforms into religious melancholy when she is raped by the rake Lovelace. She provides a major and very influential instance of (modern) nervous sensibility blended with older discourses of religious melancholy and the consumptive good death.[10] Clarissa's arrangement of a coffin with en-

---

[9] See Porter 1991: xxxviii.

[10] For two accounts of Clarissa's sensibility and its consequences see Stephanson 1988 and Lawlor, "Long Grief", 2006.

gravings that remind her of her mortality as she wastes away of consumption reworks John Donne's famous consumptive death.

Isaak Walton's *The Life of John Donne* describes Donne's own preparations for death:

> A monument being resolved upon, Dr. Donne sent for a Carver to make for him in wood the figure of an urn, giving him directions for the compass and height of it; and to bring with it a board, of just the height of his body. "These being got, then without delay a choice painter was got to be in readiness to draw his picture, which was taken as followeth.—Several charcoal fires being first made in his large study, he brought with him into that place his winding-sheet in his hand, and having put off all his clothes, had this sheet put on him, and so tied with knots at his head and feet, and his hands so placed as dead bodies are usually fitted, to be shrouded and put into their coffin, or grave. Upon this urn he thus stood, with his eyes shut, and with so much of the sheet turned aside as might show his lean, pale, and deathlike face, which was purposely turned towards the east, from whence he expected the second coming of his and our Saviour Jesus." In this posture he was drawn at his just height; and when the picture was fully finished, he caused it to be set by his bed-side, where it continued and became his hourly object till his death.
>
> (Walton 1640: 77-78)

Clarissa Harlowe's death in the eponymous novel is clearly a conscious echo of Donne's pious demise. The difference is that Clarissa's consumption is combined with a love melancholy initially prompted by a secular object, and then compounded by a rape that initiates consumption: a holy disease but also indicative of secular love thwarted (Lawlor 2006: 60). The discourse of gender dictates that the masculine consumption of the seventeenth century becomes a feminine consumption in the eighteenth. Bourgeois females in Richardson's religious framework have no option but to die if their secular love is destroyed by aristocratic rapaciousness – a trend that was to continue into the nineteenth century, in which the illusion of the 'angel in the house' would compound the problem of female purity and its defilement.

Sensibility to Romanticism

As the eighteenth century continued the fashionability of melancholy and consumption persisted due to a number of developments both cultural and medical, prime among them the concept and culture of sensibility. Albrecht von Haller (1708-77) had defined the quality of sensibility as something that resided in the centre of the nerve and that allowed the perception of exterior impulses or stimuli. Physical tissues containing nerves now could be said to possess sensibility, and the property of 'irritability' rested in the muscles and worked separately from the nervous system. Hence Haller enabled medical theory to recognise the importance of the solid parts of the body and the independence of sensibility and irritability from an allegedly separate and inviolable soul (Risse 1992: 160-63). Nerves and fibres now took on a dominant role in medical theory, and allowed the progression towards Romantic concepts of the unconscious operation of the body and the erosion of the power of reason.

Crucially for the study of representations of consumption and melancholy, sensibility became an integral aspect of the novel, poetry and drama, with sensitive and weeping heroes, from the consumptive hero of *Tristram Shandy* (1760) to the extreme melancholic sensibility of the *Man of Feeling* (1771). Heroines too were more and more defined by physical reactions to emotional events.[11] Such representations of the fashionable melancholy of sensibility and the sentimental could vary in degree. Consumption too was an index of sensibility, a sure sign of authentic artistic or spiritual suffering *à la* Keats or Novalis. Poets, writers and artists trembled with sensibility, were over-excited in their supply of nervous life force, and exhausted their energies: they lived fast and died young (literally as well as theoretically in the case of Keats and Shelley). The increased focus on the self, as opposed to the civic and social responsibilities of the earlier period, meant that Romantic melancholy intensified the idea of this disease as a marker of self-reflection, permitting contemplation of the deepest aspects of existence, and generally typifying creative genius.

At the end of our period, then, fashionable melancholy was profoundly linked with the medical theory of the nerves, and this did not cease with the advent of Romanticism and the 'Brunonian' vitalist medicine that was so influential in the representations of the period. The boom in Scottish medicine furthered the cause of 'nerve theory'.[12] Unfortunately for John Brown, his ideas and the related systems proved a failure in practice and did not persist long in medicine, although vitalism itself was a powerful discourse in the artistic sphere (Risse 1992: 165-67).

By the late eighteenth century, both melancholy and consumption had entered into a new phase of fashionability, partly informed by literary and philosophical trends such as the Graveyard School in poetry, and by a new emphasis on individual genius, both of which resulted in the emergence of the figure of the "gloomy egoist".[13] The role of medical theory of the nerves was also crucial in this continued fashionability, as it continued to mark out the sensitive individual as a person prone to melancholy, and enabled the mythology of melancholy and consumptive genius to be reactivated, although via a different physiological rationale. This new physiology of sensibility and the nerves was in some ways

---

[11] The vast literature on sensibility includes: Barker-Benfield 1992, Csengei 2011, Mullan 1988, Todd 1986, Van Sant 1993 and Vila 1998.

[12] See Porter 1988: xxxiv.

[13] See Sickels 1932.

an advantage for women, who were thought to be finer-nerved than men, but the problem was that women might also be considered as more feeble in their intellectual and physical constitutions, including the operations of the brain (Stanton 2003: 627).

Gendering Romantic Melancholy and Melancholic Self-Fashioning

Again, female writers struggled to claim part of the melancholic fashionable heritage. Charlotte Smith (1749-1806) was a female poet who suffered from depression and who used it for her poetry. She had a prosperous country childhood, but saw her early marriage as a form of slavery and proceeded to endure the deaths of several of her children, including her favourite, Augusta. These events, understandably enough, plunged her into depression and anxiety. In her *Conversations Introducing Poetry* (1804), a children's book, she baldly stated – via the character of a teacher talking to a child – the general opinion of the literary sort on the relationship of melancholy to genius: 'It has been observed, George, that almost all men of genius have a disposition to indulge melancholy and gloomy ideas; and in reading our most celebrated poets, we have evidence that it is so' (Smith 1804: 100 and quoted in Dolan 2003: 239).

Smith, via the *Elegiac Sonnets and other Essays* (which appeared in 1784 and were revised until her death) as well as her prefaces to various works, presented herself as a true melancholic and therefore a genuine poet, and attempted to forge a space for herself in the tradition of melancholic sensibility. In her first sonnet in the volume she regarded herself as both cursed and blessed by her gift: "those paint sorrow best who feel it most" (Smith 1784: 2). In her Preface to the Fifth Edition she stated starkly: "I wrote mournfully because I was unhappy" (Smith 1993: 5). Adopting the pose of the melancholic in Sonnet XXXII, "To melancholy. Written on the banks of the Arun, October 1785", Smith invoked "the pensive visionary mind" (1790: 32, l. 14) of the melancholy poet.

Charlotte Smith has prompted a critical debate about her deployment of her personal circumstances to build up a poetic image: Jacqueline Labbe has suggested that Smith's "dead child thus functions as simultaneously an instance of personal loss and an opportunity to strengthen her poetic persona, as poetry becomes the vehicle by which she expresses her grief" (Labbe 2003: 66). According to this reading, Smith was making poetic capital out of her personal tragedies, a strategy that does not look morally blameless, but Smith's financial circumstances perhaps left her with little choice. It is also true that the general discourses surrounding poetic melancholy actively encouraged her to appropriate the male tradition for her own ends. She also associated herself (via her poetry and prose) with male poets of a melancholic cast like Collins, Otway and Hayley, following a similar pattern of appropriation of male poets as the famous

Davidson sisters in America, who both died young of consumption and whose fame was largely dependent on the fact of their illness and youth rather than poetic ability.[14] As Smith herself put it in a blatant, if deliberately inelegant, piece of melancholic self-fashioning in the Frontispiece to her *Elegiac Sonnets*: 'Oh Time has Changed me since you saw me last, / And heavy Hours with Times deforming Hand / Have written strange Defeatures in my face' (Smith 1797: frontispiece).

Conclusions

We have found, then, that the role of gender in the creation, maintenance and decline of fashionable diseases is crucial, but not the only factor. Gender is one part of a historically specific complex of discourses and events: we need to re-cognise the importance of literary and philosophical traditions onto which gendered positions can be grafted – traditions which often date back to classical literature. To understand fashionable disease – or at least the ones examined here – a long historical view is required, together with a nuanced perspective on gender relations. The story I have told in this essay describes a tradition of masculine fashionable disease (usually in relation to artistic genius), but also a persistent attempt by female authors to appropriate that tradition for their own purposes.

List of Works Cited

Barker-Benfield, G. J. *The Culture of Sensibility: Sex and Society in Eighteenth-Century Britain.* Chicago: U of Chicago P, 1992.

Boswell, James. *Boswell's Life of Johnson: Together with Boswell's Journal of a Tour of the Hebrides, and Johnson's Diary of a Journey into North Wales.* Vol. 3. Ed. George Birbeck Hill. Oxford: Clarendon, 1934.

Burton, Robert. *The Anatomy of Melancholy.* 1632. Vol 1. Ed. Thomas C. Faulkner, Nicolas K. Kiessling and Rhonda L. Blair. Oxford: Clarendon Press, 1989.

Cavendish, Margaret, Duchess of Newcastle. *The Philosophical and Physical Opinions.* London, 1655.

Csengei, Ildiko. *Sympathy, Sensibility and the Literature of Feeling in the Eighteenth Century.* Basingstoke: Palgrave, 2011.

Dolan, Elizabeth A. "British Romantic Melancholia: Charlotte Smith's *Elegiac Sonnets*, Medical Discourse and the Problem of Sensibility." *Journal of European Studies* 33 (2003): 237-53.

Ficino, Marsilio. *De Vita Libri Tres.* Basel, 1549.

Gowland, Angus. "The Problem of Early Modern Melancholy." *Past & Present* 191.1 (2006): 77-120.

---

[14] See Lawlor 2004 and Lawlor 2010.

Gray, Thomas. *Letters*. Ed. Paget Toynbee and Leonard Whibley. Oxford: Oxford UP, 1935.

Hodgkin, Catherine. *Madness in Seventeenth-Century Autobiography*. Basingstoke: Palgrave, 2007.

Horwitz, Allan and Jerome C. Wakefield. *The Loss of Sadness: How Psychiatry Transformed Normal Sorrow into Depressive Disorder*. Oxford: Oxford UP, 2007.

Kleinman, Arthur. *The Illness Narratives: Suffering, Healing and the Human Condition*. New York: Basic Books, 1988.

Labbe, Jacqueline M. *Charlotte Smith: Romanticism, Poetry and the Culture of Gender*. Manchester: Manchester UP, 2003.

Lawlor, Clark. "'It is a path I have prayed to follow': The Paradoxical Pleasures of Romantic Disease." *Romantic Pleasure*. Ed. Tom Schmid and Michelle Faubert. Basingstoke: Palgrave, 2010. 109-132.

---. *Consumption and Literature: The Making of the Romantic Disease*. Basingstoke: Palgrave, 2006.

---. "'Long Grief, dark Melancholy, hopeless natural Love': Clarissa, Cheyne and Narratives of Body and Soul". *Gesnerus: Swiss Journal of the History of Medicine and Sciences* 63.1/2 (2006): 103-112.

---. "Transatlantic Consumptions: Disease, Fame and Literary Nationalisms in the Davidson Sisters, Southey and Poe." *Studies in the Literary Imagination* 36.2 (2004): 109-26.

---. and Akihito Suzuki (eds.). *Literature and Science, 1660-1834*. Part I, Vol. 2. *Sciences of Body and Mind*. London: Pickering and Chatto, 2003.

Mullan, John. *Sentiment and Sociability: The Language of Feeling in the Eighteenth Century*. Oxford: Clarendon P, 1988.

Pepys, Samuel. *The Diary of Samuel Pepys*. Vol. 9. Ed. Robert Latham and William Matthews. London: G. Bell and Sons, 1976.

Pope, Alexander. "The Rape of the Lock." 1714. *The Major Works*. Ed. Pat Rogers. Oxford: Oxford UP, 2006. 77-100.

Porter, Roy and G. S. Rousseau. *Gout: The Patrician Malady*. New Haven: Yale UP, 1998.

Porter, Roy. Introduction. *The English Malady*. By George Cheyne. 1733. Ed. Roy Porter. London: Routledge, 1991. ix-li.

---. Introduction. *An Essay, Medical, Philosophical, and Chemical, on Drunkenness, and its Effects on the Human Body*. By Thomas Trotter. Ed. Roy Porter. London: Routledge, 1988. ix-xl.

Rippl, Gabriele. "Mourning and Melancholia in England and its Transatlantic Colonies: Examples of Seventeenth-Century Female Appropriations." *The Literature of Melancholia: Early Modern to Postmodern*. Ed. Martin Middeke and Christina Wald. Basingstoke: Palgrave, 2011. 50-66.

Risse, Guenter B. "Medicine in the Age of Enlightenment". *Medicine in Society: Historical Essays*. Ed. Andrew Wear. Cambridge: Cambridge UP, 1992. 149-98.

Schiesari, Juliana. *The Gendering of Melancholia: Feminism, Psychoanalysis and the Symbolics of Loss in Renaissance Literature*. New York: Cornell UP, 1992.

Sickels, Eleanor M. *The Gloomy Egoist. Moods and Themes of Melancholy from Gray to Keats*. New York: Columbia UP, 1932.

Smith, Charlotte. *The Poems of Charlotte Smith*. 5th ed. Ed. Stuart Curran. New York: Oxford UP, 1993.

---. *Conversations Introducing Poetry: Chiefly on Subjects of Natural History. For the Use of Children and Young Persons*. London: J. Johnson, 1804.

---. *Elegiac Sonnets and Other Poems*. London: Cadell, 1797.

---. *Elegiac Sonnets and Other Essays*. 5th ed. London: Cadell, 1790.

---. *Elegaic Sonnets and Other Essays*. 2nd ed. Chichester: Dodsley, 1784.

Stanton, Judith P. *The Collected Letters of Charlotte Smith*. Indiana: Indiana UP, 2003.

Stephanson, Raymond. "Richardson's 'Nerves': The Physiology of Sensibility in *Clarissa*." *Journal of the History of Ideas* 49.2 (1988): 267-85.

Todd, Janet. *Sensibility: An Introduction*. London: Methuen, 1986.

Van Sant, Jessie. *Eighteenth-Century Sensibility and the Novel: The Senses in Social Context*. Cambridge: Cambridge UP, 1993.

Vila, Anne C. *Enlightenment and Pathology: Sensibility in the Literature and Medicine of Eighteenth-Century France*. Baltimore: Johns Hopkins UP, 1998.

Walton, Isaak. *The Life of John Donne*. London, 1640.

Felix Sprang

"Disastrous Birth-Nights":
Childbed and Child-Birth in the Nineteenth-Century Novel.
Reflections on Gender and Medicalization

One of the alluring frescoes in the Rinuccini Chapel of Santa Croce in Florence depicts the birth of Mary, Christ's mother. As a devotional image that motif is rather uncommon, even if depictions of the nativity of Mary flourish briefly in the Trecento, the most prominent example being the fresco by Giotto in the Scrovegni Chapel. There are relatively few depictions of Mary's birth because – as an apocryphal story – the birth of Christ's mother was marginalised and of little concern for theological debates. It is overshadowed by both the annunciation and the birth of Christ which clearly take pride of place in Christian iconography.[1] However, the relatively few visual presentations of the birth of Mary bring to the fore the peculiarity of the abundant images of the new-born Christ. The nativity scene, the birth of Christ, is never shown as a birth: we see the infant either presented in Mary's arms or exhibited in the manger, but there are no references to the birthing that took place in Bethlehem.

The absence of references to birthing itself is conspicuous in the very first depiction of the nativity scene dating from the fifth century, and that absence had become the norm when these images gained currency in the Quattrocento. As Gertrud Schiller has pointed out, "[t]he purpose of these early images is not to illustrate the story of the Nativity but rather to bear witness to the arrival of the divine Child, which had fulfilled both Messianic prophecies and the longings for a saviour nourished in the Late Antique period itself" (Schiller 1971: 26) Like Mary's immaculate conception, her giving birth is veiled and mystified. Mary's birth, in contrast, as shown in Giovanni da Milano's fresco, explicitly reminds us of birthing as an embodied process.[2] The monoscenic panel narrates the events immediately following Mary's birth: at the centre of the fresco, a midwife holds the baby with a nurse ready to receive it in her arms. In the background, Saint Anne is washing her hands propped up in the bed where she gave

---

[1] The intriguing iconography of Saint Anne has been discussed by Nixon 2004, von Behr 1996, Dörfler-Dierken 1992, and Ashley 1990.
[2] For a contextualization of the fresco as part of the fresco cycle see Gregori 1965. For a discussion of the fresco cycle see Poeschke 2003: 350-61, and Lavin 1990: 90-98.

birth. And in the foreground we see two women carrying the placenta covered with a cloth out into the hall.[3]

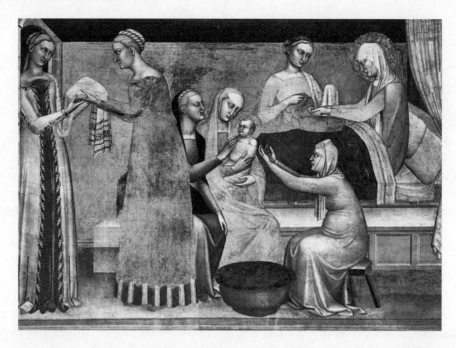

Fig. 1 Giovanni da Milano. *Birth of Mary* (c. 1365) Rinuccini Chapel of Santa Croce in Florence.

For a devotional image the fresco warrants a remarkable interest in the practice of giving birth. Later depictions, for example by the Master of the Life of the Virgin (1470), Domenico Ghirlandaio (c. 1490) or Jan Baegert (c. 1510), are very similar in their pictorial arrangement and narrative content.[4] Details may differ – sometimes Saint Anne is given broth, sometimes the bath water is poured – but with their visual references all these images give pride of place to the birthing itself: the birth is the story told in these narrative images, the protagonist is Saint Anne and not the child born. Consequently, these images can also be read as a consoling commentary on Genesis 3:16, "I will greatly multiply thy sorrow and thy conception; in sorrow thou shalt bring forth children." What these images do not visualise at all is the latter half of that verse: "and thy desire shall be to thy husband, and he shall rule over thee." What we see in these

[3] Until the late sixteenth century, secular art, for example the engravings in Jacob Rueff's *De conceptu et generatione hominis* (1554), also depicted birthing as a women's domain with compositions very similar to the template established in sacral art.

[4] For a brief survey of Byzantine frescoes depicting Saint Anne in the iconic tradition of the *virgo lactans* see Lasareff, 1938: 33.

images of Mary's birth is a sisterhood. Mary's birth is clearly depicted as a woman's affair, and most frescoes and paintings include only women. In a very few
cases, for example in Ghirlandaio's painting, Joachim is present in the background, but there can be no doubt that St. Anne is assisted and cared for by women only when giving birth.

I should like to contrast the iconography of Mary's birth, or – in line with the
ensuing argument – the iconography of St. Anne giving birth, with a recent and
on-going debate brought to the fore by the documentary *Freedom for Birth*
(2012).[5] The women's rights campaign and the film highlight the global scale of
violations of women's rights when they give birth. The main concerns that the
campaigners wish to express with this documentary were discussed in an article
in the *Observer* by Louise Carpenter under the heading "The mothers fighting
back against birth intervention" (Carpenter 2012: 30). Statistics suggest that
giving birth is indeed increasingly seen as a medical condition with caesarean
sections alone accounting for 23.8 per cent of all births at maternity units in the
U.K. in the year 2008, for example (see Bragg et al. 2010). Supported by a
grassroots movement of women who complain about patronizing and bullying
medical staff in the delivery room, and backed by a European court ruling that
criticised impediments for women who had decided to give birth at home, the
"freedom for birth" campaigners criticise the trend towards medicalising birth
and the negative effect that this trend has had on women's rights to decide how
to give birth.[6] "[E]xamples of 'foetal supremacy' over a woman's right to
choose what is or isn't done to her," Louise Carpenter explains in her report,
"have prompted a rapidly growing international pressure movement" (Carpenter
2012: 30).

---

[5] See the website www.freedomforbirth.com for details on the production of the documentary
and the campaign.

[6] In 2009 Anna Ternovszky sued her country, Hungary. As long as the risk of facing
prosecution for assisting home deliveries dissuades midwives in Hungary from agreeing to
her wish for a home birth, Ternovszky argued, her human right to decide how to give birth is
infringed. The European Court of Human Rights ruled in favour of Anna Ternovsky, and in a
joint statement the judges András Sajó and Françoise Tulkens explained that "[i]n the present
case the liberty is not self-explanatory as the expectant mother has to interact during the period of pregnancy with authorities and regulated professionals who act as figures of some kind
of public authority vis-à-vis the pregnant person, who is understandably very vulnerable because of her dependency. It is this consideration that makes us believe that a freedom may
necessitate a positive regulatory environment which will produce the legal certainty providing
the right to choose with effectiveness. Without such legal certainty there is fear and secrecy,
and in the present context this may result in fatal consequences for mother and child. The
ruling and case details for Ternovszky v. Hungary are provided online by the European Court
of Human Rights: http://hudoc.echr.coe.int/sites/eng/pages/search.aspx?i=001-102254.

The criticism voiced by the "freedom for birth" campaigners is not new –in *For Her Own Good: 150 Years of the Expert's Advice to Women* Barbara Ehrenreich and Deirdre English have pointed at the legacy of paternalism disguised as expertise, and Susan Faludi has identified a growing patriarchal sentiment in the 1980s as a *Backlash: The Undeclared War Against Woman*.[7] However, I think that the debate about women's rights to determine the birthing process often lacks a historical perspective. What I propose, then, is to look at the history of obstetrics and to consider in particular a crucial period in our literary imagination when conceptions of giving birth were shaped in the popular domain. Focusing on the English novel and a British context, I will point at a historical development that replaced women midwives with men midwives and male medical practitioners, and I will show that this development was flanked with depictions of pregnant mothers and their predicament in nineteenth-century fiction.

The historical development can be sketched if we consider two texts, Jane Sharp's *The Midwifes Book* (1671), a pragmatic textbook addressing pregnant women and midwives, and William Harris's *Lectures on Puerperal Fevers* (1845), an attempt to identify the causes for childbed fever and its treatment addressing an exclusively male audience. The two texts reflect not only that puerperal fever had become the main concern in institutionalized obstetrics; they also testify that a culture of midwifery had been replaced by an academic approach to birthing. Harris's *Lectures* with their case studies are not theoretical abstractions as criticised by Sterne, they are informed by experience. However, the *Lectures* foreground the "numerous writers" (8) discussing "facts and arguments" (10) in papers published exclusively by "Gentlem[e]n of great professional attainments" (14f.), and at the centre of the text there is a dead body with the *autopsia cadaveria*, the post mortem of a woman who has died of child-bed fever. The text presents evidence that the connection of experimental pathology and obstetrics in fact proved fatal but Harris seems to take the loss of life for granted; he seems to be positive that these inevitable losses will result in a better medical care in the future:

> Dr. Cambell says that, after dissecting a woman that died of puerperal fever, he went the same evening, without changing his clothes, to deliver a poor woman in the Canongate, who afterwards died of the same disease; in the same clothes he delivered another woman with forceps, who also died, and three others in succession shared the same fate. Doctor James Orr, after dissecting a female that died of the disease at Carron-Mills, for want of accommodation did not wash his hands carefully, and without changing his clothes, attended two females in their confinement, both of whom

[7] Ehrenreich and English voice their argument perhaps most clearly in the section "Exorcising the Midwives", 93-98; Faludi in particular in chapter 5, "Fatal and Foetal Visions: The Backlash in the Movies", 140-70, even if the focus here is on nursing rather than giving birth.

were seized with the disease and died. "It is a disagreeable declaration for me to mention", says Dr. Gordon, of Aberdeen, "that I myself was the means of carrying the infection to a great number of women […]."

(Harris 1845: 13f.)

Harris explicitly addresses the fact that physicians often unknowingly carry the infection, and he states that "when it [i.e. the malady] takes possession of the puerperal female, in its malignant form, it too often defies all the resources of our art, however skilfully directed" (27). However, the text nevertheless supports the predominant view in mid-nineteenth-century England that "medical men could manage childbirth better than ignorant untrained midwives" (Loudon 1990: 703). As Irvine Loudon explains, "by the end of the eighteenth century virtually all of the surgeon-apothecaries (the predecessors of general practitioners) had adopted 'man midwifery' as a central part of their practice" (Loudon 1990: 703). This development and its implication have been thoroughly discussed. What has caught less attention, though, is how literary texts and the popular imagination have supported that development.

Robert A. Erickson has pointed at "popular notions of how midwives and witches came together into a legendary composite figure during the seventeenth and early eighteenth centuries" (Erickson 1986: 18). This composite figure, Erickson explains, renders the midwife as an unstable and ambivalent "cunning woman": conceived as a black witch she has the "capacity for inflicting crippling *verbal* abuse and calling up diabolic forces" and "has the helpless victims, mother and unborn child, in the power of her literal grasp" (ibid.) The negative characterization competes with the "image of the good, mature, or aged midwife (or 'white witch'), a woman beyond childbearing but intimate with all that it implies, a 'hearty good woman,' merry, a 'blesser' who can 'unbind' the evil of the black witch" (ibid.).

The ambivalence about the training and moral adeptness of midwives is a subtext that can be explored in Laurence Sterne's *Tristram Shandy*. The novel reflects the social and disciplinary shifts in obstetrics and explores the predicament of women who had to give birth at a time of changing practices. It is a matter of debate whether "[t]he medical details [in *Tristram Shandy*] are an accurate reflection of the learning and practice of the day" (Porter 1989: 63) or whether the novel is a literary appropriation which "mimics medical vocabulary, and also doctors the books of physicians, reducing their prescriptions to abstractions" (Hawley 1993: 84). There can be no doubt, however, that *Tristram Shandy* reflects the hopes and anxieties of a period that saw fundamental changes in obstetrics: changes with respect to gender, changes with respect to medical practices, and changes with respect to how childbearing was conceived not only among practitioners and midwives but also among a reading public at large. Throughout the first three books of the novel the preparations for the protagonist's birth are discussed time and again. Elizabeth Shandy is adamant that the village midwife, Mrs. Wood, should be present when she gives birth while Walter Shandy insists that the birth of his child be overseen by the practitioner Dr. Slop with "his new-invented forceps" which Walter and Dr. Slop consider to be "the safest instrument of deliverance" (Sterne 2003: 136). Moreover, Walter and Dr. Slop both argue in favour of turning the child in the womb. While Walter thinks that this intervention will prevent the head from being compressed during birth, Dr. Slop proposes the method "for reasons merely obstetrical" (ibid.).[8]

Downstairs in the parlour, Walter, his brother, Sir Toby, and Dr. Slop discuss the advantages of using forceps while Elizabeth experiences labour pain in the bedroom upstairs. Dr. Slop's demonstration of the instrument goes horribly wrong when he first takes off the skin from Toby's knuckles and then crushes a melon with the forceps. Supported by Susannah, the maid, and Mrs. Wood, Elizabeth is horrified by Dr. Slop's instrument but ultimately the three women have to consent to the practitioner's authority. The baby is born with the use of Dr. Slop's forceps; mother and child survive the operation even if the child's nose is broken in the process.

Sterne's humorous account of the birthing scene glosses over the more serious issues but the novel clearly juxtaposes a medical, male gaze at the female body and a compassionate female contact with the body. According to Bonnie Blackwell, "Mrs. Wood, the midwife, represents what the novel calls simply 'the sisterhood' [...]: the beleaguered midwives of England who witnessed their unquestioned monopoly over childbirth reversed in approximately forty years, in the face of ardent propaganda in favor of the instrument-wielding man-midwife" (Blackwell 2001: 81). *Tristram Shandy* dramatizes this rivalry for authority between (male) practitioners or man-midwives and female midwives, a rivalry which allowed the male practitioners to capitalize on the prestige of their profession (see Wilson 1995: 192-94). But more generally it also sets against each other a sisterhood supportive of the woman giving birth and a masculine profession focusing exclusively on the child.[9]

---

[8] Bonnie Blackwell suggests, I think wrongly, that Walter wishes the forceps to be applied for a more speedy delivery. In my reading Walter seems more concerned about turning the child with the forceps in order to protect the child's brain. For a discussion of Walter's theory in connection with eighteenth-century studies of the anatomy of the brain see Sprang 2007: 177-79.

[9] Bonnie Blackwell discusses the detrimental effect that William Smellie's mechanical labour simulator, made from metal, wood, whale-bone and leather, had on the nine hundred students he trained, making them believe that "the man-midwife [is] the sole intrepid, hardworking body in labor" when assisting births (Blackwell 2001: 93).

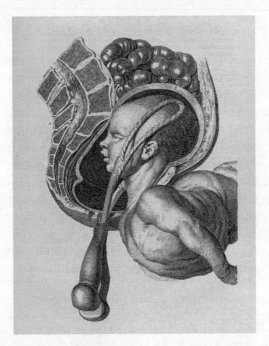

Fig 2: William Smellie. *A sett of anatomical tables, with explanations, and an abridgment, of the practice of midwifery* (1754), Tab. XXXV.

There was ardent criticism from midwives, most notably, perhaps, from Elizabeth Nihell who had published *A Treatise on the Art of Midwifery. Setting forth Various Abuses therein, Especially as to the Practice with Instruments* in 1760 – but to no avail.[10] Women were soon marginalized as obstetricians: "[f]e-male midwives in England organized and charged the male intruders with commercialism and dangerous misuse of the forceps. But it was too late – the women were easily put down as ignorant 'old wives' [...]" (Ehrenreich and English 2010: 59). I think that nineteenth-century novels played a decisive role in the decline of female midwives. While *Tristram Shandy*, on the whole, beckons us to sympathise with the sisterhood, Victorian novels largely support the dominant perspective that only man-midwives and trained obstetricians should oversee a birth. Moreover, they clearly conceptualize giving birth as a medical condition. These novels, then, paid lip service to a male expertise that demarked the dividing line between medical and 'normal' conditions of preg-nant women and of women in their puerperium (see Moscucci 1990: 50-64; O'Dowd 1994: 167-69).

[10] For a brief discussion of Nihell's treatise in connection with *Tristram Shandy* see Erickson 1986: 212.

Victorian Novels as Catalysts for the Medicalization of Childbirth

Victorian England saw a dramatic rise in maternal mortality. Historians of medicine, who have scrutinized documented evidence for birth rates, still-borns and maternal deaths, agree that death rates at the beginning of the seventeenth century were much lower than is usually presumed. David Cressy, among others, has argued that in the seventeenth century "[m]ost women survived childbirth without complications and most mothers quickly recovered" and that "early modern childbirth was not so dangerous as was feared, though the chance of death was more like one in a hundred" (Cressy 1999: 30). While it is difficult to obtain reliable statistical data for the eighteenth century, we will have to assume that the numbers rose during the experimental phase in obstetrics, partly because of the introduction of lying-in houses in the cities where infections could spread more easily (London 1750; Dublin 1757).[11] According to Irvine Loudon the situation remained unaltered throughout the nineteenth century:

> The evidence suggests that between 1870 and 1935 it was usually safest to be delivered at home by a well-trained midwife rather than in a hospital by a doctor; but it was no safer to be rich rather than poor. Although high maternal mortality was often associated with areas of poverty, the link was indirect. Socio-economic deprivation per se was not an important determinant factor in maternal mortality, but the place of delivery and the care and skill of the birth attendant were.
>
> (Loudon 2003: 183)

In fact, "hospital mortality, which was often five or even ten times as high as it was in home deliveries in the worst of slums, rose to unprecedented heights in the second half of the nineteenth century" (Loudon 1990: 704).[12]

Victorian novels tell a different story.[13] In fictional accounts dramatizing pregnancy, labour, childbirth and puerperium, the woman at home is in great danger. However, before we turn to Victorian novels we must account for a peculiar fact. With *Tristram Shandy* as a popular narrative that explores issues of birthing over 150 pages we must assume that this narrative would have in-

---

[11] Schofield concedes that mortality rates may have been as high as 3% around 1750, de Brouwere has looked into parish records and has calculated a rate of 2.9%, Dobbie suggests that the rate remained at about 1.3% throughout the period 1600-1800, and Wrigley argues that the numbers fell from 2% in 1700 to 1,1% in 1800 (see de Brouwere 2007: 343f.; Schofield 1986, Dobbie 1982, and Wrigley1997: 313-315).

[12] It was only at the end of the nineteenth century with discoveries of antiseptics by Gordon, Holmes and Semmelweiss, and, more importantly, in the early twentieth century with the implementation of stricter hygiene alongside advancements in blood transfusions that numbers decisively fell again (see Loudon 2000).

[13] The following passage is an extended version of an essay published previously (see Sprang 2013).

fluenced writers of Gothic fiction. Isobel Grundy has investigated the portrayal of childbirth by 120 women who both wrote and bore children in the period 1660-1820 and concludes that "tentatively, we can say there is less description of, and comment on, pregnancy and childbirth than on other health issues, or on death" (n. p.). According to Grundy, "the chances of dying in childbirth were probably much higher for a fictional character than for a living woman in the eighteenth century, especially if she was giving birth to a heroine" (n. p.) but childbed-death scenes are still far and between in late eighteenth-century and early nineteenth-century fiction. We know that eighteenth-century women writers Mary Wollstonecraft and Mary Brunton died of puerperal fever. And we know that Mary Shelley only barely escaped death after suffering severe perinatal bleeding. Without wishing to strain biographical readings, we may assume that Mary Shelley has raised a monument for women dying in childbed with the character Clorinda in her novel *Lodore* (1835):

> She was placed on the bed, – she still lived; her faint pulse could not be felt, and no blood flowed when a vein was opened, but she groaned, and now and then opened her eyes with a ghastly stare, and closed them again as if mechanically. All was horror and despair – no help – no resource presented itself; they hung round her, they listened to her groans with terror, and yet they were the only signs of life that disturbed her death-like state. At last, soon after the dawn of day, she became convulsed, her pulse fluttered, and blood flowed from her wounded arm; in about an hour from this time she gave birth to a dead child. After this she grew calmer and fainter. The physician arrived, but she was past mortal cure; – she never opened her eyes more, nor spoke, nor gave any token of consciousness. By degrees her groans ceased, and she faded into death: the slender manifestations of lingering vitality gradually decreasing till all was still and cold.
>
> (Shelley 1835: Vol. III, 217)

Clorinda's state is clearly described as a serious medical condition – the symptoms suggest obstetrical haemorrhage – but even in her last moments she is not reduced to a medical case. Shelley's fictional account focuses on the dying mother, and it does so with compassion. The qualifying simile "as if mechanically" (217) may hint at a criticism of Smellie's mechanical mother: Clorinda may appear like an automaton but Shelley clearly states that that is a false impression. Instead, Clorinda remains the sole focus of the passage, and her death is treated with dignity. The village doctor who feels her pulse and opens her vein is hardly present in the narrative, and the English physician who was summoned from Naples to the inn in Mola di Gaeta (Formia) arrives too late but there are no melodramatic elements that dramatize the scene as Clorinda "fade[s] into death" (217).

It cannot be proven that the increasing number of women writers with their perspective contributed to changing attitudes towards child-birth and maternal

deaths. However, it is plausible that both male and female authors shunned exploiting maternal deaths as plot elements because they felt it was improper to do
so at a time when mortality rates increased dramatically. Sterne's contemporaries and immediate successors had witnessed the terrible plight of women that
came with the medicalization of giving birth. They suspected – if only intuitively – that death rates had been lower in their parents' and grandparents'
generation, and they thus shied away from exploiting scenes of perinatal death
for their narratives.

It is equally plausible that there are no scenes of maternal deaths in novels
from that period because "[t]he typical Gothic mother is absent: dead,
imprisoned or somehow abjected, to use the term that Julia Kristeva applies to
that state of being" (Anolik 2003: 25). If "[t]he mother, like the stage of marriage is the enemy of the 'narratable'," (Anolik 2003: 27) as Ruth Bienstock
Anolik suggests, Gothic novelists employed childbed deaths to render the absent
mother plausible but they did not narrativise these deaths. With the exception of
Shelley's *Lodore*, perhaps, it is well into the nineteenth century that we
encounter fully dramatized scenes of mothers dying in childbed. Arguably,
Victorian authors had learnt to accept the high death rates – and they were less
reluctant to criticise the medical practise of attending women prior to their
giving birth and after as botched and careless. As Carolyn Dever has pointed
out, "it is far more dangerous to give birth in a fictional world that in any region,
under any conditions, within any social class in Victorian Britain" (Dever 1998:
11). In her lucid account, Dever observes that "the fictional investment of
maternal morbidity accommodates agendas ranging from the misogynist to the
proto-feminist" (Dever 1998: 17). While I share Dever's conviction that the
Victorian novelists employed maternal death as a means to justify authoritative
patriarchal structures, I think that her Freudian reading misses the point. The
function of the childbed death topos, in my opinion, is not to press home the
argument that "the *only* good mother is a dead mother" (Dever 1998: 19). Dever,
quoting from Florence Nightingale's *Introductory Notes on Lying-In Institutions*
(1871), explains that the statistical evidence is "entirely in favour of home
delivery" (Dever 1998: 12), and she points out that the Victorian novel paints a
different picture. However, the agenda that accounts for such a discrepancy, if
there is an agenda at all, I think, is primarily driven by the context of
institutionalization and medicalization, which are by default patriarchal in
Victorian Britain.

In order to identify the aesthetic and narrative choices, along with their socio-
political implications, I would like to look at five scenes that depict child-birth
and maternal deaths. I should like to start with *Oliver Twist*, Dickens's first
attempt at a full-length novel. Dating from 1838, the novel begins with a scene
that arguably set generic conventions for Victorian novels. The story of Oliver

begins with the narrator recalling the birth of the protagonist, explaining that Oliver only survived because nobody interfered in his birth. The text thus explicitly juxtaposes Oliver's survival with his mother's death: "The surgeon deposited it [the child] in her arms. She imprinted her cold white lips passionately on its forehead; passed her hands over her face; gazed wildly round; shuddered; fell back – and died" (2). The narrator admits that giving birth in a workhouse is not "the most fortunate and enviable circumstance that can possibly befall a human being" but that "it was the best thing for Oliver Twist that could by possibility have occurred" (1). At the very beginning of the novel readers are thus asked to take a double perspective – what turns out to be life-saving for Oliver is fatal for his mother. The death of Oliver's mother is rendered in melodramatic fashion, the character estranged from all hope and comfort. Readers learn very little about the birth itself but the narrator suggests that the intoxicated and elderly nurse and the parish surgeon intervene very little and leave "Oliver and Nature [to fight] out the point between them" (1). When Oliver gives out his first cry – after more than three minutes – the surgeon has already returned to his chair near the fire, and the drunk midwife "applie[s] herself to the green bottle" (3).

Dickens explores the theme of maternal death further in his novels, and in *Dombey and Son* (1846-1848) the death of Mrs. Dombey, who has just given birth to the male heir, serves as a plot element as much as a means to characterise all those involved in the first chapter: Dombey, his sister-in-law Mrs. Chick, Florence, the nurse Blockitt, the family practitioner Mr. Pilkins, and the court physician Doctor Peps. The scene also lays out the hierarchical dimension of obstetrical practice in Victorian England. The nurse and the family practitioner Mr. Pilkins attend to Mrs. Dombey, but when Fanny Dombey turns "feeverish", the court physician Doctor Parker Peps is consulted. The dialogue between Mr. Pilkins and Doctor Peps as well as their interaction tells us a lot about the social spheres that separate the general practitioner and the court physician but we learn very little about medical practice. In the end, it is the sister-in-law who gives a last (cynical) advice to Fanny "to rouse herself" (20) while both the family doctor and the court physician have given up on her. Fanny's death is a quiet death, a slipping away turned into a poetic movement in the last lines of that chapter: "Thus, clinging fast to the slight spar within her arms, the mother drifted out upon the dark and unknown sea that rolls round all the world" (21).

There is a marked difference here between the death of Oliver's mother and the death of Fanny. While the scene in *Oliver Twist* depicts the last moments of Oliver's mother in an almost grotesque fashion, Fanny is treated gracefully and given the status of a martyr in a household corrupted by greed and envy. And while the novel *Oliver Twist* discusses the social and medical circumstances of giving birth, albeit briefly, *Dombey and Son* isolates the maternal death completely from the medical context.

Dickens's poetic and dignifying description of Mrs. Dombey's death resonates with Emily Brontë's account of Catherine Linton's death in *Wuthering Heights* (1847). While Catherine's distress – torn between lover and husband, duty and humanity – is dramatized fully in the preceding chapters, Catherine's death is told in a single sentence with remarkable restraint: "About twelve o'clock, that night, was born the Catherine you saw at Wuthering Heights, a puny, seven months' child; and two hours after the mother died, having never recovered sufficient consciousness to miss Heathcliff, or know Edgar" (164). The dead mother here, like Mrs. Dombey, is an "image of perfect peace. Her brow smooth, her lids closed, her lips wearing the expression of a smile" (164).

In Elizabeth Gaskell's first novel *Mary Barton* (1848) the death of Mary's mother is a gap in the narrative that readers must fill. The last thing we are told is that John Barton asks his neighbour to attend to his wife in labour while he will go and get the town doctor. When he returns with the doctor his wife is already dead: "The cries were still for ever. John had no time for listening. He opened the latched door, stayed not to light a candle for the mere ceremony of showing his companion up the stairs, so well known to himself; but in two minutes, was in the room, where lay the dead wife [...]" (20).

In Anthony Trollope's *Last Chronicle of Barset* (1867) the narrative voice refers to the death of Major Grantly's first wife in childbed in passing. With a single sentence in chapter three readers are told that "Major Grantly had been a successful man in life – with the one exception of having lost the mother of his child within a twelve-month of his marriage and within a few hours of that child's birth" (25). Cryptic and caustic as the passage may be, it suffices to remind readers that a mother dying "within a few hours of that child's birth" is a tragedy and constitutes a serious crisis (see Bergmann 7f.).

If there is a development then in these novels with respect to how they discuss the predicament of women giving birth – it is a development of reduction. How can we account for this development? As Carolyn Dever, among others, has pointed out, Jane Austen's *Northanger Abbey* (1818), may help to explain that trajectory. At the very beginning of that novel, the narrator mocks the convention of maternal death and explains that Catherine is a very unlikely heroine because "her mother had [had] three sons before Catherine was born; and instead of dying in bringing the latter into the world, as any body might expect, she still lived on – lived to have six children more – to see them growing up around her, and to enjoy excellent health herself" (15). This *en passant* but nevertheless scathing observation may have resonated with Victorian authors when thinking about narrativising maternal deaths, and it may thus help explain why scenes of maternal mortality are so scare in Victorian novels.

At the same time, we may wish to read the reduction of fictional characters dying of puerperal fever or other complications after giving birth as well as the omission of scenes of giving birth as a gesture of the ineffable. Victorian novelists may have known only too well that their authorial gaze was incongruous with their ethical stance. "In birthgiving," Cristina Mazzoni sums up her study of *Pregnancy and Childbirth in Literature and Theory*, "the preponderant conjunction of pain, meaning, and silence is itself an ethical dimension" (Mazzoni 2002: 205). Victorian novels, then, may also offer opposition to the professional and penetrating gaze of the medical doctor, rejecting authorial scripts in the form of case studies found in obstetrical textbooks, and suggesting that these accounts are incompatible with the experience of the suffering human being.

Perinatal Death in the Novel and Peripheral Perspectives

If we wish to understand the role that Victorian novels have played for the gendering and medicalization of giving birth, we must step back and consider how maternal mortality is treated aesthetically in these novels. Generally, as Carolyn Dever has pointed out convincingly, the maternal body competes with the unfolding of the protagonist's self: "the *Bildungsroman* of narrative realism relies on maternal loss to set the young protagonist free to construct selfhood independent of parental constraint" (Dever 1998: 24). But I think that the disappearance of the mother as a character who dies in childbed tells a different story. With a trajectory from an individualized character (Oliver Twist's mother) to a type (the first wife of Major Grantly), Victorian novelists seem to lose interest in mothers dying in childbed. However, if we consider that "many nineteenth-century novels sense the potential to shift the focus away from the established center, toward minor characters, and that novels often obliquely or emphatically represent this process" (Woloch 2003: 44), narratives that only refer to mothers dying in childbed may be read as a comment on an increasingly institutionalized and male perspective. While the dead mother is forgotten as the plot unfolds in these novels, readers can turn that absence into a haunting presence. Dickens's novels in particular suggest such a reading: with Oliver's thoughts our thoughts return to his dead mother and when he feels that she sits by his side during his shivers (see 87), we feel the presence of his mother. And for Paul and his sister Florence the dead mother remains a constant companion evoked by the sea imagery that permeates the narrative. In fact, the absent mother is a crucial motif in all the novels discussed above, a motif that is perhaps often misunderstood because we fail to acknowledge how important minor characters are as aesthetic and narrative constituents of the Victorian novel. As Alex Woloch has pointed out,

> [a] full analysis of minor characters must examine not simply the specific description
> of particular characters but also how these characters are inflected into a complex
> narrative system. Such analysis highlights the intersection of description and structure,
> elucidating how particular stylistic configurations emerge out of and flow into the
> larger, dynamic construction of dominant and subordinate elements within the
> narrative totality.
>
> (Woloch 2003: 125)

Even if mothers who die from puerperal fever or haemorrhages at the beginning
of a novel must by default remain minor characters they often decisively shape
the complex narrative system. These mothers are not simply abjected, as argued
by Ruth Bienstock Anolik, and their deaths do not primarily signify, as argued
by Carolyn Dever. When we consider these fictional characters in the light of
the iconography of Mary's birth and the campaign "Freedom for Birth", the
peripheral perspective of these marginalized mothers urges us to re-assess developments in medical practice. As Jane Thrailkill has pointed out with respect
to changing conceptions of childbed fever, the peripheral perspective is an "im-
passioned defense of a medical art predicated on […] the vision that each person
constituted a unique and coherent whole, and that the study and care of human
life must be deeply rooted in individual experience" (Thrailkill 1999: 681).
Fictional mothers dying of puerperal fever urge us in particular to rethink our
notion of women giving birth as medical cases that are grouped into clusters. At
a time when "[c]ontagion seemed morally random and thus a denial of the
traditional assumption that both health and disease arose from particular states
of moral and social order" (Rosenberg 1993: 92), Victorian novels explore a
general debate: how far is disease linked to individual prepositions. As Christine
Hallett has pointed out,

> [t]here was much debate [in the early nineteenth century] about the value of
> suggestions that inflammation was a 'natural' feature of childbirth, some physicians
> arguing that it offered the obvious explanation for conditions such as puerperal fever,
> others maintaining that it did not explain why *all* women did not suffer from such
> fevers. In attempting to understand how puerperal fever could arise in some, but not
> all, women, physicians took the view that, whilst all parturient women had a natural
> tendency towards fever, only those in whom there were predisposing factors were at
> serious risk.
>
> (Hallett, 2005: 13)

The fact that characters who die of childbed fever and other complications
recede into the distance of fictional worlds in the nineteenth century may thus be
owed to how medical discourse constructed them: as victims of an amorphous
disease. In other words, the medical condition of women with puerperal fever or
severe bleeding worked against the narrativising and characterising. If we accept

this line of interpretation, novels did indeed trace the masculinization and medi-calization of giving birth – but in doing so they also subverted that process. It is undoubtedly true that Victorian novels did not provide a counter-narrative, a counter-narrative that empowered midwives and women, a counter-narrative that praised received wisdom as opposed to experimental science. The absence of empowered women in labour and empowered midwives also raises awareness about the marginalization of the woman giving birth and the women attending her.

Conclusion

In my opinion, Jane Thrailkill's final statement that "we still turn to narrative to honor individual lives, [while] we draw on the impersonal methods of modern medicine to save them" (Thrailkill 1999: 699), is correct. However, we should not forget that our reading experience affects how we construe medical practice and medicine as a domain in our culture. I hope to have shown that Victorian novels both react to changing attitudes to giving birth and direct our attention at the medicalization and masculinization of labour and the puerperium. These novels focus on the predicament of women who have to give birth when traditional midwifery was marginalized by professional obstetrics, with those attending to these women ill-prepared and without empathy. The death of the mother is certainly an intriguing topos in nineteenth-century fiction more generally, but perinatal death in the Victorian novel is not simply a means to set the protagonist free in the sense that the *Bildungsroman* stresses nurture over nature. The nineteenth-century novel presents a narrative in which labour is a medical condition that has to be overseen by men with obstetric training. At the same time, however, it exposes the shortcomings of medicine as theory and as practise. Melodramatic as well as nuanced depictions of mothers dying in childbed have shaped our notion of the dangers involved in home births at a time when giving birth at the lying-in hospitals was far more hazardous. These novels bring to the fore the despair and frustration as medical assistance either comes too late or is to no avail, a plot element that further stresses the characterization of the woman in labour as a passive, helpless patient. In that sense, dying mothers are treated as a type, a presentation that is in tune with Victorian notions of disease as contagion, and in tune with the conception of women in labour as medical cases. However, in presenting women as helpless patients vis-à-vis a hopeless medical profession, these novels challenge the medicalization and masculinization of labour.

The popularity of a recent BBC 1 series, *Call the Midwife*, I think is owed to the unbroken currency of these Victorian narratives as templates for women in labour. Based on a memoir by Jennifer Worth, the series is set in a nursing convent in the Poplar district, East London, in the 1950s, and it highlights the service that the sisters as midwives bring to the poor community. With a predominantly female cast, the programme evokes the sisterhood that we see in Giovanni da Milano's fresco and it indulges in a nostalgia centred on working class values. With elements of girly gossip and romantic love plots, the series is not a call for women's rights in birthing. The setting in the after-war years, however, reminds contemporary audiences of the period of relative empowerment before women had to assume more traditional roles.[14] With the peculiar status of a convent in a society exploring jazz music that the series exploits for its appeal, midwifery as active sisterhood is implicitly idealized as something belonging to a nostalgic past. In moments of crisis, Dr. Patrick Turner, the resident physician, takes over, and the London Hospital with its male surgical ward is represented as a (modern) alternative to the home birth assisted by the nuns and sisters.

The narratives coined in Victorian novels and the nostalgia evoked in *Call the Midwife* are part of the paradoxical attitude to birthing that prevails today. Caught between the horrors of childbed death and the ideal of a "natural" birth at home, these narratives have shaped not only the popular imagination but also obstetric discourse. With caesarean sections accounting for nearly a quarter of all births in Britain, there can be no doubt that in our collective memory giving birth has been transformed into a medical condition. We should remind ourselves that nineteenth-century novels have played a decisive role in our conception of giving birth. There is no call in these novels for a "natural" birth that categorically rejects medical intervention, and we should not construe these novels as guidelines to make choices in the non-fictional world. Instead, we should read these novels as reminders that pregnant women and women in labour are vulnerable and often find their perspective marginalized by authoritative professionals. The novels thus raise serious issues about the male gaze on the female body and the construction of knowledge in the domain of giving birth. The profession has begun to address this problem, and maternity wards increasingly place the mother with her particular needs at the centre (see Jordan). In order to facilitate this process we must raise awareness of the cultural construction of pregnancy, labour, the puerperium and lactation. *Call the Midwife*, for all its nostalgia, may raise awareness if we bear in mind nineteenth-century trajectories of medicalization and masculinization. Victorian novels have played their part in rendering this trajectory visible; they are crucial for understanding conceptions about birth that prevail today. I will not suggest that these novels should be shelved in maternity wards. If one wish is granted at the

---

[14] The character Sister Monica Joan, born into a titled family, one of the first trained women midwives in the 1890s, and now living at the convent in her 90s, establishes a connection between Victorian and postwar Britain, between the suffrage campaign and, for example, the Six Point Group. For continuities and disruptions of feminism in Britain see Caine.

end of this paper, I would wish that Giovanni da Milano's imaginary sister visit all maternity units today offering her services to paint a scene of birth, a fresco for our times.

List of Works Cited

Anolik, Ruth Bienstock. "The Missing Mother: The Meanings of Maternal Absence in the Gothic." *Modern Language Studies* 33 (2003): 24-43.

Ashley, Kathleen M. *Interpreting Cultural Symbols: Saint Anne in Late Medieval Society.* Athens: University of Georgia Press, 1990.

Austen, Jane. *Northanger Abbey.* London: Penguin, 2003.

von Behr, Johann. *Die Pisaner Marientafel des Meisters von San Martino und die zyklischen Darstellungen der Annenlegende in Italien von 700 bis 1350.* Frankfurt: Lang, 1996.

Bragg, Fiona, David A Cromwell, Leroy C Edozien, Ipek Gurol-Urganci, Tahir A. Mahmood, Allan Templeton, and Jan H. van der Meulen "Variation in Rates of Caesarean Section among English NHS Trusts after Accounting for Maternal and Clinical Risk: Cross Sectional Study." *British Medical Journal* 341.777 (2010): c5065. Published online 2010 October 6. doi: 10.1136/bmj.c5065

Blackwell, Bonnie. "'Tristram Shandy' and the Theater of the Mechanical Mother." *ELH* 68.1 (2001): 81-133.

Brontë, Emily. *Wuthering Heights.* London: Penguin, 1995.

de Brouwere, Vincent. "The Comparative Study of Maternal Mortality over Time: The Role of the Professionalisation of Childbirth." *Social History Medicine* 20.3 (2007): 541-62.

Caine, Barbara. *English Feminism 1780-1980.* Oxford: Oxford UP, 1997.

Carpenter, Louise. "The mothers fighting back against birth intervention." *Observer on Sunday*, 16 December 2012. Magazine section, 30.

Cressy, David. *Birth, Marriage and Death. Ritual, Religion and the Life-Cycle in Tudor and Stuart England.* Oxford: Oxford University Press, 1999.

Dever, Carolyn. *Death and the Mother from Dickens to Freud: Victorian Fiction and the Anxiety of Origin.* Cambridge: Cambridge UP, 1998.

Dickens, Charles. *Oliver Twist, or, The Parish Boy's Progress.* Ed. Philip Horne. London: Penguin, 2003.

Dickens, Charles. *Dombey and Son.* London: Penguin, 2002.

Dobbie, B. M. Willmott. "An Attempt to Estimate the True Rate of Maternal Mortality, Sixteenth to Eighteenth Centuries." *Medical History* 26 (1982): 79-90.

Dörfler-Dierken, Angelika. *Die Verehrung der heiligen Anna in Spätmittelalter und früher Neuzeit.* Göttingen: Vandenhoeck & Ruprecht, 1992.

Ehrenreich, Barbara and Deirdre English. *Witches, Midwives, and Nurses: A History of Women Healers.* New York: Feminist P at the City U of New York. 2010.

---. *For Her Own Good: 150 Years of the Expert's Advice to Women.* London: Pluto Press, 1979.

Erickson, Robert A. *Mother Midnight: Birth, Sex, and Fate in Eighteenth-Century Fiction (Defoe, Richardson, and Sterne).* New York: AMS Press, 1986. 18.

Faludi, Susan. *Backlash: The Undeclared War Against Women.* London: Vintage, 1990.

Gaskell, Elizabeth. *Mary Barton, A Tale of Manchester Life.* London: Penguin. 1996.

Gregori, Mina. *Giovanni da Milano alla Cappella Rinuccini.* Milano: Fabbri, Skira, 1965.

Grundy, Isobel. "Delivering Childbirth: Orlando Project Encoding." n.p, n.d., http://www.ualberta.ca/ORLANDO/publications/Childbirth.htm. Last accessed on 16 February 2012.

Hallett, Christine. "The Attempt to Understand Puerperal Fever in the Eighteenth and Early Nineteenth Centuries: The Influence of Inflammation Theory." *Medical History* 49.1 (2005): 1-28.

Harris, William. *Lectures on Puerperal Fevers*. Philadelphia: T. & G. Town, 1845.

Hawley, Judith. "The Anatomy of *Tristram Shandy*." *Literature & Medicine During the Eighteenth Century*. Ed. M. M. Roberts and R. Porter. London: Routledge, 1993. 84-100.

Jordan, Brigitte. "Authoritative Knowledge and Its Construction." *Childbirth and Authoritative Knowledge: Cross-Cultural Perspectives*. Ed. Robbie E. Davis-Floyd and Carolyn F. Sargent. Berkeley: U of California P, 1997. 55-78.

Lasareff, Victor. "Studies in the Iconography of the Virgin." *The Art Bulletin* 20.1 (1938): 26-65.

Lavin, Marilyn Aronberg. *The Place of Narrative: Mural Decoration in Italian Churches, 431-1600*. Chicago: U of Chicago P, 1990. 90-98.

Loudon, Irvine. "Maternal Mortality: 1880–1950. Some Regional and International Comparisons." *Social History of Medicine* 1.2 (2003): 183-228.

---. *The Tragedy of Childbed Fever*. Oxford: Oxford UP, 2000.

---. "Obstetrics and the General Practitioner." *British Medical Journal* 301.6754 (1990): 703-7.

---. "Obstetric Care, Social Class, and Maternal Mortality." *British Medical Journal* 293.6547 (1986): 606-8.

Mazzoni, Cristina. *Maternal Impressions. Pregnancy and Childbirth in Literature and Theory*. Ithaca: Cornell UP, 2002.

Moscucci, Ornella. *The Science of Woman: Gynaecology and Gender in England, 1800-1929*. Cambridge: Cambridge UP, 1990.

Nixon, Virginia. *Mary's Mother: Saint Anne in Late Medieval Europe*. University Park: Pennsylvania State UP, 2004.

O'Dowd, Michael J. *The History of Obstetrics & Gynaecology*. New York: Parthenon, 1994.

Porter, Roy. "'The whole secret of health': Mind, Body and Medicine in *Tristram Shandy*." *Nature Transfigured: Science and Literature, 1700-1900*. Ed. J. Christie and Sally Shuttleworth. Manchester: Manchester UP, 1989. 61-84.

Poeschke, Joachim. *Wandmalerei der Giottozeit in Italien 1280 – 1400*. München: Hirmer Verlag 2003.

Rosenberg, Charles. *Explaining Epidemics and Other Studies in the History of Medicine*. Cambridge: Cambridge UP, 1992.

Schiller, Gertrud. *Iconography of Christian Art*. Vol. 1. Greenwich: New York Graphic Society, 1971. 26.

Schofield, Roger. "Did the Mothers Really Die? Three Centuries of Maternal Mortality in the 'World We Have Lost'." *The World We Have Gained*. Ed. Lloyd Bonfield, Richard Smith and Keith Wrightson. Oxford: Blackwell, 1986. 231-60.

Shelley, Mary. *Lodore*. London: Richard Bentley, 1835.

Smellie, William. *A sett of anatomical tables, with explanations, and an abridgment, of the practice of midwifery, with a view to illustrate a Treatise on that subject, and Collection of cases*. London: [s.n.], 1754.

Sprang, Felix. "*Tristram Shandy* und die *Anthropologia nova* – Systematik in Literatur und Medizin." *Medizinische Schreibweisen*. Ed. Nicolas Pethes and Sandra Richter. Tübingen: Niemeyer, 2007. 171-87.

---. "'Let me see the child and die.' The Medicalization of Childbirth in Eighteenth- and Nineteenth-Century Novels." *The Writing Cure*. Ed. Jarmila Mildorf and Alexandra Lembert-Heidenreich. Münster: Lit Verlag, 2013. 135-53.

Sterne, Laurence. *The Life and Opinions of Tristram Shandy, Gentleman*. Ed. Melvyn New and Joan New. London: Penguin, 2003.

Thrailkill, Jane F. "Killing Them Softly: Childbed Fever and the Novel." *American Literature* 71.4 (1999): 679-707.

Trollope, Anthony. *The Last Chronicle of Barset*. London: Penguin. 2002.

Wilson, Adrian. *The Making of Man-Midwifery: Childbirth in England, 1660-1770*. Cambridge: Harvard UP, 1995.

Woloch, Alex. *The One Vs. the Many: Minor Characters and the Space of the Protagonist in the Novel*. Princeton: Princeton UP, 2003.

Worth, Jennifer. *Call the Midwife*. Twickenham: Merton, 2002.

Wrigley, Edward Anthony. *English Population History from Family Reconstitution, 1580-1837*. Cambridge: Cambridge UP, 1997.

www.freedomforbirth.com

Anne-Julia Zwierlein

"The texture of her nerves and the palpitation of her heart": Vocation, Hysteria, and the 'Surplus Female' in Nineteenth-Century Literature and Medical Discourse

During the nineteenth century, medicine became ubiquitous in British (and Western) public and professional culture. Medical manuals and tracts became accessible to large publics and played an important role in establishing physical norms for all stages and conditions of life – birth, childhood and adolescence, sexuality and procreation, disease, ageing, and death. Lawrence Rothfield speaks of the nineteenth-century 'medicalization' of the everyday (144). In Britain, the Medical Reform Act of 1858 introduced an official register of physicians; their training became standardized, and hospitals were given a key role. Among the numerous medical discoveries were bacteria, chloroform, and antiseptics, as well as technological advances such as the discovery of the x-ray. New branches of medical science, psychology, neurology and sexuology, defined new types of disease and new patients. Michel Foucault (1963) and Georges Canguilhem (1966) have argued that from the nineteenth century onwards, the 'sane' and the 'normal' were collapsed, and physicians and literary writers alike became interpreters and diagnosticians of the 'social body'.

Nineteenth-century literary texts reflected medical concerns, often in graphic detail. Medical explanations were also modified, criticized or confronted with competing discourses, such as mythological or religious concepts of identity. The desire to pierce bodily surfaces and uncover the invisible and hidden, and medicine's shift in focus from the individual to the collective, all characterize nineteenth-century medical research and the literary modes of realism and naturalism. These developments were especially relevant where psychiatry and the phenomenon of 'hysteria' were concerned. In the field of psychology, nineteenth-century literary texts frequently described the experiences that science was trying to explain. Robert L. Stevenson's *Dr Jekyll and Mr Hyde* (1886) and Oscar Wilde's *Dorian Gray* (1891) define new fields of psychological enquiry, the split self and the multiple personality; specifically female diseases such as hysteria were paramount in sensation novels, Wilkie Collins's *The Woman in White* (1860) or Mary Elizabeth Braddon's *Lady Audley's Secret* (1862) which introduced shocking crime into seemingly peaceful, feminized domestic settings. Along with Charlotte Brontë and George Eliot, sensation novels established as a

literary figure the new patient type of the hysterical female. One of the precursors of the detective novel in terms of its emphasis on narratological problems of evidence and perspective, the sensation novel frequently offers a central detective figure who pursues the criminal's secrets with a dogged persistence that turns into "monomania": the detective figure's own sanity is
repeatedly doubted by himself, or slandered by others.[1] There is a thin line between Robert Audley's morbid melancholy and obsessive pursuit of his cause,
classifiable as male hysteria, and the 'officially' mad and hysterical Lady
Audley who ends her days in an insane asylum. Hysteria, indeed, was fashionable during the nineteenth century; Peter Melville Logan claims that this
"nervous disorder [...] became the leading category of illness, accounting for
two-thirds of all disease" (Logan 2007: 1). While I will keep in mind – and view
– the phenomenon of male hysteria, in what follows I will investigate two
famous hysterical women, Gwendolen from George Eliot's *Daniel Deronda*
(1874-6) and Sue from Thomas Hardy's *Jude the Obscure* (1895), emphasizing
the nineteenth century's shifting explanations for exceptional neuroses and the
link, in both cases, with the eternal nineteenth-century questions of 'work' and
'vocation'.

Hysteria and the Readability of Symptoms

As Susan Sontag suggests, illness in literature can either "impinge from outside
the self as penalty or emanate from within the self as expression" (Sontag 1992:
105). Fred Vincy's illness in *Middlemarch*, similar to Pip's in *Great
Expectations* or Eugene's in *Our Mutual Friend*, are rites of passage which
allow the subject to recover in time "to live a healthier, happier, organically
stabilized life" (Rothfield 1992: 105). However, depictions in Victorian narratives of chronic illnesses and especially hysteria serve a different function:

> Chronic, developing pathology [...] – Rosamond's [...] or Gwendolen Harleth's hys-
> teria, for instance – pertains to a second kind of narrative, one in which the temporality
> of plot is [...] articulated upon the temporality of the body, its organic growth and
> decay, its duration of illness, its descent toward death, its complicated finitude: the
> narrative, in short, of a pathological organicism.
>
> (Rothfield 1992: 105-6)

Nineteenth-century psychiatry, with its research into psychosomatic diseases,
read bodily symptoms as expressions of psychic processes. Sigmund Freud's
and Josef Breuer's *Studien zur Hysterie* (1895/96; translated into English by
James Strachey) show that a multiplicity of ambivalent symptoms were

---

[1] Compare Walter Hartright in *The Woman in White* and Robert Audley in *Lady Audley's
Secret*.

connected with the disease. Indeed, many physicians at the time regarded hysteria as "a wastepaper basket of medicine where one throws otherwise unemployed symptoms", as Charles Lasègue had it (see Scull 2009: 107). Symptoms like aphasia or memory loss underlined the danger that diagnosis might be constructing rather than revealing the disease's aetiology. Hysteria was always closely connected with sexuality, witness the term's origin in the Greek word for 'uterus'; thus Freud, in tracing hysterical states to sexual causes, was going back to Greek Hippocratic medicine. Dorothea's mildly hysterical symptoms in *Middlemarch* are tied to medieval traditions through their association with female visionary states and mysticism. Hysteria was also linked to anxieties about a general social decline and biological degeneration. Richard von Krafft-Ebing in *Psychopathia Sexualis* (1886; English translation 1892) and Max Nordau in *Entartung* (1892-93; English translation: *Degeneration*, 1895) painted images of emaciated, unnaturally exalted and sexually 'perverted' hysterics, symbols of an exhausted, degenerated age.

A common feature in medical vocabulary was the close discursive link between 'hysteria' and 'simulation' or dissembling; in 1853 Robert Brudenell Carter described how following a primary disturbance the hysteric could develop secondary and tertiary attacks, sometimes even deliberately induced by the patient through recall of the original emotions; while simulating illness, he suggested, they often "adopt[ed] into their performance symptoms inadvertently suggested by their medical attendant or by illnesses they had witnessed in other people" (Scull 2009: 68-69).[2] Jean-Martin Charcot, whose public performances of female patients' hysteria at the Paris Salpêtrière made him famous, called the hysterical patient "la grande simulatrice" (qtd. in Fischer-Homberger 1975: 125), and a colleague of his described hysterical females contemptuously as "veritable actresses":

> The hysterics who exaggerate their convulsive movement [...] make an equal travesty and exaggeration of the movements of their souls, their ideas, and their acts [...] in a word, the life of the hysteric is nothing but one perpetual falsehood; they affect the airs of piety and devotion, and let themselves be taken for saints while at the same time abandoning themselves to the most shameful actions.
>
> (Scull 2009: 107-108, n.3)

Charcot, however, believed "that hysteria was a genuinely organic disorder, a disease rooted firmly in the higher nervous system, and in these respects part of the broader spectrum of neurological disorders" (Scull 2009: 108), and he emphasized that hysteria could also afflict men.

The enigmatic nature of the disease seems to have fascinated Victorian writers. Sensation novels used representations of hysteria to question identity

[2] See Carter 1853: 46 and *passim*.

concepts: "Writers exploited the contested aetiologies of [hysteria] which they found in medical knowledge in order to incorporate uncertainty and inconsistency into their narratives of physiological and psychological collapse" (Wood 2001: 115).[3] This also holds true for Eliot: Rothfield has commented on "Eliot's [...] extreme (and [...] historically determinate) sense of medicine's innate uncertainty" which led her to stress "the ethical imperative for medicine and medical realism" (Rothfield 1992: 106). The uncertainty about the cause-symptom relation is integral to sensation novels where suspicions are always, possibly, the result of obsessive delusions. Even though the central criminal female is usually classified as 'insane' with less hesitation, the lucid, cold logicality of insane minds takes centre-stage; in Collins's *Armadale* (1866), for instance, Lydia Gwilt even 'poses' as the inmate of an insane asylum in order to pursue her murderous plans. Again, hysterical states of mind, in their very obsessiveness, uncannily resemble sharp-sighted rationality – and the simulation and role-playing they entail can be seen as exaggerated versions of the conventional role-playing that Victorian society and etiquette demanded especially of females.

Daniel Deronda: Vocation, Hysteria, and "superfluous girls"

Eliot's *Daniel Deronda* narrates Gwendolen's life story alongside Daniel's. While the male protagonist, whose status as an outsider "helped to intensify his inward experience" (*DD* 152)[4], for a long time remains hampered by a "too reflective and diffusive sympathy" (*DD* 308), he finally finds his vocation – a crucial concept in all Eliot novels – and an external channel for his energies by reconnecting with his Jewish roots. Gwendolen's energies, by contrast, remain directed to the inside, becoming increasingly self-destructive. Depicting Gwendolen's 'hysteria', Eliot engages in great detail with neurology and psychology; while she was writing the novel, her partner Lewes was working on *Problems of Life and Mind*, which contained a complex description of the human nervous system. As Jane Wood remarks, Gwendolen's nature is divided between her courage ("nerve") and her hypersensitive vulnerability ("nervousness") (Wood 2001: 141). The inexplicable "gusts and storms" (*DD* 235) she experiences become partly explicable for the reader through contextual information, although the narrator's comments on Gwendolen's prehistory and psychological condition remain inconclusive. The phenomenon of "unconscious sensibility" as described by Lewes manifests itself in Gwendolen's sudden mood changes: "She

---

[3] The novels themselves were famously called "feverish productions" by Margaret Oliphant, and their popularity was seen as "indicative of a certain morbid condition in the public mind" (anon. 1863: 188).

[4] Eliot, George. *Daniel Deronda*. Ed. Graham Handley. Oxford: Oxford UP, 1988 (=*DD*).

wondered at herself in these occasional experiences, which seemed like a brief remembered madness, an unexplained exception from her normal life" (*DD* 51).[5] Her nervous condition translates small external changes into large internal turmoil. Vivacious and assertive in social situations, she is often plagued by irrational fears:

> What she unwillingly recognized [...] was that liability of hers to fits of spiritual dread [...]. She was ashamed and frightened [...] in remembering her tremor on suddenly feeling herself alone, when, for example, she was walking without companionship and there came some rapid change in the light. Solitude in any wide scene impressed her with an undefined feeling of immeasurable existence aloof from her, in the midst of which she was helplessly incapable of asserting herself. The little astronomy taught her at school used sometimes to set her imagination at work in a way that made her tremble; but always when some one joined her she recovered her indifference to the vastness in which she seemed an exile; she found again her usual world in which her will was of some avail [...].
>
> (*DD* 52)

Gwendolen experiences her own physicality as alien and unstable – indeed, she experiences a frequent terrifying detachment from her own body. As Athena Vrettos argues, her disease is narrated through spatial metaphors; she is "obsessed with privacy, persistently seeking structures to contain emotional and pathological secrets" (Vrettos 1995: 61). While her "neurosis remains stubbornly impenetrable to both Deronda's hermeneutic powers and her own" (Vrettos 1995: 62), her desire for locked spaces corresponds with her fear of wide horizons. Again, Vrettos comments that Gwendolen's "moments of immobility in open spaces [...] can be compared to the exaggerated postures of Charcot's hysterics" (Vrettos 1995: 64).

In the context of Eliot's oeuvre, Gwendolen's nervous hypersensitivity links her to Latimer in the novelette "The Lifted Veil" (1859): his psychophysically abnormal condition enables him to read the thoughts and feel the emotions of other people – and he is therefore subjected to a continual onslaught of impressions which others routinely suppress. In terms of Victorian gender politics, he is therefore feminized. Such highly suggestible organisms – usually female – were extreme versions of what Victorian physiological psychologists saw as physical inscriptions of experiences into the organism, as Lewes stated in *Studies in Animal Life*: "Nothing leaves us as it found us. Every man we meet, every book we read, every picture or landscape we see, every word or tone we hear, mingles with our being and modifies it" (Lewes 1862: 37). While Latimer, as Sally Shuttleworth explains, is "entirely open to his surrounding medium; he cannot police his boundaries" (Shuttleworth 2001: xxii), Gwendolen, too, suffers

---

[5] See Lewes' theory of "unconscious sensibility" (Lewes 1860: 2:58-60), and William B. Carpenter's similar depiction of "unconscious cerebration" (Carpenter 1874: 101).

because of her extreme sensitivity; impressions are physically inscribed, scorched or burnt into her body; while in theory there is also the possibility of her being impressed with salutary, positive suggestions, this is overruled in the text by a pervasive sense of her passivity and helplessness. Like Latimer, Gwendolen experiences visions and premonitions; she sees Grandcourt's death on a painting even before she has meet him. When he falls from his boat into the sea, her visions and outside reality finally coincide: "'I saw my wish outside me.'" (*DD* 596) Eliot's representation of Gwendolen's visions is linked to the question of how 'external' stimuli are translated into 'internal' perceptions – and where to draw the line between a healthy and a diseased process of translation. Lewes had treated this question when inquiring into the function of nerves as transmitters between the body and what he calls 'spirit' (Wood 2001: 136). In a letter to Harriet Beecher Stowe of 24 June 1872, Eliot wrote that as science advances the distinction between subjectively created visions and visions induced by external stimuli seems increasingly problematic:

> It seems difficult to limit – at least to limit with any precision – the possibility of confounding sense by impressions, derived from inward conditions, with those which are directly dependent on external stimulus. In fact, the division between within and without in this sense seems to become every year a more subtle and bewildering problem.

(Eliot 1869-73: 280)

Gwendolen's psychological development is characterized by such an impossibility of distinguishing between external and internal impulses – which ties in with physicians' observations on secondary and even tertiary attacks of hysteria. To complicate matters further, the individual's "inward conditions" were also seen by some physiological psychologists, among them Lewes and Spencer, as the inherited "residue of past experiences" (Lewes 1878-9: 270) (for example, one's ancestors'). Sometimes, according to Spencer, "the impulses produced out of that [distant and hitherto unrealized past] become more vivid than those of immediate sentient life" (Spencer 1855: 584).

Work (if not vocation), the eternal Victorian topic, was sometimes offered as a solution: John Foster's famous *Essays in a Series of Letters* (1805), for example, which can be counted as an important Victorian cultural document because they had reached 30 editions by 1846, contain an essay "On Decision of Character", whose observations on will-power – or lack of it – are pertinent to Gwendolen's case. The question of vocation is central to Foster's canonical essay, which, together with Samuel Smiles's *Self-Help* (1859), expressed some deep-held Victorian convictions about determination and work ethics: "It is a poor and disgraceful thing, not to be able to reply, with some degree of certainty, to the simple questions, What will you be? What will you do?" (Foster 1819:

98-90). Foster's warning that such people, victims of their own indecision, are inferior even to animals, can be read as a comment on Gwendolen's psychological subjection to Grandcourt:

> You will often see a person anxiously hesitating a long time between different, or opposite determinations, though impatient of the pain of such a state, and ashamed of its debility. A faint impulse of preference alternates toward the one, and toward the other; and the mind, while thus held in a trembling balance, is vexed that it cannot get some new thought, or feeling, or motive, that it has not more sense, more resolution, more of any thing that would save it from envying even the decisive instinct of brutes.

> (Foster 1819: 89-90)

Gwendolen's martyrdom during her marriage is anticipated in Foster's warning, "An infirm character practically confesses itself made for subjection" (Foster 1819: 97). Indeed, Gwendolen is horrified when she realizes she cannot tell how she is going to reply to Grandcourt's marriage proposal: "This subjection to a possible self, a self not to be absolutely predicted about, caused her some astonishment and terror" (*DD* 114). Foster briefly discusses the question of a physiological basis for such a lack of will-power, eventually reaffirming the customary link between a strong bodily and mental constitution.[6]

The lack of a useful occupation, and not William James's "evolutionary arguments for women's arrested intellectual development" (Wood 2001: 151), is prominent among the multiple 'causes' offered by the text for Gwendolen's condition. When the narrator calls her and her sisters, with sad irony, "four superfluous girls" (*DD* 196), this implicitly hints at Henry Maudsley's explanation of (female) hysteria as the outcome of lives marked by prohibition and constraint: While "some practitioners in the medical profession believed that women had a fixed stock of energy which would be rapidly depleted, with disastrous consequences for childbearing, if women's weak brains were taxed with a lot of mental work" (Purvis 1991: 3)[7], Maudsley emphasized that women's lack of intellectual achievement was an acquired deficit: "Through generations her character [...] has been made feeble by long habit of dependence; by the circumstances of her position the sexual life has been undesignedly developed at the expense of the intellectual" (Maudsley 1867: 203).[8] Horatio Bryan Donkin likewise postulated in 1892 that the multiple restrictions imposed on females lead to stunted physical and mental growth, even producing psychological deformities:

---

[6] See Foster 1819: 103-6.
[7] See as another example Spencer 1896: 107-8.
[8] But in his later works Maudsley did biologize gender difference, see Maudsley 1874: 468-9.

Apart from whatever fundamental difference of nerve-stability there may be between the sexes, […] the girl usually meets with far more obstacles to uniform development and consequent nervous control than the youth. […] there are in the surroundings and general training of most girls many hindrances to the retention or restoration of a due stability, and but few channels of outlet for her new activities. […] 'Thou shalt not' meets a girl at almost every turn. The exceptions to this rule are found in those instances where girls and women of all conditions, owing to the influence of good education or necessity, or both, have regular work and definite pursuits.

(Donkin 1892: 621)

Eliot uses Gwendolen as a case study of such a female, weakened in body and mind, suffering from "nerves". Her education has provided only cultural commonplaces for drawing-room conversation, and her mother was unable to check her egotism; she is thus a helpless prey to her own nervous condition. Moreover, she lacks a useful occupation, like the protagonist in Charlotte Perkins Gilmans' well-known short story "The Yellow Wallpaper" (1892), who is diagnosed by male physicians as suffering "temporary nervous depression – a slight hysterical tendency", and has to undergo a "rest cure" which, in fact, reinforces her neurotic symptoms by depriving her of what she herself thinks she needs, "congenial work, with excitement and change" (Gilman 1990: 762). According to Daniel's diagnosis, Gwendolen suffers from the narrowness of her existence; in contrast to his own mission, founded on the Jewish "inheritance that has never ceased to quiver in millions of human frames" (*DD* 458), and to Dorothea's epiphanic recognition in *Middlemarch* that she "was part of [the] involuntary, palpitating life" (Eliot 1996: 741) around her, Gwendolen remains a victim of "the texture of her nerves and the palpitation of her heart" (*DD* 384). Again, the difference between her and 'healthy' individuals resides in the fact that for her, it is not the outside which "quivers" or "palpitates" but her own inside. She is unable to emerge from the depths of her hysterical condition.

After Daniel has ceased to be available as a guiding figure, she returns to her mother, a development which equals the resumption of her earlier position as an egotistical, spoiled child. Losing Daniel reduces Gwendolen "to a mere speck" (*DD* 689). There is no cathartic moment as with Dorothea, no "progress toward a state of active, involved life" (Kearns 1987: 223). Indeed, we last see Gwendolen in the grips of yet another fit of hysteria:

[…] her mother came in and found her sitting motionless. […] "[…] but don't be afraid. I am going to live", said Gwendolen, bursting out hysterically. […] Through the day and half the night she fell continually into fits of shrieking, but cried in the midst of them to her mother, "Don't be afraid. I shall live. I mean to live."

(*DD* 879)

Again, Gwendolen is "sitting motionless", recalling countless earlier moments of such frozen hysterical postures. "The end of Eliot's novel thus remains radically unresolved, for Gwendolen has embraced Deronda's moral vision without eradicating her own nervous symptoms. In essence, Deronda's narrative closes while Gwendolen's is abandoned" (Vrettos 1995: 78-79). Instead of illustrating the mid-century self-help ideal and Carlylean work ethics, her trajectory reduces her to her biology, anticipating the fragile, hysterical female figures of the *fin de siècle* – a time when gender differences were increasingly 'biologized' – and 'pathologized'.

Jude the Obscure: Vocation, Hysteria, and Being "too menny"

Still, work ethics and self-help do remain positive concepts for Eliot which she at least implicitly opposes to the failed life trajectory of creatures such as Gwendolen. In Thomas Hardy, especially his negative novel of formation *Jude the Obscure* (1895), the humanistic ideal of a free process of development in varied interchange with one's surroundings, as defined by Goethe, Humboldt and their English interpreters Arnold and Mill, is dismissed as utopian. In fact, in this last of Hardy's novels, biological heredity and social restrictions have destroyed the individual's capacities for development. Hardy himself describes the theme of his novel as follows: "[I]t is concerned first with the labours of a poor student to get a University degree, & secondly with the tragic issues of two bad marriages, owing in the main to a doom or curse of hereditary temperament peculiar to the family of the parties" (Hardy 1980: 93). The relevant contexts of theories of degeneration, scientific determinism, and atavism have often been discussed: The protagonists Jude and Sue are forced, in Maudsley's phrasing, to "liv[e] [their] forefathers essentially over again" (Maudsley 1916; 267), because "No one can escape the tyranny of his organization; no one can elude the destiny that is innate in him, and which unconsciously and irresisibly shapes his ends" (Maudsley 1873: 76). Both are 'too finely tuned' for their surroundings, as they themselves diagnose. Already during his childhood Jude is sensitive and 'not a survivor'; his pity and empathy for weaker creatures – "he was a boy who could not himself bear to hurt anything" (*J* 11) [9] – is not seen as a virtue, as in John Ruskin's praise of "gentleness to all brute creatures" (Ruskin 1903-12: 143), but presented by the narrator, with some regret, as a disadvantage in the universal struggle for survival – in fact, as a pathological trait, as "morbid". [10] In contrast

[9] Hardy, Thomas. *Jude the Obscure*. Ed. Patricia Ingham. Oxford: Oxford UP, 1996 (= *J*).
[10] See *J* 9. Shuttleworth compares Jonathan Hutchinson's article "On Cruelty to Animals", *Fortnightly Review* (1876), where a consideration of plants and animals is represented as exaggerated sensitivity: "Yet this is surely morbid, and is far less to be desired than the more robust type of character, which pursues happiness with energy and shuts its eyes to unavoidable pain" (Shuttleworth 2002: 135).

to Eliot's novels, Hardy does not present the boy Jude's sense of a harmonious union with nature as an epiphany; it is not a solution or a path towards a meaningful, altruistic way of life.

While Jude experiences his life as a harsh incongruence of body and spirit, "the appalling consequences for the self of disinterested pursuit of knowledge" in a gross, worldly environment, it is his body, including his sexual desires, which destroys his loftier ambitions (Levine 2002: 203). Sue's trajectory is characterized by the same dilemma in different ways. According to Hardy's gender-specific technique of "differential embodiment", she is more strongly associated with her body than Jude is – albeit *ex negativo*: she is "so ethereal a creature that her spirit could be seen trembling through her limbs, […] one who, to him, was so uncarnate as to seem at times impossible as a human wife to any average man." (*J* 195) In early reviews Sue was repeatedly pathologized and classified as either hysterical or frigid – for instance by R.Y. Tyrrell, Classical Philologist at Trinity College, Dublin, who called Hardy's description of Sue's personality as "all this minute registry of the fluctuations of disease in an incurably morbid organism" (Tyrell 1970: 295). D.H. Lawrence in his study about Thomas Hardy (1914) also analysed Sue's underdeveloped sexuality as her major deficit.[11] According to these reductionist readings, Sue could be seen as another literary example of the 'intellectual woman' as described by physician Thomas S. Clouston and others, a woman who endangers her attractiveness to men as well as her reproductive capacities by intellectual exertions.[12] She could thus be seen to represent the social phenomenon of the 'New Woman', invented, derided and celebrated during the 1890s – and indeed, like these proto-feminists she shows a desire to determine her own sexuality rather than 'sell' it to a man via marriage contract.[13] Jude himself adopts this perspective when insisting on Sue's individual freedom after her marriage to Phillotson: "'Wifedom has not yet assimilated and digested you in its vast maw as an atom which has no further individuality.'" (*J* 197) In a retrospective interpretation of his own novel, a "Postscript" from 1912, Hardy calls Sue "the first delineation in fiction […] of the woman of the feminist movement – the slight, pale 'bachelor' girl – the intellectualized, emancipated bundle of nerves that modern conditions were producing" (*J* xxxviii). The attempts of this 'ethereal' creature to extricate herself from conventional gender roles and the burden of her ancestral past are doomed to fail; Sue feels "crushed into the earth by the weight of so many previous lives" (*J* 213). Her sexual ambivalence, "her strange ways and curious uncon-

---

[11] See Andrew Radford, *Thomas Hardy and the Survivals of Time*, Aldershot 2003, 188: "As her surname implies and Lawrence explains in his *Study of Thomas Hardy* (1914), the bride in this 'fine-nerved, sensitive girl' is fatally constrained by the head."
[12] See Clouston 1886.
[13] On Sue as a 'New Woman' see Simpson 1991 and Horlacher 2006: 178-92 and 235-40.

sciousness of gender" (*J* 154), cannot surmount social conventions and gender roles.

Work and meaningful occupation, still implicitly a solution for Eliot, has ceased to be one here: both Jude and Sue work all their lives. While Jude, apprenticed to a stonemason, is unable to enter his chosen profession and pursue what he perceives as his real 'vocation' because he is rejected by the university authorities after years of autodidactic studies, Sue is given formal training as a pupil teacher, a profession she herself has chosen. However, her work is not configured as liberating and meaningful, but as confining her, literally, inside enclosed spaces: her entire educational course is metaphorically linked to her confinement within the teacher training institution and her subjection to a rigid discipline and daily routine. To punish herself for the death of her children, Sue eventually surrenders, masochistically, to her legal husband Phillotson, who is physically repulsive to her, in order to tame her "rebellious flesh" (*J* 363). As with the *fin-de-siècle* hysterics observed by Charcot in Paris, this can be read as her ventriloquizing the laws of patriarchy and misogyny – or as her attempting, again in a manner comparable to historical hysterics, to refine herself out of (bodily) existence in order to circumvent those laws altogether. Adopting an extreme, fundamentalist Christian ritual, self-flagellation, and lying motionless on the church floor for hours, Sue finally relinquishes her idea of a harmonious life in accordance with one's nature. Hardy's famous notebook observation, 7 April 1889, "that the human race is too extremely developed for its corporeal conditions, the nerves being evolved to an activity abnormal in such an environment" (Hardy 1989: 227), seems to resound in his description of these two protagonists. Sue in fact maintains in similar words that: "at the framing of the terrestrial conditions there seemed never to have been contemplated such a development of emotional perceptiveness [...] as that reached by thinking and educated humanity." (*J* 361) Education and self-culture have thus ceased to be helpful in 'getting on in life' – they only reinforce the incongruence between thinking human beings and their physical conditions. The connection between Eros and Thanatos in *Jude the Obscure* has been seen as a Freudian description of the death drive; not only "Little Father Time", who kills himself and his step-siblings because, in a precocious Malthusian nightmare, he thinks they are "too menny", but also Jude and Sue themselves illustrate the desire of an organism for the original state of catatonia, of non-existence and death.[14] Eliot and Hardy thus share the diagnosis of an increasing lack of orientation in a time of social transition, a time when the individual ceases to matter, submerged in statistics,

---

[14] See Jude's quotation of the doctor's words: "The doctor says there are such boys springing up amongst us – boys of a sort unknown in the last generation – the outcome of new views of life. They seem to see all its terrors before they are old enough to have staying power to resist them. He says it is the beginning of the coming universal wish not to live." (*J* 355)

the collectivism of demography and – possibly – degeneration. In Hardy, disease and gender have been firmly placed within a biologistic, evolutionary framework.

Coda: Vocation, Hysteria, and the 'Surplus Female'

Marriage laws during Victorian times equalled an implicit prohibition to work, at least where females of the upper and increasingly the middle classes were concerned. Thus marriage came close to being the only legitimate goal of female biographies and the only source of financial provision for women. Nineteenth-century feminists frequently suggested a refusal to marry as the only possibility for females to retain the capacity for independent action; in 1856, Eliot, among many others, signed a petition to parliament, initiated by Barbara Bodichon, that demanded the right for married women to retain their own property and potential professional earnings.[15] Dinah Maria Mulock Craik in "A Woman's Thoughts about Women" (1858) emphatically claims about her ideal character of a successful – and unmarried – woman: "she has not married – not wasted a day, not an ounce of her talents" (Craik 1999: 375), and radical feminist Mona Caird famously described Victorian marriage laws and marriage itself as "an insult to human dignity" (Caird 2000: 79). The position of a woman within marriage, she claimed, resembled that of a parasite, forced to live a degraded, secondary life through her husband. Nineteenth-century debates about demography and the 'surplus female', reminiscent of the "superfluous girls" from *Daniel Deronda*, resulted in drastic suggestions such as William Rathbone Greg's in "Why Are Women Redundant?" (1862) to convey 'old maids' to the colonies, where they would be more useful than in Britain. While he describes the participation of unmarried women in the labour market as their "hav[ing] to carve out artificial and painfully-sought occupations for themselves" (Greg 1999: 158), questions about female work were linked by early feminists to visions of vocation and a meaningful pursuit in life. Eliot's *Middlemarch* likewise sees the question of 'vocation' as central, using it as the leitmotif of the entire plot, its male and female life trajectories, occupations, and marriages. *Daniel Deronda* implicitly endorses the medical theory that a lack of occupation produces neuroses and hysteria, diametrically opposed to theories about the benefits of a "rest cure". Hardy in *Jude the Obscure*, by contrast, shows us a grim, deterministic world in which people are "superfluous" or "too menny", leading "unnecessary li[ves]" (*J* 11), subjected to the dictates of their social class and biological inheritance. They cannot redeem themselves by their own efforts, by 'self-help' or a meaningful occupation: Sue's hysteria is generated despite her work-filled life.

[15] See Paxton 1991: 34.

Is there anything beyond failure in Gwendolen's or Sue's fate? Following Julia Kristeva's suggestion, we might ask whether writing "strategies that [call] the unity of the subject into question", as depictions of hysteria unquestionably do, can possibly enable women "to say something new within the language inherited from patriarchy" (McGrath 2002: 16). It has often been suggested that the manifestations of hysteria, the role-playing, secrecy and opacity, rather than being male attributions, were also concrete 'weapons' in a power struggle between the sexes, undermining patriarchy's laws of coherence, logicality, and orthodoxy. Thus Freud's "conceptualization of hysteria as an incoherent or interrupted narrative history" could point us towards potentially subversive ruptures in both Eliot's and Hardy's novels: the lack of closure in these hysterical females' narratives, their "narrative contradiction, incoherence, repetition, displacement, impediment, amnesia, and conflict" could, as Vrettos has argued in a different context, "offer ways of understanding cultural processes at work" (Vrettos 1995: 11). Thus perhaps, along with Kristeva, we might ask whether the very incoherence of hysteria could be seen as liberating – and whether female trajectories such as Gwendolen's or Sue's are pronounced failures only because they are contending with conventional expectations about work and vocation, self-help and success. But then again, 'success' was male in nineteenth-century culture – and hysteria, whatever its physiological grounding, seems to be an extreme, and logical, reaction to the phallic narrative that defines women as more 'suggestible' or 'impressionable' than males, i.e., as receptacles. Women, according to this narrative, are folding up into themselves rather than directing their energies to the outside world in following professional pursuits or vocations – but, of course, they were legally barred from most professions, and 'vocation', too, was male. Hysteria thus crystallizes the illogicalities of the Victorian cultural moment, and is legible as a self-defeating protest.

List of Works Cited

Anon. "Novels and Novelists of the Day." *North British Review* 38 (1863): 168-90.

Caird, Mona. "Marriage." *The Fin de Siècle: A Reader in Cultural History, c. 1880-1900*. Ed. Sally Ledger and Roger Luckhurst. Oxford: Oxford UP, 2000. 77-80.

Carpenter, William B. *Principles of Mental Physiology, with their Applications to the Training and Discipline of the Mind, and the Study of its Morbid Conditions*. London, 1874.

Carter, Robert Brudenell. *On The Pathology and Treatment of Hysteria*. London: Churchill, 1853.

Clouston, T. S. *Science and Self-Control: A Lecture to Students of the Edinburgh University*. Edinburgh, 1886.

Craik, Dinah Maria Mulock. "A Woman's Thoughts about Women." *Victorian Prose: An Anthology*. Ed. Rosemary J. Mundhenk and LuAnn McCracken Fletcher. New York: Columbia UP, 1999. 371-75.

Donkin, Horatio Bryan. "Hysteria." *A Dictionary of Psychological Medicine*. Vol. 1. Ed. Daniel Hack Tuke. London, 1892. 619-21.

Eliot, George. Letter to Harriet Beecher Stowe. 24 June 1872. *The George Eliot Letters*. Vol. 5. Ed. Gordon S. Haight. New Haven: Yale UP, 1957-78. 279-82.

---. *Daniel Deronda*. Ed. Graham Handley. Oxford: Oxford UP, 1988.

---. *Middlemarch*. Ed. David Carroll. Introd. Felicia Bonaparte. Oxford: Oxford UP, 1996.

Fischer-Homberger. *Die traumatische Neurose: Vom somatischen zum sozialen Leiden*. Bern: Huber, 1975.

Foster, John. "On Decision of Character." *Essays in a Series of Letters*. 6th ed. London, 1819. 89-166.

Gilman, Charlotte Perkins. "The Yellow Wallpaper". *Heath Anthology of American Literature*. Vol. 1. Lexington: Heath, 1990. 761-73.

Greg, William Rathbone. "Why Are Women Redundant?" *Victorian Prose: An Anthology*. Ed. Rosemary J. Mundhenk and LuAnn McCracken Fletcher. New York: Columbia UP, 1999. 157-63.

Hardy, Thomas. Letter to Edmund Goss. 10 November 1895. *The Collected Letters of Thomas Hardy*. Vol. 6. Ed. Richard Little Purdy and Michael Millgate. Oxford: Clarendon Press, 1980. 93.

---. *The Life and Work of Thomas Hardy*. Ed. Michael Millgate. London: Macmillan, 1985.

---. *Jude the Obscure*. Ed. Patricia Ingham. Oxford: Oxford UP, 1996.

Horlacher, Stefan. *Masculinities: Konzeptionen von Männlichkeit im Werk von Thomas Hardy and D. H. Lawrence*. Tübingen: Narr, 2006.

Kearns, Michael S. *Metaphors of Mind in Fiction and Psychology*. Lexington: UP of Kentucky, 1987.

Levine, George. *Dying to Know: Scientific Epistemology and Narrative in Victorian England*. Chicago: U of Chicago P, 2002.

Lewes, George Henry. *The Physiology of Common Life*. Vol. 2. Leipzig, 1860.

---. *Studies in Animal Life*. London, 1862.

---. *The Study of Psychology*. Vol. 2. London, 1878-9. 270.

Logan, Peter Melville. *Nerves and Narratives: A Cultural History of Hysteria in Nineteenth-Century British Prose*. Berkeley: U of California P, 1997.

Maudsley, Henry. *The Physiology and Pathology of the Mind*. London, 1867.

---. *Body and Mind: An Enquiry into Their Connection and Mutual Influence, Specially in Reference to Mental Disorders*. London: Macmillan, 1873.

---. "Sex in Mind and Education." *Fortnightly Review* 15 (1874): 468-9.

---. *Organic to Human: Psychological to Sociological*. London: Macmillan, 1916.

McGrath, Lynette. *Subjectivity and Women's Poetry in Early Modern England*. Aldershot: Ashgate, 2002.

Paxton, Nancy. *George Eliot and Herbert Spencer: Feminism, Evolutionism, and the Reconstruction of Gender*. Princeton: Princeton UP, 1991.

Purvis, June. *A History of Women's Education in England*. Milton Keynes: Open UP, 1991.

Radford, Andrew. *Thomas Hardy and the Survivals of Time*. Aldershot: Ashgate, 2003.

Rothfield, Lawrence. *Vital Signs: Medical Realism in Nineteenth-Century Fiction*. Princeton: Princeton UP, 1992.

Ruskin, John. "Fors Clavigera". *The Works of John Ruskin: The Library Edition*. Ed. E. T. Cook and Alexander Wedderburn. Vol. 3. London, 1903-12. 132-45.

Scull, Andrew. *Hysteria: The Biography*. Oxford: Oxford UP, 2009.

Shuttleworth, Sally. Introduction. *The Lifted Veil and Brother Jacob*. By George Eliot. Ed. Sally Shuttleworth. London: Penguin, 2001. xi-l.

---. "'Done because we are too menny': Little Father Time and Child Suicide in Late-Victorian Culture." *Thomas Hardy: Texts and Contexts*. Ed. Philip Mallett. Houndmills: Palgrave Macmillan, 2002. 133-55.

Simpson, Anne B. "Sue Bridehead Revisited." *Victorian Literature and Culture* 19 (1991): 55-66.

Spencer, Herbert. *The Principles of Psychology*. London, 1855.

---. *Education: Intellectual, Moral, and Physical*. 2nd ed. New York, 1896.

Tyrrell, R. Y. *Fortnightly Review* (1896): 857-64. Repr. *Thomas Hardy: The Critical Heritage*. Ed. Reginald Gordon Cox. London: Routledge, 1970. 291-99.

Vrettos, Athena. *Somatic Fictions: Imagining Illness in Victorian Culture*. Stanford: Stanford UP, 1995.

Wood, Jane. *Passion and Pathology in Victorian Fiction*. Oxford: Oxford UP, 2001.

Anna Farkas

"Killing no Murder": Puerperal Insanity and Infanticide
in Late-Victorian British Literature

As Josephine McDonagh has shown in her book *Child Murder and British Culture, 1720-1900* (2003), child murder was a pervasive and powerful cultural trope in Britain in the eighteenth and nineteenth centuries. The murder of a child by its own mother is to this day considered a particularly shocking crime, as news-media coverage attests on a regular basis. It is not surprising, therefore, that there is also a long tradition of literary representations of this crime. The literary narrative of child murder in the nineteenth century has been shown to be tied up with the legal discourses surrounding a particularly harsh seventeenth-century statute, which dictated conceptions about the profile and motivation of the perpetrator even after its repeal, fixing illegitimacy as the decisive factor.[1] What has not been considered so far, however, is how not only legal practice, but also literary representation concerning this crime changed with the rise of a powerful new medical discourse in the latter part of the century. Puerperal insanity, severe mental disturbance after childbirth, was first classified in the 1820s, and soon became widely accepted as a prevalent complication of pregnancy and child birth, which was associated with the increased danger of the mother doing violence either to herself or her child. Invariably, this influenced the prosecution of child murder cases, as the increased popularity of the insanity defence in the second half of the century shows (see Smith 1981: 148-153). In the 1880s and 1890s the literary representation of child murder was changing accordingly, the focus was no longer on sexual morality, but the crime became associated with disease. Due to its perceived unnaturalness it also remained an ideological battleground for conceptions of femininity and maternity. In this chapter, I will first trace the transformation of the dominant discourse of infanticide in the nineteenth century and then turn to two late-Victorian texts, the novel *Mrs. Keith's Crime* (1885) by Lucy Clifford and the play *Alan's Wife* (1893) by Florence Bell and Elizabeth Robins, which exemplify the altered focus of the literary representation of child murder at the end of the nineteenth century.

Concerns about the moral and economic implications of a rising rate of illegitimacy in early-modern England led to the passing of a draconian statute

---

[1] See, for example, McDonagh 2003: 1-13; Thorn 2003: 13-42; Krueger 1997.

for the prosecution of child murder in the English parliament in 1624: "An Act to prevent the Destroying and Murthering of Bastard Children."[2] This law determined the gender and marital status of child murderers and also inscribed the likely motivation and a typical scenario for the crime: unmarried women killed their illegitimate children to avoid retribution from the community. In order to deter likely offenders and discourage extramarital sex, the law facilitated a murder conviction by making the concealment of the death of an illegitimate child sufficient grounds for capital punishment. Similar laws followed in Scotland and Ireland in 1690 and 1707. The law remained in force until 1803 and continued to shape the literary representation of child murder even after its repeal, as can be seen from the example of two prominent nineteenth-century novels, Walter Scott's *The Heart of Midlothian* from 1818 and George Eliot's *Adam Bede* from 1859.

In both texts, the action is situated within the range of the relevant statute – *The Heart of Midlothian* opens with the Porteous riot in 1736, and the beginning of *Adam Bede* is very precisely dated to "the eighteenth of June, in the year of our Lord 1799" (Eliot 2008: 5) – and they both reproduce the profile of the typical child murderer as it was established by the law: Effie Deans in *The Heart of Midlothian* and Hetty Sorrel in *Adam Bede* are female and unmarried. In *The Heart of Midlothian*, Effie Deans, the younger daughter of a Scottish Lowlands farmer, is imprisoned in Edinburgh under the suspicion of child murder. Seduced by a wanted criminal, she has hidden her pregnancy and given birth in secret. When she recovers from the delivery, the child is gone, and she is indicted under the 1690 statute. This law was even more severe than its English counterpart as it stipulated that the concealment of pregnancy and birth alone was sufficient evidence for a murder conviction if the mother could not produce the child afterwards. As she is unable to prove that she did *not* kill the child, she is sentenced to death and only reprieved when her older sister walks all the way from Scotland to London to procure a pardon from Queen Caroline. The novel exposes the fallibility of the statute – Effie's child is revealed not to be dead at all – but does not materially diverge from its narrative of illegitimacy. Effie has been led astray from her strict Protestant upbringing and is now trapped, not just by the walls of the prison, but also by her shame.

The same is true for Hetty Sorrel in *Adam Bede*, another retelling of the classic scenario of child murder. Impregnated and abandoned by her lover, the dairymaid Hetty hides her pregnancy from her family and ends up giving birth in the house of a stranger. At that point she has despaired of assistance from the baby's father, whom she could not locate, and only wants to go back to her old life. But she also fears her family's scorn should it become known that she has

---

[2] For a detailed treatment of the background to the passing of this law, see Jackson 1996: 29-59.

born an illegitimate child, so she decides to "get rid of it" (406) and abandons the baby in the wood, where it soon dies. Hetty is sentenced to death for child murder, but is reprieved at the last minute when her sentence is commuted to transportation. This sensational ending is necessary for the dramatic arc of the plot, but it would actually have been rather improbable as the outcome of an actual court case at the time, as juries in the second half of the eighteenth century had become very reluctant of convicting under the 1624 statute, even if the evidence was as clear as it is in *Adam Bede*. By the turn of the century, the law was considered unenforceable, which led to its repeal in 1803.

Medical evidence had long played a role in child murder trials, but in the eighteenth and early- to mid-nineteenth centuries it was primarily forensic medicine focusing on the body of the child.[3] This changed in the nineteenth century with the formal categorisation of puerperal insanity and the growing importance of the insanity defence. In her recent book, *Dangerous Motherhood: Insanity and Childbirth in Victorian Britain* (2004), Hilary Marland identified the obstetrician Robert Gooch, who maintained a private practice and also attended at lying-in hospitals in London, as the one who 'named' and influentially described the disease in 1820, following on from numerous unsystematic accounts of women experiencing episodes of mental disturbance after childbirth that went back to the early modern period (see Marland 2004: 28-64).[4] Puerperal insanity occupied a territory that was contested by two medical disciplines, obstetrics, which had developed from midwifery, and alienism, the forerunner of psychiatry, which was quickly growing in importance. Obstetricians and alienists clashed on a number of points, particularly the location of treatment – the private home or the asylum – but they agreed on the key characteristics: the prevalence – puerperal insanity was a common problem which affected rich and poor women alike – the severity of the symptoms – the patient was likely to try and harm herself and/or her child – and the overall prognosis – with proper treatment, there was a good chance of a complete recovery (see ibid).

Representatives of both disciplines stressed the violence of the patients' mania, particularly regarding behaviour that violated conventional norms of femininity. In a series of lectures on midwifery and the diseases of women and children Gooch had given at St. Bartholomew's Hospital in London, which were published posthumously, he observed the following: "When puerperal mania does take place, the patient swears, bellows, recites poetry, talks bawdry, and kicks up such a row that there is the devil to pay in the house: it is odd that

---

[3] For the role played by coroners in Victorian infanticide trials, see Behlmer, 1979. See also Krueger 1997: 283-86.

[4] I am deeply indebted to Hilary Marland's excellent history of puerperal insanity for bringing the range of medical authors who wrote on this topic in the nineteenth century to my attention.

women who have been delicately brought up and chastely educated, should have such rubbish in their minds" (Skinner 1831: 290). This was later echoed by John Charles Bucknill and Daniel H. Tuke in their influential handbook *A Manual of Psychological Medicine*, which first appeared in 1858: "although the patient may have been remarkable previously for her correct, modest demeanour, and attention to her religious duties, most awful oaths and imprecations are now uttered, and language used which astonishes her friends" (Bucknill and Tuke 1968: 237). But the violence was not just verbal. In 1882, Thomas Coulston, who had gained considerable clinical experience over the course of twenty years as superintendent of various lunatic asylums in England and Scotland, strongly emphasised the infanticidal tendency of women suffering from puerperal insanity: "One of the most joyous times of life is made full of fearful anxiety, and the strongest affection on earth is then often suddenly concerted by disease into an antipathy: for the mother not only 'forgets her sucking child,' but often becomes dangerous to its life" (Coulston 1882: 493). Infanticide was thus written into the medical discourse on puerperal insanity, providing scientific back-up for a legal practice that had been rapidly growing in importance as the nineteenth century progressed: the insanity defence in child murder trials.

Even in the seventeenth and eighteenth centuries when the 1624 statue was in full force, women accused of child murder were occasionally pardoned on the grounds of temporary insanity, but then it tended to be applied to the few married women who were indicted for the crime, as Dana Rabin has shown: "Infanticide by married women was considered so shocking and so unlikely that the only motive assigned to it was insanity" (Rabin 2002: 76). Growing sympathy for the plight of unmarried women, which eventually rendered the 1624 statute unenforceable as juries refused to convict under it, led to increased attention to the defendant's state of mind in the late eighteenth century, regardless of her marital status. Although the association of child murder with illegitimacy continued in the nineteenth century, and particularly engaged the public during the supposed 'infanticide epidemic' of the 1860s, the attitude towards infanticidal women had changed dramatically.[5] The widespread acceptance of the medical discourse on puerperal insanity, especially regarding its prevalence and the severity of the mental disturbance associated with it, led to a recasting of infanticide from the realms of law and morality to those of disease, and resulted in the abolishment of capital punishment for this crime, in practice if, initially, not on principle. The last woman to be executed for child murder in England died in 1849 and, after lengthy discussion in parliament, the first

---

[5] For the on-going concerns about unmarried motherhood in Victorian England, see Higginbotham 1989.

Infanticide Act was passed in 1922, which defined infanticide, the killing of a new-born child, as a form of manslaughter.[6]

In the second half of the nineteenth century, medical and legal discourses had embraced a new narrative of child murder which emphasised the pathology, not the moral depravity or criminality of the murdering mother. It is not surprising, therefore, that the literary representation of child murder changed, as well, in the late-nineteenth century. The association with illegitimacy ended. The children who are killed by their mothers in British literature of the 1880s and 1890s are the product of legitimate marriages. For example, Lucy Clifford's Mrs. Keith and Florence Bell's and Elizabeth Robins's Jean Creyke are both widows. *Mrs. Keith's Crime* and *Alan's Wife*, which continue the child murder narrative from earlier works in this tradition, shift the focus away from questions of sexual morality. Disease takes the place of seduction in the exculpatory framework of late-Victorian literary representations of child murder.

Disease is everywhere in *Mrs. Keith's Crime*. The *Contemporary Review* identified the novel's "curious interest in disease" as the marker of its modernity, an example of "the influence of that change by which, in our day, science has been made the mould of literature" (Wedgwood 1885: 750). The ravaging progress of disease through the life of the eponymous Mrs. Keith drives – one could say constitutes – the plot. Having lost her husband in a bathing accident on the beach before the beginning of the action, she quickly also loses the older of her two children, a perfectly healthy boy, through scarlet fever. Only her five-year old daughter Molly remains. But the novel's very first sentence, "Surely he is mistaken?", is already ominous. (Clifford 1897: 3) It relates to a doctor's assessment of Molly's health. She is consumptive. Only a warmer climate could save her. So Mrs. Keith takes Molly to Southern Spain, where her decline is temporarily arrested, but not ultimately reversed. The majority of the text is taken up with the minute chronicling of her symptoms. About half way through, it is confirmed that Molly cannot live and soon her mother's health also fails. The crisis comes when Mrs. Keith is told by the resident doctor that she will likely predecease her daughter, leaving the child to the mercies of the unsympathetically drawn locals: "Let that cruel woman tend her, let strange hands smooth her pillow, and cold hearts watch her die? Oh no,— no,— no, I cannot, and it shall not be, for to-night, when they leave us alone, I will *kill* her" (332). The killing is presented as a necessary, even a humane act, due to the inevitability of disease and the unfriendliness of the surroundings.

Alan's Wife draws more immediately on the contemporary discourse of puerperal insanity, while also bringing another type of bodily incapacitation into

[6] For an overview of these developments, see Jackson 2002: 1-17; Rose 1986: 70-78. For a detailed assessment of the background to the two infanticide acts, see Ward 1999.

play, disability. The heroine, Jean Creyke, worships her husband for his "health and strength" and expects the child she is carrying to become "just such another as his father" (Bell and Robin 1893: 10 and 17). But when Alan is suddenly killed in an accident, and her son is born disabled, she faces a very different reality. Unlike Molly, the baby's survival is not in doubt, but he will grow up to be "a cripple [...] [who] won't walk and run like other boys" (25). Jean herself is listless and shows little interest in the child. According to the late-Victorian understanding of the disease such behaviour was typically associated with puerperal insanity, as T. S. Coulston's description in his *Clinical Lectures on Mental Diseases* shows: "The mother looks self-absorbed and dull. She does not take such notice of the baby as is usual, or such interest in what is going on" (Coulston 1882: 493). When Jean is left alone with her son, she decides to kill him because she fears that his disability would make him suffer later in life, and she cannot be sure to be able to protect him from such pain. The murder stuns both Jean's mother and Colonel Stuart, the representative of the law, who is trying to find an explanation for an act that seems incomprehensible to him: "I can't help feeling that there must be some extenuating circumstances" (39). What he is thinking of becomes clear when he asks Jean's mother: "Do you think her mind was at all affected at the time?" (40). Jean's mother then urges her daughter to make a confession along those lines: "Honey, tell his worship how you came to do it. Tell him you hadn't your wits right; that you didn't know what you were doing to the little bairn!" (42). The medico-legal discourse concerning the link between puerperal insanity and infanticide is here inscribed into the text of the play, including the habitual leniency towards infanticidal women in judicial practice. Child murder is once again framed by disease, but this time not physical, but mental illness.[7]

Jean, however, rejects this reading, which would rob her of her agency. Instead, she elevates the killing to a supreme act of maternal love and personal virtue.[8] She ignores her mother's plea and refuses to speak until the very end of the play when she is goaded into finally explaining herself by the accusation that she has committed a crime, "Crime! [...] I've had courage just once in my life – just once in my life have I been strong and kind – and it was the night I killed my child!" (47). Mrs. Keith expresses the same sentiment in very similar language: "Oh, what strange things are sometimes called crimes – what false things are called courage. [...] Oh, brave hearts, that love and bear, do not say

[7] The play has been read in the context of the broader category of hysteria before, but except for a brief mention of Jean's "realist performance of puerperal insanity" by Katherine Kelly, the specific historical circumstances of the play's portrayal of mental illness have not been explored (Kelly 2004: 545). For readings linking the play with hysteria, see Diamond 1997: 3-39; Townsend 2000: 110-115; Ehnenn 2008: 97-133.

[8] Josephine McDonagh has pointed out that Jean "draws on the traditional lexicon of child murder" (McDonagh 2003: 179).

that I have no courage when I quench the life in my sweet one's eyes tonight. I cannot leave her here alone; I am not cold or cruel enough for that" (340). Both works plead what one reviewer identified as the theme "'killing no murder'" ("Recent Novels" 1885: 3). What distinguishes them is their treatment of disease, in relation to both mother and child.

A potential eugenic subtext in both works specifically relates to the physical impairment of the children. Jean's enthusiastic praise of her husband Alan as a type of virile superman has led Rebecca Cameron to argue for the play's "entrenchment in contemporary eugenics [...] [which] adds an unsavoury dimension to [Jean's] motive for killing her child" (Cameron 2004: 94).[9] Cameron also acknowledges, however, that Jean "performs the act through, not despite, a sense of duty to her child. The act itself is framed in terms of Christian duty as well as maternal self-sacrifice" (ibid.), effectively refuting a simplistic interpretation like Catherine Wiley's representation of Jean as a "character who murders a child she cannot love because it is physically imperfect" (Wiley 1990: 433). The text explicitly states the opposite: "They say I don't love you – I don't care for you at all! Yes, yes, I do, dear, yes, I do!" (30). Jean's glorification of physical strength and vitality in the first of the three scenes and her undeniable discomfort and dejection at the boy's disability in the second do, however, provide a basis for a eugenic reading. I would nevertheless stipulate that this would have to make allowances for the complexity of the play to be successful. *Mrs. Keith's Crime* takes a much clearer position in this debate. Here proto-eugenic ideas are attributed to the unsympathetic Spanish landlady, the 'cruel woman' Molly's care would fall to if Mrs. Keith succumbed to her illness before her daughter, as Catherine Hancock has pointed out (Hancock 2004: 310). Earlier in the narrative, when confronted with a "deformed boy", Manuela is reported to have said that "it was a pity he was allowed to live; the deformed and the sick ought to die," marking her out as "a disciple of Darwin" (162). A "eugenic murder" (McDonagh 2003: 179), like the one McDonagh sees in *Alan's Wife*, is, therefore, the nightmare Mrs. Keith believes herself to be saving Molly from when she "kills her child to save its life" ("Recent Novels" 1885: 3). The rejection of eugenic thought as barbaric is unequivocally expressed.

Each text's outlook is determined by the central subjectivity's proximity to disease. Mrs. Keith, who knows herself to be terminally ill and whose daily life has long been entirely preoccupied with the management of disease, her child's and her own, believes herself to be surrendering to its overwhelming force by killing her child, but argues that under these exceptional circumstances normal rules should not apply. In *Mrs. Keith's Crime*, "disease [....] appears as the

[9] See also McDonagh: "the play naturally caused something of a stir for its treatment of a eugenic theme" (McDonagh 2003: 179). For a different perspective, see Kelly 2004: n. 30 557.

tragic Fate [...] questioning the authority of traditional precepts," as the critic for the *Contemporary Review* observed (Wedgwood 1885: 751). Jean, on the other hand, who is jolted out of a state of glorified health and bodily perfection by her husband's accident, rejects the narrative of disease that is offered to her in the guise of an insanity defence because she believes that this would diminish the moral quality of her act. Like Mrs. Keith, she conceives of the killing as the ultimate proof of maternal devotion. By refusing to collaborate with the sympathetic authorities, who want to save her life, she insists on fully realising her sacrifice: "I had to do what I did, and they have to take my life for it. I showed him the only true mercy, and that is what the law shows me!" (47-48).

The two texts' different takes on the link between disease and infanticide also shaped their reception in the contemporary press. *Mrs. Keith's Crime* was repeatedly criticised for its 'morbid' theme, but that was really only what was to be expected, as Edward Delille explained in an essay on Clifford in the *Novel Review* a few years after the novel's first publication: "The theme of Mrs. Clifford's first long story, 'Mrs. Keith's Crime,' has been condemned as morbid. It is a tendency peculiar to the English mind to regard as morbid, or objectionable, or unhealthy – vague words expressing vaguer ideas – any writing in which feelings of a painful nature are analysed or described" (Delille 1892: 285). Its alleged morbidity appears not to have frightened the book-buying public, however, as the novel went through four editions in as many years. Overall the critical response, both on its first, anonymous, publication, and subsequent new editions, was largely positive. The *Athenaeum* praised its "pathos, humour, subtle characterisation, and brilliant dialogue" ("Novels of the Week" 1885: 661). What is striking is the critics' eagerness to absolve Mrs. Keith of her crime. The *Daily News* wrote that "the crime of Mrs. Keith, [...] is surrounded by many absolving circumstances" ("Recent Novels" 1885: 3). The *Pall Mall Gazette* even suggested that the book's title was altogether misleading: "The reader will be apt to open it expecting some commonplace tale of sensational wickedness and remorse," and suggested the alternative title "'A Mother's Tragedy'" instead ("Mrs Keith's Crime" 1885: 5). Clearly the representation of disease in the novel as an irresistible force succeeded in not only winning the critics' sympathy for the protagonist's suffering, but actually led them to condone the controversial remedy she chooses, an outcome the first-person narrator is openly vying for.

It is, in fact, remarkable how little the positive reviews dwelled on the representation of disease and the murder itself.[10] The *Graphic*, for example, warned its readers that "the situation to which [the novel] leads up [...] is

[10] One exception was *John Bull*, whose reviewer complained that "little Molly is, like his late Majesty King Charles II., an unconscionable time in dying" ("New Novels" 1885: 350).

hideous to the last extreme", but then teasingly refused to reveal what it is ("New Novels" 1885: 639). Instead, it gave only the following statement as a plot synopsis: "The motive of this remarkable book is the passionate love of a mother for her child" (ibid). By contrast, the infanticide in *Alan's Wife* was inevitably named and persistently medicalised. *The Times* described the play as a *"study in puerperal mania"* ("Independent Theatre" 1893: 4), the *Gentleman's Magazine* identified "obstetrics [as] the principal motive" (McCarthy 1893: 633), and the well-known theatre critic A. B. Walkley portrayed Jean as "a poor wretch, maddened by horrible misfortune, her brain still dizzy with the pangs of childbirth" (Walkley 1893: 512). *Mrs. Keith's Crime* was also repeatedly invoked in reviews of *Alan's Wife*. The *Observer* compared the two directly to demonstrate what was wrong with the play:

> Like the heroine of Mrs. Clifford's singularly pathetic, albeit morbid novel, Alan's wife, or rather his widow, kills her child; but, unlike Mrs. Keith, the unhappy woman commits her crime because she is suffering from a terrible mental disease, and is not responsible for her actions. There is nothing of the inevitable about this particular manifestation of insanity, whereas in *Mrs. Keith's Crime* we are made to feel that given the circumstances the catastrophe was not to be avoided.
>
> ("At the Play" 1893: 7)

The remarkable contradiction concerning the relative pathology of child murder in *Mrs. Keith's Crime* and *Alan's Wife* that is expressed here makes it apparent to what extent the critics were responding to the representation of disease in the two texts. Mrs. Keith, who embraces the overwhelming power of disease, is excused; Jean, who resists it, is not 'responsible for her actions', but is still somehow at fault. Her mental illness, though 'terrible', is somehow less 'inevitable' than Mrs. Keith's physical illness. By insisting on the medical framing of the killing in the text that appears to challenge it, the critics were reinforcing the established link between child murder and disease.

The reviews also demonstrate that gender was an integral part of this debate. While, according to the *Pall Mall Gazette*, the story of Mrs. Keith was "in its whole conception and execution [...] womanly," and her decision to kill her child under the circumstances "pardonable, however shocking" ("Mrs. Keith's Crime" 1885: 5), the *Era* found Jean to be "without maternal instinct, and, consequently [...] a monster" ("Independent Theatre" 1893: 8). The two protagonists, and by extension the novel and the play as a whole, were judged on the basis of their realisation of the maternal ideal. Moreover, through their maternity, Mrs. Keith's and Jean's femininity was assessed. Edward Delille described Mrs. Keith, whose plea to have the killing of her child recognised as the ultimate act of maternal devotion was successful, as "a sorely-tried, suffering, and loving woman, with a simple woman's mind and heart [...] very sympathetically human" (Delille 1892: 288). By contrast, Jean, who makes the same demand on the audience of *Alan's Wife*, was pronounced a faulty literary construction by the *Graphic*. She is not a real woman at all, because "poor women, who, like the playwright's Jean Creyke, have the misfortune to give birth to a cripple child, do not suffocate their offspring in the cradle [...] the natural mother looks into the cradle with eyes that are blind to deformities" (Thomas 1893: 499). The violence of the critics' response to *Alan's Wife* is best explained with the play's provocative evocation, but ultimate rejection of a recently established cultural paradigm, the link between female insanity and infanticide. The representation of child murder on the stage was in itself a daring experiment in the London theatre of the 1890s, a strain for the susceptibilities of the critical establishment. And while the influence of the discourse of puerperal insanity guaranteed that a woman who killed her child would at least be regarded as pitiable, not simply wicked, the denial of temporary insanity in the absence of other extenuating circumstances in such a case left only the conclusion that she must, in fact, be "a monster, with whom we can feel no sympathy whatsoever" ("Independent Theatre" 1893: 8).

In the 1880s and 1890s female writers in Britain and America, who are now often identified as 'New Woman writers', were tackling controversial topics. One result of this was an increase in the number and complexity of the literary representations of female insanity. These texts have primarily been read through the lens of hysteria, but as a number of them are more specifically situated in the contemporary medical discourses of puerperal insanity, I would argue that they can profit from a more precise historical reading. One of the best-known accounts of female insanity of the time, the short story *The Yellow Wallpaper* by the American author Charlotte Perkins Gilman, which was first published in 1892, places the diagnosis of the mental disturbance experienced by the protagonist in the context of childbirth. *The Yellow Wallpaper* focuses on the protagonist's relationship with her physician husband, not her child, as she descends into psychosis, but other texts of the period follow the pattern established by contemporary medical and legal discourses and link female insanity with infanticide. In Sarah Grand's *The Heavenly Twins* from 1893 an attempted suicide/infanticide is linked to pregnancy and embedded in a complex history of one character's depressive illness. And in 1895, the Independent Theatre Society, the avant-garde theatre company which had produced *Alan's Wife* two years before, mounted another play that made explicit reference to puerperal insanity, and stressed the inevitability of the disease's link with child murder in a powerful gothic twist.[11] These texts complicated a literary narrative

---

[11] *Salvé* (1895) by Aimee Beringer focuses on an elderly couple, who have fallen on hard times through the profligacy of their only son, who left them to settle his debts when he emigrated to Australia years before. It is revealed that the mother suffered an episode of

of child murder in Britain that had been fairly stable for about two hundred years by removing illegitimacy as the default motivation for the crime, and instead placing infanticide in the framework of disease. They also tested the boundaries of contemporary discourses of gender, as the furious debate about the limits of femininity and maternity in the wake of the first publication and production of *Mrs. Keith's Crime* and *Alan's Wife* showed.

List of Works Cited

Sources before 1900

"At the Play." *Observer*. 30 April 1893. 7.

[Bell, Florence and Elizabeth Robins.] *Alan's Wife. A Dramatic Study in Three Scenes. First Acted at the Independent Theatre in London*. London: Henry & Co., 1893.

Beringer, Mrs Oscar. *Salvé*. 1895. TS LCP 53570 P. British Lib., London.

Bucknill, John Charles and Daniel H. Tuke. *A Manual of Psychological Medicine*. 1858. New York and London: Hafner, 1968.

Clifford, Mrs W. K. *Mrs. Keith's Crime: A Record*. 6th ed. London: T. Fisher Unwin, 1897.

Coulston, T. S. *Clinical Lectures on Mental Diseases*. London: J. A. Churchill, 1883.

Delille, Edward. "Mrs. W. K. Clifford." *Novel Review* 1.4 (July 1892): 285-93.

Eliot, George. *Adam Bede*. Ed. Carol A. Martin. Oxford: Oxford UP, 2008.

"The Independent Theatre." *Era* 6 (May 1893): 8.

"The Independent Theatre." *The Times*. 01 May 1893. 4.

"'Mrs. Keith's Crime.'" *Pall Mall Gazette*. 8 June 1885. 5.

McCarthy, Justin Huntly. "Pages on Plays." *Gentleman's Magazine* (June 1893): 632-38.

"New Novels." *Graphic*. 20 June 1885. 639.

"New Novels." *John Bull*. 30 May 1885. 350.

"Novels of the Week." *Athenaeum*. 23 May 1885. 660-61.

"Recent Novels." *Daily News*. 29 Sept. 1885. 3.

Skinner, George (ed.). *A Practical Compendium of Midwifery: Being the Course of Lectures on Midwifery, and on the Diseases of Women and Infants, Delivered at St. Bartholomew Hospital by the late Robert Gooch, M. D.* London: Longman, Rees, Orme, Brown, and Green, 1831.

Thomas, W. Moy. "New Plays." *Graphic*. 6 May 1893. 499.

W[alkley], A. B. "The Drama: 'Alan's Wife.'" *Speaker*. 6 May 1893. 512.

Wedgwood, Julia. "Contemporary Records: Fiction." *Contemporary Review* 48 (1885): 749-57.

puerperal insanity after the birth of her child. Ignoring her husband's premonitions, she leaves the house to make a last appeal to the landlord who is threatening their eviction. In her absence the prodigal son returns, but does not immediately reveal his identity to her when she returns. Instead he shows her the gold he has brought with him. Driven to desperation, she stabs her son for his gold, only recognising him as he lies dying. When she realises whom she has killed, she goes mad and reverts to the time after her son's birth when she was suffering from puerperal insanity.

Sources after 1900

Behlmer, George E. "Deadly Motherhood. Infanticide and Medical Opinion in Mid-Victorian England." *Journal of the History of Medicine* 34 (1979): 403-27.

Cameron, Rebecca S. "Ibsen and British Women's Drama." *Ibsen Studies* 4.1 (2004): 92-102.

Diamond, Elin. *Unmaking Mimesis: Essays on Feminism and Theater*. London: Routledge, 1997.

Ehnenn, Jill R. *Women's Literary Collaboration, Queerness, and Late-Victorian Culture*. Aldershot: Ashgate, 2008.

Hancock, Catherine R. "'It was Bone of her Bone, and Flesh of Her Flesh, and She Has Killed it': Three Version of Destructive Maternity in Victorian Fiction." *Literature Interpretation Theory* 15 (2004): 299-320.

Higginbotham, Ann R. "'Sin of the Age': Infanticide and Illegitimacy in Victorian London." *Victorian* Studies 32.3 (1989): 319-37.

Jackson, Mark. *New Born Child Murder: Women, Illegitimacy and the Courts in Eighteenth-Century England*. Manchester: Manchester UP, 1996.

---, "The Trial of Harriet Vooght: Continuity and Change in the History of Infanticide." *Infanticide: Historical Perspectives on Child Murder and Concealment, 1550-2000*. Ed. Mark Jackson. Aldershot: Ashgate, 2002. 1-17.

Kelly, Katherine E. "*Alan's Wife*: Mother Love and Theatrical Sociability in London of the 1890s." *Modernism/Modernity* 11.3 (2004): 539-60.

Krueger, Christine L. "Literary Defences and Medical Prosecutions: Representing Infanticide in Nineteenth Century Britain." *Victorian Studies* 40.2 (1997): 271-94.

Marland, Hilary. *Dangerous Motherhood: Insanity and Childbirth in Victorian Britain*. Basingstoke: Palgrave Macmillan, 2004.

McDonagh, Josephine. *Child Murder and British Culture, 1720-1900*. Cambridge: Cambridge UP, 2003.

Rabin, Dana. "Bodies of Evidence, States of Mind: Infanticide, Emotion and Sensibility in Eighteenth-Century England." *Infanticide: Historical Perspectives on Child Murder and Concealment, 1550-2000*. Ed. Mark Jackson. Aldershot: Ashgate, 2002. 73-92.

Rose, Lionel. *The Massacre of the Innocents. Infanticide in Britain, 1800-1939*. London: Routledge & Kegan Paul, 1986.

Smith, Roger. *Trial by Medicine: Insanity and Responsibility in Victorian Trials*. Edinburgh, Edinburgh UP, 1981.

Thorn, Jennifer. Ed. *Writing British Infanticide. Child-Murder, Gender, and Print, 1722-1859*. Newark: U of Delaware P, 2003.

Townsend, Joanna. "Elizabeth Robins: Hysteria, Politics and Performance." *Women, Theatre and Performance: New Histories, New Historiographies*. Eds. Maggie B. Gale and Viv Gardner. Manchester: Manchester UP, 2000. 102-20.

Ward, Tony. "The Sad Subject of Infanticide: Law, Medicine and Child Murder." *Social and Legal Studies* 8.2 (1999), 163-80.

Wiley, Catherine. "Staging Infanticide: The Refusal of Representation in Elizabeth Robins's *Alan's Wife*." *Theatre Journal* 42.4 (1990): 432-46.

Ingrid Gessner

Of He-Nurses and She-Doctors: Gendered Accounts of Yellow Fever in Postbellum American Literature[1]

Introducing Yellow Fever

The disease of yellow fever is not indigenous to North America, but vector and virus originated in Africa and entered the New World through the slave trade; yellow fever first occurred in Spanish Florida in 1649-1650 (Swagerty and Dobyns 1983: 279, quoted in Patterson 1992: 855).[2] In 1693 Boston and other towns were infected when ships from the West Indies brought it to then British North America (Krieg 1992: 49). The probably best documented (and thus textually represented) yellow fever epidemic struck the then-capital of the United States, Philadelphia, in 1793. Between four and five thousand residents, or 8-9 percent of the city's population, died.[3] In the late eighteenth century Benjamin Rush and James Caldwell, the editors of *The Medical Repository*, a magazine that combined medical and natural historical topics with occasional poetry entries, deliberately called the disease "West-India and American yellow fever" and categorised it as one of "our epidemics" (Rush 1803: 156; Caldwell 1802: 16; quoted in Arner 2010: 458). In literary and medical writing, yellow fever, and the threat connected to it, served to define and unite the American nation.

---

[1] I would like to thank Katharina Boehm for her astute comments on an earlier version of this article.

[2] Epidemiologist Robert Desowitz describes a "concatenation of conditions" (Desowitz 1997: 99) that "led to near simultaneous outbreaks of a previously unknown disease in Havana, Barbados, Guadeloupe, St. Christopher, and Mexico's Yucatan peninsula. We know that those conditions included the importation of African slaves to work plantations and presumably the accidental inclusion of the Aedis aegypti mosquito in the holds of ships whose sailors and cargos of slaves carried the flavivirus that causes yellow fever. Once in the New World the virus prospered, as did its mosquito carrier, in European settlements across the tropical and subtropical latitudes" (Koch 2011: 73-74).

[3] Charles Brockden Brown's gothic novel *Arthur Mervyn* (1799/1800), Matthew Carey's *Short Account of the Malignant Fever* (1793), and Philip Freneau's poem "Pestilence" (1793), among many other medical and historical texts describe the Philadelphia epidemic as a crisis situation for the young nation and also testify to the cultural significance of the disease threat. Medical discourse operated on a similar plane.

Yellow fever that accounts for the most severe epidemic outbreaks of disease in the nineteenth-century United States struck irregularly. Sometimes communities were afflicted yearly by epidemics in the summer and early fall, then yellow fever completely disappeared and did not come back for decades. By the 1840s yellow fever had retreated from northern port cities to southern ones, and, by the 1870s, reached cities further inland connected through a growing system of rail transportation.[4] Several outbreaks of yellow fever during the 1870s culminated in the devastating 1878 epidemic during which twenty thousand people, or 10 percent of the population, died in the lower Mississippi Valley (Patterson 1992: 857–58; "Major U.S. Epidemics" 2007). Yellow fever's horrifying symptoms – including jaundice, bleeding from nose and mouth, stool stained dark with blood, and copious black vomit – together with a high case-fatality rate of up to 50 percent and higher created panic and fear incomparable to other diseases.[5] With mortality rates of 8-10 percent of the population during major epidemics a certain congruence of perceived and actual threat can be asserted. However, not every yellow fever epidemic was equally devastating, whereas the perceived threat remained. The last major outbreak of yellow fever in the United States occurred in New Orleans in 1905. Today we know that yellow fever is an acute viral disease transmitted to humans by the bite of the female *Aedes aegypti* mosquito; unspreadable through human contact and noncontagious. Until the arthropod vector in the disease transmission was confirmed in 1900 medical and literary writing on yellow fever equally relied on speculation and fictionalisation.

While tied to concerns of nation and race, yellow fever is neither an explicitly gendered nor a sexually transmitted disease, yet questions of gender become foregrounded in nineteenth-century US-American yellow fever narratives in the postbellum era. In this article on cultural and gendered representations of yellow fever I situate myself in the Reconstruction and immediate post-Reconstruction period that is characterised by a need for reconciliation and wish to restore national unity. Three narrative representations of catastrophic yellow fever epidemics in the 1870s portray Northern physicians and nurses who went south to offer relief: Wesley Bradshaw's popular sentimental novella *Angel Agnes or, The Heroine of the Yellow Fever Plague in Shreveport* (1873), and his tale *Mattie Stephenson: The Sweet Young Martyr of Memphis* (1873) both detail the 1873 epidemic. The 1878 yellow fever epidemic that overtook many southern states is represented in Elizabeth Stuart Phelps's realist short story "Zerviah

---

[4] See Humphreys 28, 61 on the role of the railroad. Margaret Humphreys also observes that a "new anxiety about regional disparities" between North and South could be detected in the writings of medical southerners (Humphreys 1999: 46).

[5] Very high mortality rates, however, may indicate that milder cases were not recognized as yellow fever. Survivors of yellow fever gain lifetime immunity (Patterson 1992: 855).

Hope" (1880).[6] It features the first of Phelps's actively and successfully practicing female doctors, who is partnered with a male nurse serving as title character. All three narratives follow doctors and nurses from Pennsylvania, Illinois, and New York as "volunteers to the fever district" ("ZH" 78). While *Angel Agnes* and *Mattie Stephenson* rely on a conventional male doctor/female nurse-setup, the sex of physician and nurse are reversed in Phelps's story, thus inverting the conventional pattern of male dominance and female subordination. In her study on the *Romance of Reunion* Nina Silber has observed that northerners in the reconstruction period "began to fashion an image of reunion that built upon sentimental values and developed an explicit vision of gender and power" (Silber 1993: 64).[7] Silber's finding regarding this "image of marital reunion" that is tied to the "language of romantic and sentimental reunion" offers itself to be tested in the three discussed texts, all of which testify to the fact that "the yellow fever epidemic prompted repeated expressions of the senti-mental view of reconciliation" between North and South (Silber 1993: 65). Following the rhetoric of sentimental fiction the nurses in all three stories die a martyr's death. Agnes Arnold, weak from exhaustive caregiving, accidentally falls and dies of a broken spine; Mattie Stephenson succumbs to the fever, and Zerviah Hope dies after aiding a freedman. I aim to show how *Angel Agnes*, *Mattie Stephenson*, and "Zerviah Hope" both represent and redefine existing patriarchal structures as well as present "human fellowship – food, physician, purse, medicine – that spoke from the heart of the North to the heart of the South" ("ZH" 81) as strategies to heal a nation still divided, yet united by the common threat of yellow fever. In all three narrative enactments of restoration the role of the medical woman as an "agent of healing between the North and South" (Wegener 2005: 2) becomes apparent.

Wesley Bradshaw, *Angel Agnes or, The Heroine of the Yellow Fever Plague in Shreveport* (1873)

The 1873 Shreveport epidemic, during which at least sixteen percent of the city's population died, still ranks as one of the worst yellow fever outbreaks in the United States.[8] It provides the setting for Wesley Bradshaw's sentimental

[6] In the following, for simplicity's sake, I will use *AA* for *Angel Agnes, or, The Heroine of the Yellow Fever Plague in Shreveport*, *MS* for *Mattie Stephenson: The Sweet Young Martyr of Memphis* and "ZH" for "Zerviah Hope".

[7] Although many northerners – in light of the political chaos and turbulence of Reconstruction – "remained skeptical about the likelihood of a genuine reconciliation," the "bonds of matri-mony" or the "image of inter-sectional romance" (real and imagined) seemed to offer one way to stabilize the bond of union (Silber 1993: 40).

[8] I am basing the mortality rate of 16.5 percent on Patterson (*Statistics of Population* 1872: Table 3: 155). Carrigan estimates the case fatality rate for the Shreveport epidemic at 26

novella *Angel Agnes or, The Heroine of the Yellow Fever Plague in Shreveport* that presents the story of Agnes Arnold, the daughter of a wealthy Philadelphia businessman, who reads about the devastating yellow fever epidemic and decides to go to Shreveport to offer her assistance.[9] Laura Laffrado reads the act of enlisting for (female) volunteer nursing as "a culturally sanctioned, asexual substitute for marriage" (Laffrado 2009: 97).[10] In fact, as a letter by her fiancé diminishes prospects of marriage, Agnes chooses the substitution of volunteer nursing. The disease functions as a testing ground for virtue, dedication, and goodness; in other words, morality is offered as a means to control yellow fever and reunite North and South under the epidemic's threat.

Bradshaw had made a name for himself with popular historical fictions of the Civil War. His brand of sensational literature (*Maud of the Mississippi*, 1863; *General Sherman's Indian Spy*, 1865; *The Angel of the Battlefield*, 1865) democratised the war in that it obliterated distinctions in rank, class, or between men and women by fantasising about female heroines with access to high-ranking generals. Bradshaw's literary debut *Pauline of the Potomac, Or General McClellan's Spy* (1862) features such a heroine whose father on his deathbed sends her off to the Civil War and thus symbolically dedicates his daughter's life to save the union.[11] In *Angel Agnes*, Bradshaw employs the successful formula of his Civil War narratives with an initial family disruption that leaves an orphaned female heroine destined to fight, in this case, yellow fever: "During the late war, fond fathers sent their sons to the battlefield, not that they wished to have them slaughtered, but willing that, for the sake of their cause, they should take the risk" (*AA* 7). It is by the same reasoning that Mrs. Arnold approves of her daughter's wish to go to the diseased city of Shreveport.[12]

The novella follows in the tradition of sentimental fiction with its focus on marginalised groups who lack power, such as mothers, children, and blacks, but

---

percent (Carrigan 1994: 106; 111). The devastating progression of the epidemic was covered (not always accurately and often with a sensationalist bent) in newspapers across the nation (for example, "The Yellow Fever: Subscriptions for the Aid of Shreveport" 1873; "Yellow Fever: Relief Contributions" 1873).

[9] This echoes the real presence and assistance of Northern volunteers, many of whom fell victim to the disease and were buried at Shreveport.

[10] Laffrado argues this in the context of Louisa May Alcott's *Hospital Sketches* (1863). On Louisa May Alcott's *Hospital Sketches* see also Young 69-108.

[11] See Fahs for a brief analysis of Bradshaw's Civil War writings (Fahs 2003: 241-45).

[12] The narrative addresses veteran readers directly, and even puts the female heroine's emotional strength above that of the veterans: "Reader, if you are a man, possibly you have been in the army, and then possibly you have been in a column, to which has been assigned the task of storming a well-served battery of pieces. If so, you may remember the feelings that were within your heart as you left the last friendly cover of woods […]. To Agnes Arnold going into Shreveport, the emotions must have been very much like yours in front of that battery. Yet there was no fluttering of her pulse" (*AA* 8).

who are symbolically empowered to serve as social models while true emancipation is withheld. Sentimental strategies furthermore include suffering (sick
or dying) children and infants;[13] as well as partings (Agnes leaving her mother)
and reunions (with her ex-fiancé, who then dies). The saintlike, 'angelic'
Agnes[14] is never infected by the fever. Like her namesake she is chaste and also
becomes a virgin martyr like Saint Agnes who is frequently depicted with a
lamb at her side (*agnus*). Agnes's work ethic and superior moral goodness is
offered as a means of controlling the disease. The narrative thus reverts to the
notion of character as the main idea of redemption and control.

When the district's physician pays a visit to the house under Agnes' care, he
is astonished in light of the recovery of the fever victims. He attributes the
recoveries to Agnes's "faithful and intelligent nursing" and admits to the
ineffectual modes of treatment of his own profession. These treatments fail "in
nearly eighty per cent. of every hundred" (*AA* 14). He also procures the view
that it was not the medicine offered by the doctors but "the methods and means
used by the natives" (*AA* 11), in this sense a southern treatment, which made the
difference in disease control. Prompted to elaborate on the efficiency of what the
doctor terms "grandmother remedies" (*AA* 14) Agnes rejects this denotation and
instead attributes her treatment to a Spanish gentleman from Havana. The text
thus presents a treatment supposedly originating in Cuba as most successful.[15]
With his promise that he shall not fail to try it, the physician remains the one to
authorise Agnes's yellow fever treatment and actions. In the narrative the
successful 'Spanish' therapy[16] is also conveyed to a black undertaker by Agnes.
Like Agnes the black man is fulfilling his part in fighting the epidemic, albeit on
a lower social scale. By dictating the steps of her treatment to the black man, she
assumes an authority that is not necessarily medical. The black man exclaims: "I
knowed it was magic – somethin' like that, and not medicine at all!" (*AA* 13).
The hierarchical social structure of African American undertaker, female nurse,
and male doctor is solidified in the text. In providing a potential "Spanish" colo-
niser's recipe for the treatment the narrative not only suggests a non-white
remedy for the disease, but also concedes superiority to the "Spanish" disease

[13] In reality children were less likely to be struck by yellow fever or suffered from milder
cases.
[14] Apart from the title, we learn from the sick Sister Theresa that Agnes's patients call her
'Angel Agnes'; Theresa prays that "God and the saints keep [her] an angel, as [she] is now, "
which also foreshadows Agnes's untimely death (*AA* 19).
[15] This is remarkable because the origin of the Shreveport yellow fever epidemic at the time
was traced to Cuba ("Yellow Fever at Shreveport" 1873). Yet the question of origin or the
concept of transportability – which was most probably known to Bradshaw – never comes up
in the novella that focuses on treatment and healing.
[16] The 'Spanish' therapy entails putting the patient's feet in hot and very strong mustard water
and then applying salt mackerel to the fever patient's feet.

treatment. It thus at least questions a WASP-ish identity construction that partly rests on a contrast to Catholic Spain.

Agnes dies of a broken spine and severe internal injuries she sustains from a fall due to fatigue after caring too extensively for one of her many patients, a 12-month infant She wishes to be buried next to her intended husband, George Harkness, who – despite their broken engagement – had followed her South and succumbed to the fever earlier in the story. In this way, the two Northerners are reunited in death in the South. What makes Agnes so powerful in the dying scene is her inevitable martyr's death: it is she who dictates what is to be done in a "most composed manner" (*AA* 27). This temporary reversal of power relations, a popular strategy of sentimental fiction, is also significant in terms of my argument of female emancipation, since Agnes is the one in control, not only in her dying hour,[17] but also when she is caring for her patients. At one point the male doctor endorses her superior quality as nurse and expresses his wish for her companionship and nursing care which he believes could only be possible if he were a woman: "Miss Arnold, you are worth all our nurses; and really I'm afraid all us physicians also put together. [...] I really begin to wish I was a woman myself so that if I should get the fever I might have you to nurse me well again. When Agnes tells him to "never mind about the being a woman" (*AA* 20) and promises to come should he fall sick with the fever, she points toward the possibility of a companionship across gender and professional divisions (physician-nurse). Since it was not uncommon anymore at the time that female nurses cared for male patients, the physician seems to refer to the professional divide. A future female emancipation might be hinted at, but is not finally redeemed as the strong Agnes has to die a martyr's death.

Wesley Bradshaw, *Mattie Stephenson: The Sweet Young Martyr of Memphis* (1873)

In 1873 yellow fever not only struck Shreveport on the Red River, but also travelled up the Mississippi as far as Memphis, Tennessee, a town with a population of about 50,000 at the time. Of the 15,000 persons who stayed in Memphis during the epidemic, approximately 7,000 fell ill, and 2,000 died (Carrigan 1994: 111); the destructive force was thus comparable to that of the Shreveport disaster. Wesley Bradshaw's tale *Mattie Stephenson: The Sweet Young Martyr of Memphis* (1873) recounts the plight of young Martha Stephenson. With the death of the protagonist announced on the first page the text presents an account of Mattie's brave deeds and untimely death during the Memphis yellow fever epidemic. Owing to her extreme youth, the sanctification of this child martyr already sets in during her heroic nursing practices and is

---

[17] "I have no fear of death, I am prepared for it"; "Come, Death, O come" (*AA* 27).

completed through her sickness and death. The narrative, however, is not only a fictionalised eulogy but a sequel to *Angel Agnes*.

In the first lines of *Mattie Stephenson,* Agnes serves as a contrastive foil to characterise Mattie. Agnes is "exceedingly lovely," "very rich," and "engaged to be married," while Mattie is "passably pretty," "poor," and "not yet entrammelled in love" (*MS* 19). Mattie's volunteering is motivated "from pure childlike love and inborn bravery of heart" (*MS* 19). Refusing to be paid for her services despite her lack of money to buy clothes marks her as altruist and selfless. While these qualities echo those of Agnes, the reference to duty (also in relation and reference to a male military one) is more prominent in the earlier story. Agnes formulates it as a "duty to go and do what little [she] can toward alleviating the distress of those stricken sufferers" (*AA* 7). Despite the slight differences, the sentimental pattern readers know from *Angel Agnes* is again applied: this time with a marginalised poor protagonist as social role model (and again with suffering sick children and dead infants complementing the sentimental cast). Furthermore, the formal development from unified tale in *Angel Agnes* to a more hybrid, yet also reductive, approach of a hagiography with documentary elements in *Mattie Stephenson* intensifies the focus on the sanctification already prevalent in *Angel Agnes*.

Upon her arrival from New England[18] Mattie experiences the literally contaminated atmosphere in the city of Memphis as "frightful, and almost suffocating" (*MS* 20).[19] Yet seemingly unaffected by the real and symbolic spreading of fear Mattie takes on her first engagement,[20] taking care of a sick woman in childbirth. The contrast of the two females – the "shy young girl" (*MS* 20) and the agonising woman in labour – could not be greater. Mattie's actions convey that she is neither afraid to face the woman's pain nor of the possibility to contract the disease.[21] Despite the obvious differences of the two women, their femaleness is stressed to establish a bond between innocent Mattie and the

[18] Newspapers spread news of the southern yellow fever disaster to the North and helped attract northern sympathy. Newspaper reports serve as trigger to volunteer for both Agnes Arnold and Mattie Stephenson. Mattie cuts short her visit in New England to continue on to Memphis (*MS* 19).

[19] "All over the place, wherever she turned her eyes, there arose clouds of smoke from burning tar and pitch, used as disinfectants. Men were engaged in scattering chloride of lime, phenol, carbolic acid &c., in all directions" (*MS* 20). These measures were undertaken in the belief that the distributed substances might work as disinfectants. Although the means of transmission for yellow fever was not known at the time, these measures might have worked to some extent to keep the mosquitoes, who served as vectors, away from their next victims.

[20] She reports to the office of the Howard Association, a (secular) association that was originally founded in New Orleans. See Carrigan 346-50 on the association that was organized during the 1837 New Orleans yellow fever epidemic and incorporated in 1842.

[21] She calms "the patient's terror and excitement" (*MS* 21) by laying her cheek against the woman's forehead "without the slightest fear" (*MS* 21).

sick woman who "began prematurely that sorrow which, for the sin of Eve, God adjudged all womankind should suffer" (*MS* 22); together they endure and accomplish the 'labour' of childbirth. When the woman delivers two babies, "one dead and the other dying [...] both as yellow as gold" (*MS* 22-23), Mattie – probably due to her extreme youth and inexperience – fails to understand that the mother too is dying and is not able to respond to her encouraging words: "[T]he maternal ear was deaf, the mother's soul was summoned, and she heeded not the kind words and soothing voice" (*MS* 23). Refusing to take a break after this dramatic experience of initiation Mattie "at once entered the sick room again" (*MS* 23). When her next patients quickly recover under her care, Mattie's maturation is completed when she is textually elevated from "heroic girl" to "bright, ministering angel from heaven," "child saint," and "real handmaiden of God" (*MS* 23, 24): "[F]rom house to house, and from case to case, did young Mattie Stephenson flit, [...] nursing the sick, and, in her humble way, administering consolation to the dying, whispering the last word of piety and Christian hope into the many ears and hearts as the dark river flowed at their feet and engulfed them" (*MS* 23).

Providence is cited as the cause and consolation for her early death. Mattie's last patient is a man whose physical size is put in clear contrast to her delicacy. His corporeality provides a foil for Mattie's immateriality. Already more spirit than body her transformation from heroic child to incorporeal saint is thus reinforced through focusing on the vulnerability of Mattie's body: "Mattie, through over-exertion with him, reduced her system so much, that she fell an easy victim to the contagion" (*MS* 24). Since direct transmission of yellow fever was already widely contested in the 1870s, it might safely be assumed that the word contagion takes on wider metaphorical meaning here, as a symbol for the inexplicability of the disease's spreading. Mattie is diagnosed with yellow fever and taken to the hospital on the day her last patient dies. The "Sisters of Charity and Mercy, Howards, priests and clergymen of all denominations" assemble at the infirmary, vying "with each other in their kindness to the stricken girl" (*MS* 24). Mattie's passing away is described as "placid" and "peaceful" as "they had never seen before in a yellow fever patient," and her last words – "God bless you all, I am going home" (*MS* 24) – ring familiar in reference to the deathbed scene of Little Eva in Harriet Beecher Stowe's *Uncle Tom's Cabin*. The deathbed scene, circulating in the culture at large and employed here by Bradshaw, presents a "version of the ethic of sacrifice [...] that the highest human calling is to give one's life for another," writes Jane Tompkins (Tompkins 1985: 128).

On the day of Mattie's death a box with clothing and items suitable for the sick arrives from Towanda, Illinois (*MS* 27); it does not only reveal Mattie's identity but exemplifies Northern generosity to the South. The equal generosity of the people of Memphis, the expensive casket and the enormous attendance of

Mattie's funeral, could be interpreted as desperate longing for redemption in light of the perceived power of the dead young Mattie Stephenson. The redemption of the unregenerate through the power of the dead or dying as a major trope of nineteenth-century popular literature has not only been pointed out by Tompkins (Tompkins 1985: 128). Mattie's sacrificial death provides a means for the southern city's society to realign its values and stabilise the group's coherence in light of the crisis of yellow fever.

In the eulogy, reprinted as part of the narrative, a certain Reverend Boggs reminds the congregation of what Mattie did for the sick mother in childbirth, the first yellow fever patient whom she attended. She was a "slender, shy girl" and did the work others were not able to do because "[t]error had broken the tenderest ties of life; men had nerved themselves to face the danger by strong drink; women, otherwise ready with their sympathy and aid in that hour of agony, whose bitterness only a woman can know, stood aloof, with pale faces and parted lips" (*MS* 28). With this example, the reverend likens Mattie to the Good Samaritan, who – as an outsider – acted while most others shied away out of terror and fear. The reader also learns that the dead mother and Mattie now rest not very far from each other, which textually reunites the mother, an immigrant to the southern United States from Scotland, and the girl from Illinois and also stresses both women's sacrifice.

The tale ends with a supposedly authentic reprinted resolution of the Howard Association to not only lament the death of Mattie Stephenson and sympathise with her family, but also to erect a monument in Mattie's honour.[22] It is not so much the image of marital reunion that realigns North and South in the visual memorial marker and the sentimental tale, but the sacrifice of this young northern girl who will forever stay in the South, physically buried there and spiritually immortalised.

Elizabeth Stuart Phelps, "Zerviah Hope" (1880)

Elizabeth Stuart Phelps's short story "Zerviah Hope" that was first published in *Scribner's Monthly* in 1880 features the devastating 1878 yellow fever epidemic as well as Phelps's first actively practicing woman doctor with the telling name of Dr. Marian Dare. It focuses on the self-sacrifice of the title character, a male nurse with the gender-ambiguous name of Zerviah Hope (Morris 1993: 141; Wegener 2005: 12).[23] The story is set in the small South Carolina town of

---

[22] The monument was to be erected "in honor of her memory, and in justice to ourselves, and as an example to her race, [...] to mark the spot where she sleeps, and that her epitaph shall tell this sublime and beautiful story of her life" (*MS* 29).

[23] Zerviah was King David's older sister. While she is hardly described in 2 Samuel 17:25, her three sons are mentioned as David's soldiers; they are referred to with the matronymic

Calhoun ("ZH" 78) during this particularly devastating yellow fever epidemic. It begins with a steamship departing from its course to permit a group of "[p]hysicians from New York" to disembark as "[v]olunteers to the fever district" ("ZH" 78). A "short passenger" who has made no acquaintances on board the ship and is only later identified as the story's title character inquires about the lady whom he presumes to be a nurse. He learns that "[s]he's a she-doctor. […] There ain't a nurse aboard." When Zerviah Hope further stipulates that many nurses are probably to be found in Calhoun, it is the woman doctor who is the first of the three doctors to speak in the story. Exhibiting "a quick and clear-cut, but not ungentle voice" and speaking "in a business-like tone" she informs him that there are no nurses and that the place is perishing; she thus indirectly invites Zerviah to join them ("ZH" 78).

The medical field found itself in a major period of transition in the 1870s: not only did the germ theory of transmission (also with respect to yellow fever) slowly take hold, but the increasing number of women doctors also influenced the outlook of the profession. In 1849, Elizabeth Blackwell had become the first woman to receive a medical diploma in the United States; others, like Dr. Marie Zakrezweska had followed. As the Civil War ended, several hundred women had begun practicing medicine (Wegener 2005: 1), and Phelps accompanied their rise in several of her writings and "culturally, socially, and professionally" helped legitimate the "figure of the American medical woman" (Wegener 2005: 2). Two of Phelps's short stories: "Our Little Women" (1872) and "Hannah Colby's Chance" (1873) show the transformation of two young women into professional physicians (see Masteller 1984: 138). Her novel *Doctor Zay* (1882) represents Phelps's best-known treatment of the character of a woman doctor.[24] Like "Zerviah Hope" the novel is an example of role reversal drawing attention to the gendered patterns and power struggles in doctor-patient relations. Yet Phelps's interest in the topic was already apparent in the 1860s and 1870s when she engaged the topic in several essays. In an 1867 essay in *Harper's New Monthly Magazine* Phelps's commented on the still difficult but increasingly trodden path of women doctors, by rhetorically asking "What Shall They Do?": "Be a doctor? and be sure that you could be few things more womanly or more noble. The brave pioneers? God bless them for it!? have broken the way for you. It is an easier way now than the path of the idle or the ill-paid" (Phelps 1867: 523). Phelps in her essays argued against the sceptics and in favour of more

connotation of "Zerviah's sons." David relies on his sister's sons' protection and advice, yet also recognizes them to be motivated by evil. David's false trust in them leads him to conspire with one of them in evil doing.

[24] Two novels that also have a woman doctor as central character were issued in short sequence of Phelps's short story and her novel *Doctor Zay* (1882), William Dean Howells's *Dr. Breen's Practice* (1881) and Sarah Orne Jewett's *A Country Doctor* (1884).

women to receive a medical degree based on the economic success of already practicing medical women ("pecuniary value") and on their skill and professionalism (Phelps 1871: 1; Phelps 1873: 28–29).[25]

In her journalistic prose, Phelps did not only foster the education of women doctors, but also argued for their coeducation which would provide for the training of men and women "under identical disciplinary conditions" (Phelps 1874: 1), much in the vein that separate is indeed not equal.[26] Phelps convictions are equally reflected in her imaginative writings. In "Zerviah Hope" the two male doctors accompanying Dr. Dare stand for opposing views regarding female physicians. One of them, Dr. Frank, has attended a course of lectures with the female doctor and "spoke to her with an air of *camaraderie*" ("ZH" 78). Despite his sceptical views regarding the medical education of women the proven excellence of this particular woman doctor influences his conviction: he respects Dr. Dare as someone who has "outranked him at graduation" ("ZH" 78) and also recognises her as a "lady" whose family he knows. Thus, Dr. Dare's professional distinction as well as her status as a woman of higher societal rank is confirmed. The other physician, Dr. Remane, more clearly represents the prevalent view of the time: he "never consulted with doctresses" ("ZH" 79). Despite the differences a male/female fellowship between the three physicians is confirmed early in the story and in light of the unifying effect of the impending disaster: they lean toward each other wishing each other well before separating and individually confronting the crisis and the patients it brings forward ("ZH" 79). The signs of human fellowship are equally represented in the marriage plot-induced relationship between North and South, or more precisely in northern dispatches of "food, physician, purse, medicine – that spoke from the heart of the North to the heart of the South, and upheld her in those well-remembered days" ("ZH" 81).

It is the yellow fever crisis that seems, as one critic puts it, to submerge "[a]ll sex-based hierarchies of the day" (Wegener 2005: 11). Phelps moves the gender question to the foreground with her choice of characters and the characterisation of her main figures, the male and female physicians who are entering "the afflicted region of Calhoun," that seems almost completely shut off and shunned from the rest of the world:

> The quarantine laws tightened. Vessels fled by the harbor mouth under full sail, and melted like helpless compassion upon the fiery horizon. Trains upon the Shore Line

[25] Phelps furthermore identified the need for medical women assisting women patients who were often reluctant to "disclose symptoms to male practitioners" and thus welcomed the possibility to consult same-sex doctors (Morantz-Sanchez 1985: 52).
[26] In Phelps's articles the Boston University School of Medicine serves as the model for her argument; her close acquaintance Dr. Mary Briggs Harris attended the school and enabled Phelps to personally observe the class and its training.

shot through and thundered past the station; they crowded on steam; the fireman and his stoker averted their faces as they whirled by. The world turned her back upon Calhoun, and the dying town was shut in with her dead.

("ZH" 80)

When a "glum passenger" – later identified as Zerviah Hope – asks to be landed as well, no one notices him at first, until Dr. Dare invites him into the space of their boat: "There's room for you" ("ZH" 79). Tellingly, the woman doctor provides another example of her attentiveness. She seems to intuitively grasp the effect isolation and constant fear of infection has on the people when observing their "negro boatman" Scip: "There is a kind of terror for which we find that animals, as well as men, instinctively refrain from seeking expression. [...] Dr. Dare wondered if all the people in Calhoun would have that look" ("ZH" 78).

All three physicians master the trek from the landing dock to the afflicted city alone, a fact that seems most important to the woman doctor. When Dr. Frank asks Dr. Dare whether he can serve her in any way, she thanks him but confirms her self-reliance. For Dr. Marian Dare this incident represents

the first moment when the consciousness of her sex had made itself oppressive to her since she ventured upon this undertaking. She would have minded presenting herself to the Relief Committee of Calhoun, accompanied by gentlemen upon whom she had no claim. She walked on alone, in her gray dress and white straw hat, with her luggage in her own sufficient hand.

("ZH" 79)

When the "reticent passenger" approaches her to inquire about "the best way [...] to offer [him]self as a fever nurse in this place," she commends him for not going to Savannah. And after assessing for herself that "[p]lainly, this poor fellow was not a gentleman," she even allows the volunteer nurse what she could not allow her fellow in profession before, to carry her heavy bag ("ZH" 79). After being told that she will need him as a nurse the next morning, he introduces himself as Zerviah Hope, and Dr. Dare takes down his name in her note-book ("ZH" 79). The exchange confirms the woman doctor's independence from her male peers but also shows her acceptance of Zerviah as her inferior aide. It thus promotes a reversal of conventional gender roles, the subordination of the male nurse under the female doctor.

The first part of the story entitled "Prelude" ends with a direct address to the reader that assures the truthfulness and authenticity of the tale ("ZH" 80).[27] The first-person intervention also clarifies that readers are not to expect a romantic

[27] "I have nothing further to say about the story before I tell it, except that it is true" ("ZH" 80).

tale or a marriage plot, as the "story does not deal with love or ladies" nor includes "tender passages between the fever-physicians." The passage also establishes the figure of the woman doctor as a brave human being and as a scientist, but it mainly reveals her function as key to an understanding of the short stories' male title character, namely "that certain missing fragments in the history of the person known as Zerviah Hope we owe to her. She hovers over the tale with a distant and beautiful influence, pervading as womanly compassion and alert as a woman's eye" ("ZH" 80). Vision on a literal (observing Zerviah as well as her patients empathetically) and a metaphorical level (seeing Zerviah's potential as nurse) plays an important role in the story. In this sense, the woman doctor's vision is not reduced to the medical gaze (theorised by Foucault in a French cultural context), but she 'sees' both body and identity (in Zerviah's case) (Foucault 1973).[28]

In the course of the story Zerviah takes care of the worst yellow fever cases, and those most discarded by society that might qualify as Other: "[h]e sought the neglected, and the negroes. He braved the unclean, and the unburied" ("ZH" 81), and Dr. Dare watches him with a slight touch of emotionality. Asked by Dr. Frank about her "fancy to the fellow," she insists on her professionalism and curtly replies that she's "been in practice too long to take sudden fancies. There is no profession like ours, Doctor, for putting the sympathies under double picket guard" ("ZH" 80). If there is a nod to the marriage plot it is certainly muted in the story. For Zerviah, Dr. Dare is the only uninfected person he speaks to: "He was always pliable to the influence of a woman's voice or to womanly manner. He had, in the presence of women, the quick responsiveness and sudden change of color and sensitiveness of intonation which bespeak the man whose highest graces and lowest faults are likely to be owing to feminine power" ("ZH" 81). His possession or at least responsiveness to female gender characteristics is what secures Zerviah's "remarkable success as a nurse. He was found to be infinitely tender, and of fine, brave patience" ("ZH" 81). Yet, it is only the combination of male and female traits that characterise Zerviah as the ideal nurse. Similar to a reference in *Angel Agnes* soldierly qualities are accredited to the volunteer nurse, as well as almost super-human or angelic qualities are conferred upon him, complete with halo and an incorporeal, but radiant presence:

> He went to his task as the soldier goes to the front under raking fire, with gleaming eyes and iron muscles. The fever of the fight was on him. He seemed to wrestle with disease for his patients, and to trample death beneath his feet. He glowed over his cures with a positive physical dilation, and writhed over his dead as if he had killed them. He

[28] Lawrence Rothfield has theorized the "medical gaze" in a British context for the nineteenth century (Rothfield 1992).

seemed built of endurance more than mortal. It was not known when he slept, scarcely
if he ate. His weariness sat upon him like a halo. He grew thin, refined, radiant. In
short, he presented an example of that rare spectacle which never fails to command
spectators – a common man possessed by an uncommon enthusiasm.

("ZH" 81)

Again at this point in the narration, the narrator confirms credibility of the
story by pointing to the people who knew Zerviah Hope, even without being
personally known by him: "I have been told that, to this day, many people
personally unknown to him […] were unable to speak it because of choking
voices. I have often wished that he knew this" ("ZH" 81). Communication as
another means of transmitting information seems to break down. While on a
literal level the inability to speak refers to people's reverence, the possibility to
communicate or transmit the disease is referenced as well. It is curtailed by an
absence of communication. Furthermore, the foreboding character of these lines
of knowing or rather not knowing, of not being able to profess his good
reputation, is confirmed when Zerviah not much later finds out that his secret
has leaked. As it turns out, Zerviah has taken the job as nurse to atone for a
murder he has committed and was convicted for. It is Dr. Dare who confronts
him about what she refers to as "a hateful rumor" ("ZH" 83).

Due to the reversal of conventional gender roles as a result of the inverted
pattern of male dominance, communication in this situation again fails. Zerviah,
who has committed the murder out of love for a woman, professionally respects
Dr. Dare and although he craves for her compassion he does not want to take
advantage of what he perceives a female quality and cannot utter his remorse:

He wanted to go on speaking to this woman [Dr. Dare], not to defend or excuse
himself, not to say anything weak or wrong, only to make her understand that he did
not want to excuse himself; in some way, just because she *was* a woman, to make her
feel that he was man enough to bear the burden of his deed. He wanted to cry out to
her, "You are a woman! Oh, be gentle, and understand how sorry a man can be for a
deadly sin!" but his lips were parched. He moved them dryly; he could not talk.

("ZH" 83)

Dr. Dare, in return, expresses her faith in him and sends him back to his
patients. The muted or at least one-sided way of communication between the
two might also again point toward a means to control the spread (or communication) of the disease. Frederick Wegener has pointed out that "Dr. Dare's
reaffirmation of his human worth deepens the kinship [Zerviah] senses between
them" (Wegener 2005: 12). The exchange equally affects her and her understanding of and reliance on their relationship, yet she instinctively hides the
physical and physiological female side of herself: "She drew her veil; there was

unprofessional moisture on her long, feminine lashes" ("ZH" 84). The people of Calhoun take somewhat longer than Dr. Dare to re-align the image they had pieced together in their heads and are only able to recognise Zerviah again for what he did, when they find out that he has put all of his nurse's wages into the relief-contribution boxes of the local charities. Relief committee members are subsequently searching for him and require Dr. Dare's help in locating him; yet, they learn that she has contracted the fever and Dr. Frank is taking her cases.

While Dr. Dare is sick with the fever, Zerviah, who does not know about her plight, is called to Scip's hut. The spatial distance between female doctor and male nurse is amplified by the mode of narration. Zerviah finds himself physically outside of town, unreachable and alone in "a hard place for a man to die" ("ZH" 85), and this is reflected in the self-reflexive figural narrative style, as well as the reference to each single day that conveys time's slow passing among the sick: "It was Monday, but no one came. It was Tuesday, but the nurse and the plague still battled alone together over the negro. Zerviah's stock of remedies was as ample as his skill. He had thought he should save Scip. He worked without sleep, and the food was not clean. He lavished himself like a lover over this black boatman; he leaned like a mother over this man who had betrayed him" ("ZH" 86). The intimate connection and absolute dedication conveyed in the description of the patient-nurse relationship stands out as we, for example, never witness anything similar between any of the three doctors and their patients.[29] At one point Dr. Dare is seen by Zerviah mixing medicines while her patients are waiting in line, but there is no direct interaction between them.

Zerviah fervently battles for the black man's life ("ZH" 85) but loses him only to realise that he has "*got it*" ("ZH" 86). The negro boatman and the male nurse remain the only yellow fever victims of the story whose suffering and death the reader witnesses, and although the narrow-minded Dr. Remane also dies, his passing is not further elaborated on. So while, in fact, as Phelps writes "black and white, poor and rich, clean and foul, saint and sinner" ("ZH" 80) died alongside each other, the focus of the story remains on the suffering outsiders or Others. The emphasis of the passage of disease realisation is on Zerviah and the absence of Dr. Dare:

> His professional experience gave him an excruciating foresight of his symptoms, and their result presented itself to him with horrible distinctness. [...] His trained imagination had little mercy on him. He weighed his chances, and watched his fate with the sad exactness of knowledge. [...] "They would have come if they had known. They would not have let me *die* alone. I don't think *she* would have done that. I wonder where she is?"
>
> ("ZH" 87)

---

[29] See Furneaux for a theoretization of male nursing, gentleness and homosocial bonding in nineteenth-century Britain (Furneaux 2009).

The fact that Dr. Dare does not know where Zerviah is in the week they are both ill and of Zerviah knowing that she would have saved him had she only known only strengthens the bond between them.

Zerviah is trapped inside the hut and inside his diseased body, his vision is restricted: "Through the wooden shutter, Zerviah could see the lights, and the lonely palmetto, and the grave" ("ZH" 87). His dying wish is for "a great, white, holy frost [...] for these poor devils that have borne so much!" ("ZH" 87). Yet, before Zerviah's death "a little party from the city rode up, [...] Dr. Frank was with them, and the lady, Marian Dare." Her first name is given, and—in an equally intimate manner—her name is not connected to her being a doctor but with a female noble character (Maid Marian). She seems fragile, "pale, and still weak," after recovering from the fever ("ZH" 88). The narrative suggests that Zerviah sees her before his eyes close: "She knelt beside the bed, and put her hand upon his eyes. [...]. Let us hope that they knew her before they closed" ("ZH" 88). The importance of vision and of seeing is stressed again here, but the factuality of the recognition is only revealed later. In the postscript to the story we learn that "he rested, after her hand had fallen on his eyes" ("ZH" 88). Zerviah is, as Wegener suggests thus "redemptively linked to her once again at the end." Their association "as fellow healers from the North" has a "restorative function" (Wegener 2005: 13). Wegener argues that the story manifests what historian Paul H. Buck in the 1930s has called the "'bond of sympathy underlying the hostility of the divided sections'" and thus aligns itself "with the work of those who 'wrote of the sections at last united and truly reconciled by the generosity of deed and attitude of the North'" (Wegener 2005: 13).

It is in fact the released convict, the 'Other', whose generosity the people of Calhoun most openly appreciate and remember in the end. He has killed a man because he believed this act to save the woman he loved. In turn, he has lost everything and suffers for what he did wishing to repent for his sins by becoming a nurse. As a trope this also alludes to the plight and story of the South and Southerners who have fought and lost for the cause of the Confederacy. So, the immediate connection and bond between the suffering people of Calhoun and their Northern beneficiaries is established through the male nurse, the released convict, the 'Other' in many respects. In a second step it is extended through Zerviah's personal bond to Dr. Dare. Her (female) emotionality, mostly professionally retained or actively hidden in the course of the story, comes to the fore at the moment of his confession and at the crucial instance of his death, to (re)establish the special bond (between physician and nurse, man and woman, North and South). After witnessing Zerviah's death "[s]he came out, and tried to tell about it, but broke down, and sobbed before them all" ("ZH" 88). Explicitly referred to as "a martyr's death," ("ZH" 88) the sanctification of Zerviah even conjures up a possible connection to Abraham

Lincoln who wanted to reconcile North and South. The redemptive act is complete as the frost puts an end to the disease and the story.

> In the morning, when they all awoke, these of the sorrowing city here, and those of the happy city yonder; when they took up life again with its returning sunrise, – the sick and the well, the free and the fettered, the living and the dead, – the frost lay, cool, white, blessed, on his grave.
>
> ("ZH" 88)

Conclusion

According to Nina Silber "the language of romantic and sentimental reunion reached a crescendo" in the aftermath of the "profound misery and devastation of the 1878 yellow-fever outbreak" (Silber 1993: 65). This language is visible in Bradshaw's writing, yet also, in a more refined way, in Phelps's story.

With *Angel Agnes* Bradshaw constructs a popular story which offers certain redeeming venues based on sentimental strategies of victimisation and power reversal and with a female heroine who takes control of her life when her engagement is severed by her fiancé in the North. She helps the afflicted in the South where she dies a martyr's death to redeem the latter. In terms of gender dynamics in the story, the male doctor remains the authority by offering approval of Agnes's treatment, yet she also partially assumes that authority by lecturing inferiors on the Spanish therapy. The novella thus at least temporarily reverses ingrained gender norms of the time as well as a prerogative of medical interpretation and treatment of diseases: by making the effective cure non-white – but Spanish colonialist – in origin and administered by a woman. *Angel Agnes* thus also puts forth a vision of female emancipation and a medical profession that acknowledges the role of women (nurses in this case).

Mattie Stephenson repeats the pattern of *Angel Agnes* and similarly remains a sentimental tale of virtue, dedication and selflessness. Mattie's sacrificial deeds as well as her final sacrifice are offered as remedy and means of redemption for the larger disease. The visual marker put up in her memory as well as Bradshaw's fictionalisation of her story imaginatively serves to reunite North and South. Nina Silber's image of 'marital reunion' is translated into one of spiritual adoption and veneration of this girl from the North by citizens of the South.

The possibility of a companionship across gender and social divisions that is only hinted at in *Angel Agnes* is carried through in Phelps's realist short story. Although the relationship between Zerviah Hope and Dr. Marian Dare is never presented as one carried out on equal terms, its representation serves to establish the special bond between physician and nurse, man and woman, North and South. During the yellow fever crisis, North and South are doubly reunited by the help and assistance received from the North provided by the characters of Zerviah Hope and, in extension, Dr. Marian Dare, yet also by the bond of kinship established between the two unequal partners in the course of the narrative. The conventional marriage plot is muted by an equally sentimental plot of healing. In this sense, the fictionalisation of the catastrophic experience of yellow fever in all three texts serves to destabilise conventional patterns of dominance and thus – at least from a Northern literary perspective – enables national healing.

List of Works Cited

Arner, Katherine. "Making Yellow Fever American: The Early American Republic, the British Empire and the Geopolitics of Disease in the Atlantic World." *Atlantic Studies* 7.4 (2010): 447-71.

Bradshaw, Wesley. *Angel Agnes, or, The Heroine of the Yellow Fever Plague in Shreveport.* Philadelphia, PA: Old Franklin Publishing House, 1873.

---. *Mattie Stephenson: The Sweet Young Martyr of Memphis.* Philadelphia: Old Franklin Publishing House, 1873.

---. *The Volunteer Nurse! The Lovely Young Martyrs of Memphis, Grenada, New Orleans, Shreveport! The Yellow Fever Plague in the South! Being the Romantic, Heart-Touching History of Two Lovely Young Ladies.* Philadelphia: Old Franklin Publishing House, 1878.

Caldwell, Charles. *A Reply to Dr. Haygarth's Letter to Dr. Percival, on Infectious Fevers [...].* Philadelphia: Thomas and William Bradford, 1802. Early American Imprints. 2nd Ser. No. 1981.

Carrigan, Jo Ann. *The Saffron Scourge: A History of Yellow Fever in Louisiana, 1796-1905.* Lafayette: Center for Louisiana Studies, University of Southwestern Louisiana, 1994.

Desowitz, Robert S. *Who Gave Pinta to Santa Maria? Torrid Diseases in a Temperate World.* Harcourt Brace, 1997.

Fahs, Alice. *The Imagined Civil War: Popular Literature of the North and South, 1861-1865.* Chapel Hill: U of North Carolina P, 2003.

Foucault, Michel. *The Birth of the Clinic: An Archaeology of Medical Perception.* New York: Pantheon Books, 1973.

Furneaux, Holly. *Queer Dickens : Erotics, Families, Masculinities.* Oxford: Oxford UP, 2009.

Humphreys, Margaret. *Yellow Fever and the South.* Baltimore, MD: Johns Hopkins UP, 1999.

Koch, Tom. *Disease Maps: Epidemics on the Ground.* Chicago: U of Chicago P, 2011.

Krieg, Joann P. *Epidemics in the Modern World.* New York: Twayne Publishers, 1992.

Laffrado, Laura. *Uncommon Women: Gender and Representation in Nineteenth-Century U.S. Women's Writing.* Columbus: Ohio State UP, 2009.

"Major U.S. Epidemics." *Information Please Database, Pearson Education.* 2007. Web. 29 Sept. 2011.

Masteller, Jean Carwile. "The Women Doctors of Howells, Phelps, and Jewett: The Conflict of Marriage and Career." *Critical Essays on Sarah Orne Jewett.* Ed. Gwen L. Nagel. Boston: Hall, 1984. 135-47.

Morantz-Sanchez, Regina. *Sympathy and Science: Women Physicians in American Medicine.* New York: Oxford UP, 1985.

Morris, Timothy. "Professional Ethics and Professional Erotics in Elizabeth Stuart Phelps' *Doctor Zay*." *Studies in American Fiction* 21.2 (1993): 141-52.

Patterson, K. David. "Yellow Fever Epidemics and Mortality in the United States, 1693-1905." *Social Science & Medicine* 34.8 (1992): 855-65.

Phelps, Elizabeth Stuart. "Shall We Have a New England College?" *New England Medical Gazette* 8 (1873): 27–30.

---. "The Experiment Tried." *Independent* 5 Mar. 1874: 1-2.

---. "What Shall They Do?" *Harper's New Monthly Magazine* Sept. 1867: 519-23.

---. "What They Are Doing." *Independent* 17 Aug. 1871: 1.

---. "Zerviah Hope." *Scribner's Monthly* Nov. 1880: 78-88.

Rothfield, Lawrence. *Vital Signs: Medical Realism in Nineteenth-Century Fiction*. Princeton, NJ: Princeton UP, 1992.

Rush, Benjamin. "Facts Intended to Prove the Yellow Fever Not Be Contagious, and Instances of Its Supposed Contagion Explained Upon Other Principles." *Medical Repository* 6.2 (1803): 155-71.

Silber, Nina. *The Romance of Reunion: Northerners and the South, 1865-1900*. Chapel Hill: U of North Carolina P, 1993.

Statistics of Population, Tables I-VIII Inclusive. Washington: Govt. Print. Off., 1872.

Swagerty, William R., and Henry F. Dobyns. *Their Number Become Thinned: Native American Population Dynamics in Eastern North America*. 1st ed. Knoxville, TN: University of Tennessee P and Newberry Library Center for the History of the American Indian, 1983.

"The Yellow Fever: No Cases in Little Rock—Subscriptions for the Aid of Shreveport and Memphis—The Quarantine on the Railroads." *Daily Arkansas Gazette* 7 Oct. 1873: col. D.

Tompkins, Jane P. *Sensational Designs: The Cultural Work of American Fiction, 1790-1860*. New York: Oxford UP, 1985.

Wegener, Frederick. "'Few Things More Womanly or More Noble': Elizabeth Stuart Phelps and the Advent of the Woman Doctor in America." *Legacy* 22.1 (2005): 1-17.

"Yellow Fever at Shreveport." *Daily Evening Bulletin* 30 Sept. 1873: col. D.

"Yellow Fever: The Plague at Memphis and Shreveport—Relief Contributions." *Milwaukee Daily Sentinel* 25 Oct. 1873: col. D.

Young, Elizabeth. *Disarming the Nation: Women's Writing and the American Civil War*. Chicago: U of Chicago P, 1999.

Martin Decker

"You half-baked Lazarus": Masculinity and the Maimed Body in Sean O'Casey's *The Silver Tassie*

Apart from its experimental, late-expressionist second act, the aspect most frequently addressed regarding Sean O'Casey's 1928 war play *The Silver Tassie* is the troublesome history of the play's rejection by the Abbey Theatre and the accompanying public controversy between O'Casey and William Butler Yeats, then one of the directors of the theatre. Yeats, who generally discounted the First World War as a literary subject because, in his eyes, its vastness denied the possibility of real tragic and heroic agency and reduced its countless participants to a state of helplessness (McDonald 2002: 116 f.),[1] accused O'Casey of having produced a fundamentally flawed dramatic work. "The mere greatness of the world war has thwarted you," writes Yeats in a letter to O'Casey in April 1928, claiming that O'Casey was in fact "not interested in the great war; you never stood on the battlefields or walked its hospitals, and so write out of your opinions" (Yeats 1954: 741). O'Casey, whose Dublin trilogy had previously ensured the Abbey Theatre's financial as well as artistic survival, retaliated briskly:[2]

> I am afraid your statement [...] is not only an ignorant one, but it is a silly statement too. [...] Do you really mean that no one should or could write or speak about a war because one has not stood on the battlefields? [...]
> But I have walked some of the hospital wards. I have talked and walked and smoked and sung with the blue-suited wounded men fresh from the front. I've been with the armless, the legless, the blind, the gassed and the shell-shocked; one with a head bored by shrapnel who had to tack east and tack west when [*sic*] before he could reach the point he wished to get to; with one whose head rocked like a frantic moving pendulum. Did you know 'Pantosser' and did you ever speak to him? Or watch his funny, terrible antics, or listen to the gurgle of his foolish thoughts? [...] And does war consist only of hospital wards and battlefields?

(O'Casey 1975: 271-2)

[1] Already in 1915, Yeats proclaimed his refusal to write about the Great War in "On Being Asked for a War Poem": "I think it better that in times like these / A poet keep his mouth shut [...]" (Yeats 2008: 9, ll. 1-2).
[2] The controversy resulted in *The Silver Tassie* being first performed not in Dublin but in London in October 1929. The first performance of the play at the Abbey Theatre took place in August 1935 and caused a public outcry, mostly due to its depiction of Dublin women as morally depraved and materialistic. See Welch 1999: 120.

In his reply, O'Casey refutes Yeats's misguided criticism and stresses his awareness of the horrific realities of the Great War. Furthermore, he points to his
intimate knowledge of and relation to those who have "stood on the battlefield"
and left it permanently impaired, Irish soldiers returning from the front having
lost limbs, blinded, traumatised both physically and mentally. It is, I will argue
in this essay, this theme of physical disability and ability, of a certain socio-
economy of bodies, the dynamics and hierarchies of bodily strength and fitness,
which also pervades *The Silver Tassie*. As I will attempt to show, the play demonstrates that war in fact consists of more than "hospital wards and
battlefields" – in his work, O'Casey embeds the great European conflict in a
Dublin civilian working-class milieu dominated by the idolisation of hyper-
masculinity and a culture of violence, drastically exposing the forces of social
and sexual marginalisation that befall those who have become disabled, or,
rather, who have been practically emasculated by injuries suffered on Europe's
battlefields.

Disability, Gender and Culture

My reading of O'Casey's play is based on theoretical concepts of disability and
gender, two fields linked by their shared focus on the body. Disability studies
today understand 'disability' in an expanded sense (Tervooren 2003: 47), seeing
it as a concept closely related to disease as well as ageing – phenomena that
affect and transform bodies, or, rather, that change the way bodies are perceived,
categorised and charged with meaning. Disability studies, like gender studies,
view the body as a social fact, inextricably connected to culture, perception,
language, knowledge and social interaction (Dederich 2007: 58). Consequently,
disability is understood as historically and culturally determined and it is defined
against essentialist medical discourses which identify disability as the outcome
of a neutral, ahistorical and asocial bodily defect in need of repair. It is only, the
philosopher and physician Georges Canguilhem argues, this culture of
diagnostics and evaluation that attributes abnormality to the disabled body –
Canguilhem sees disability, disease and ageing as part of a normative
physiology and not as abnormal pathological conditions and he generally dis-
trusts the legitimacy of medical and biological claims of norms and normality
(Canguilhem 1974: 155 f.), thereby formulating a fundamental attitude of disability studies.

However, though closely related, disability and disease fundamentally differ
concerning the decisive factor of the permanence of impairment. While the pains
and limitations inflicted upon the body by disease frequently can be overcome,
disability excludes the possibility of healing; it is, like 'sex' and 'race', a
permanent biological condition the affected individual cannot escape. As a

consequence, a lasting 'contamination' of the disabled person's identity can be observed. Disability seems to enter and overshadow every aspect of personality, causing an equation of physical impediment and the social persona (Mitchell and Snyder 1997: 1-3) – the disabled person is exclusively perceived and interacted with in regards of his or her disability. Missing limbs, crutches, wheelchairs, eye-patches or also involuntary utterances and movements of the body become lasting signifiers of a profound abnormality and otherness. In 'ableist' societies, where the intact body defines the "baseline of humanness" (Siebers 2009: 159), the disabled person is only granted, unlike those affected by disease, a permanently "diminished state of being human" (Campbell 2001: 44). Tobin Siebers even suggests that the feelings of sympathy and grief which are directed at the disabled[3] "expose the idea that they are dead – even though they may insist that they are not dead yet" (Siebers 2009: 161).

Disability studies not only examine social responses to bodily difference but also investigate how disability and ability are constructed in literary and other cultural discourses, how texts present and make use of disability and promote certain perspectives and ideas about it. The literary presentation of disability evidently has been subject to change, however, until the twentieth century, disability was presented predominantly in a rather negative light (Davis 2001: 532). It seems that literature reflected common attitudes that connected the disabled condition with individual guilt or impurity, disability bringing about a state of imbalance and disorder that needs to be rectified.

The function of disabled characters in literature, according to David Mitchell and Sharon Snyder, is twofold: on the one hand, disability serves as a means of characterisation and, on the other hand, as a metaphorical device (Mitchell and Snyder 2006: 205) – in both cases, the experience of the impairment itself is not in the focus of representation but its symbolic and metaphorical value, disability becoming an artistic tool, a "narrative prosthesis" (Mitchell and Snyder 2006: 206) for the author, and a vehicle for the emotions of the able-bodied reader. Accordingly, disability is frequently used to express inner turmoil, moral corruption and fear and disabled characters are employed to personify existential tragedies, social conflict, human guilt and divine punishment as well as the follies of politics, evoking predictable emotional responses of readers, ranging from disgust to compassion. Furthermore, Mitchell and Snyder stress the disruptive potential of disabled bodies in texts. Disabled bodies are featured as "dynamic entities that resist or refuse the cultural scripts assigned to them" (Mitchell and Snyder 2006: 206), exposing and challenging the standards of

---

[3] Of course we have to keep in mind that disability has not always been met with compassionate and sympathetic reactions but also with sensationalism, rejection, repulsion or even the demand for the elimination of the disabled as in nineteenth- and twentieth-century discourses of social Darwinism, eugenics and racial hygiene.

'normality' assumed by the able-bodied majority. In this way, disability also becomes a signifier of unpredictability in a culture of control and conformity which lends the disabled character an uneasy or even uncanny appearance. In this manner, disability in literature can serve to elucidate the make-up of cultures and societies and the mechanisms of collective experience, acquiring an epistemological function (Dederich 2007: 110).

The connection of aspects of disability and aspects of gender becomes obvious when we set the already mentioned notion of disabled people as inhabiting a "diminished state of being human" in relation to the traditional notion of women as diminished or even 'deformed' men. From this perspective, both the disabled and the female body are placed in the same position of inferiority within a "hierarchy of value that attributes completeness to some bodies and deficiency to others" (Rosemarie Garland-Thomson quoted in Samuels 2011: 55). This relationship between bodies, values and norms is also a central concern in the theory of Judith Butler, most prominently in *Bodies that Matter*, where she, similar to the able-bodied/disabled hierarchy assumed by Garland-Thomson, identifies "a domain of abjected bodies, a field of deformation" that "fortifies [...] regulatory norms", asking which bodies "matter", which bodies appear to be worth protecting, saving and grieving (Butler 1993: 16).[4]

Another intersection of disability and gender, also pointing at another central aspect in Butler's theory, the performativity of gender, can be found in Raewyn Connell's model of hegemonic masculinity, which postulates a dynamic hierarchy of various different masculinities. According to Connell, masculinity "is almost always thought to proceed from men's bodies" (Connell 1995: 45) and she argues that the "constitution of masculinity through bodily performance means that gender is vulnerable when the performance cannot be sustained – for instance as a result of physical disability" (Connell 1995: 54). Connell convincingly suggests that the intact male body is the central prerequisite for enacting 'true' masculinity, a concept that values strength, potency and control and denies weakness, dependence and vulnerability – the very attributes conventionally assigned to the disabled as well as to women. The relationship between masculinity and disability obviously is not just one of mere incompatibility; in

---

[4] However, rather surprisingly, Butler's concepts are comparatively absent in the existing research on disability despite the obvious parallels between the concepts of the disabled body and Butler's concepts of the body. While some appreciate Butler's model of bodies as subject to oppressive discursive power, claiming that Butler offers "the disabled [...] social and political resources for contesting moralities external to [them] that exclude and 'define' [them] in oppressive ways" (Stocker 2001: 31), others demand a more careful and critical reception of Butler's ideas, voicing doubts about the seamless exchangeability of 'impairment'/'disability' and 'sex'/'gender' (Samuels 2011: 55 f.), also suggesting that the disabled body is more strongly physically determined and less susceptible to transformation than the body in Butler's concept.

fact, masculinity as an ideological and psychological process relies on the absolute separation from and superiority to the otherness embodied by the disabled (Shakespeare 1999: 58). The response of disabled men to the emasculating, disempowering effect of their condition is, as will be shown in *The Silver Tassie*, fraught with difficulty.

Disability, the Great War and Ireland

A fundamental change of the common reaction to the otherness of the disabled was brought about by the First World War. This conflict reached an unprecedented, hitherto unthinkable dimension of death, destruction and physical mutilation. The number of soldiers wounded and irreparably maimed was immense, which shows, for example, in the fact that in the late 1930s about 222,000 British officers and more than 419,000 servicemen in other ranks received disability pensions (Bourke 1996: 33). The war produced a whole generation of physically and mentally traumatised men – as a consequence, disabled persons became a common public sight, a mass phenomenon, which also led to a drastic change of the general perception of disability. For example, before the Great War, limblessness was a condition suffered largely by the poor, by factory and dock workers and professional militaries. The countless maimed veterans of the Great War, however, were conscripts rather than professional soldiers and came from all kinds of social backgrounds (Bourke 1996: 37). Thus, the war "magnified the experience of deformity" (Bourke 1996: 31) and in the course of this reformulation also the perspective on those who were disabled by accident or from birth changed. Disability was no longer predominantly perceived as a divine punishment, 'bad luck' or a monstrosity to be met with fascination or disgust. The response to the wartime mutilated was one of empathy and gratitude and included, at least until the end of the 1920s, the acknowledgment of a national responsibility to care for them (Bourke 1996: 31). This altered sentiment, as well as the economic need to restore the employability of the disabled, contributed to the post-war period becoming the starting point of modern concepts of rehabilitation and prosthetic technology (Dederich 2007: 103 f.).

Still, we must keep in mind that the above mentioned perspective on the war disabled as a national cause is a British point of view. *The Silver Tassie*'s principal setting, however, is working-class Dublin and the common Irish attitude towards the Great War and its Irish participants was generally a negative one and evidently differed from British reactions to the conflict and its victims. The Irish contribution to the war effort itself was substantial. Even without enforced conscription, more than 150,000 Irish soldiers were on active duty by April 1916, two thirds of them having volunteered already at the outbreak of the war

(Brown 1993: 226). Yet, their service was not based on a colonial sense of duty but it was mainly the result of grim economic and social circumstances at home, "the king's shilling being preferable to starvation and disease in the tenements of Dublin whatever the risks," as Terence Brown remarks (Brown 1993: 226). Many also found the motivation to join up in the prospect of Home Rule, which was promised by the British government as a reward for Ireland's part in the Great War.

The general opinion in Ireland on the role of Irish soldiers in the Great War was suspicious and conditional (Gregory and Paseta 2002: 2) from the start and turned into a verdict of outright treason (Kosok 2007: 55) after British forces, among them also Irishmen, violently terminated the Easter Rising of 1916, the revolutionary insurrection intended to overthrow British rule, which eventually became a near-sacred event in Irish historical consciousness (Phillips 2010: 115 and McNulty 2010, 66f.) and the founding myth of the Irish Free State. Consequently, the Irish involvement in the Great War turned into a national taboo, a subject ignored, belittled or even scorned for decades. There was no public support for Irish veterans whatsoever (Kiberd 1996: 259) which shows, for example, in the absence of an official Irish culture of Great War commemoration until the end of the 1990s. The Great War was practically written out of Irish history by the state ideology of the Irish Free State, which included the denial of any responsibility for Irishmen disabled during military service. The domestic disruptions brought about by Ireland's struggle for independence simply "were more immediate realities [...] than the sufferings of men who had taken a historical wrong turning that led them to a foreign field" (Brown 1993: 229). Consequently, returning servicemen encountered severe difficulties in re-adapting to a generally hostile Irish society. This shows, for example, in a 1919 report of the City of Dublin War Pensions Committee that notes that "when these men came back disabled and broken down in some cases they found that their own relatives had changed their views on public affairs and matters were extremely uncomfortable for the unfortunate man [...] the public in its resentment is inclined to threaten the disabled man" (W. G. Fallon quoted in Bourke 1996: 70). It is this sentiment of wilful ignorance or even aggression towards disabled Irish soldiers that takes centre-stage in the two closing acts of *The Silver Tassie*, however, as I will show in the following, the play relates this rejection not explicitly to nationalist fervour but to a discriminative ideology of masculinity and fitness.

Rival Bodies in *The Silver Tassie*

From the start, the working-class environment of *The Silver Tassie* is portrayed as a world governed and fascinated by masculinity, men's bodies and male strength. O'Casey seems to share this fascination when we take into account how meticulously and colourfully he describes the bodily appearance of his characters in the stage directions. For example, Sylvester, Harry Heegan's father, is "a stockily built man of sixty-five; he has been a docker all his life since first the muscles of his arms could safely grip a truck, and even at sixty-five the steel in them is only beginning to stiffen" (5);[5] Susie Monican is "a girl of twenty-two, well-shaped limbs, challenging breasts, [...] undeniably pretty, but her charms are almost completely hidden by her sombre, ill-fitting dress" (6), and Mrs. Heegan, Harry's mother, is "stiffened with age and rheumatism; the end of her life is unknowingly lumbering towards a rest: [...] everything she has to do is done with a quiet mechanical persistence. Her inner ear cannot hear even a faint echo of a younger day" (6 f.).

This particular attention to the body implied in the stage directions is con-firmed in the beginning moments of the play. While waiting for the return of the victorious footballer with the trophy, Sylvester and his friend Simon revel in memories of Harry, revealing an almost pathological obsession with the physical, with violence and masculinity. Only in his early twenties, Harry has obviously acquired a legendary status in his community. The praise of his body, his physical power and aggression is euphoric, for example, when Sylvester recounts full of admiration how he has "seen him do it, mind you. I seen him do it. Break a chain across his bisseps!" (7). Another anecdote concerning Harry's strength even verges on homoerotic reverie, Sylvester presenting the story of Harry beating up a policeman, which rather evokes the image of a romantic mating ritual than a street brawl:

> An' the hedges by the road-side standin' stiff in the silent cold of the air, the frost beads on the branches glistenin' like toss'd-down diamonds from the breasts of the stars, the quietness of the night stimulated to a fuller stillness by the mockin' breathin' of Harry, an' the heavy, ragin' pantin' of the Bobby, an' the quickenin' beats of our own hearts [...].
>
> (8)

Harry's supreme status evidently is a result of his superior ability of violent self-assertion and the absence or inefficiency of any other authorities like fathers or the law. In the social environment described in the play, masculinity is primarily defined by strength and fitness, male hierarchies are worked out by violent contests and, consequently, the strongest and most reckless men inhabit the highest positions, epitomising hegemonic masculinity.

Observing civilian disablement in Britain in the first decades of the twentieth century, Joanna Bourke notes that the "deliberate injuring of another man was

---

[5] All quotations from the play refer to the following edition: Sean O'Casey. "The Silver Tassie." *Collected Plays*. Vol. 2. London: Macmillan, 1964. 1-111.

part of growing up. [...] To be 'decorated' or 'well-painted' with blood was a manly accomplishment. It trained men for war, and could sometimes be as damaging to the male body" (Bourke 1996: 35-37). The play seems to confirm this observation also for Ireland. Football, the game that enables Harry Heegan to cement his leading position, offers a perfect peacetime arena for such feats. The parallels between football and violence, particularly the violence of war, are frequently played out in *The Silver Tassie*, visually most remarkably when Harry enters the stage for the first time, sporting "khaki trousers, a military cap stained with trench mud" combined with "a vivid orange-coloured jersey with black collar and cuffs" (25), his football shirt. Also, Harry's description of his decisive goal abounds with belligerent imagery and jargon: "seeing in a *flash* the goalie's hands sent with a *shock* to his chest by the *force* of the *shot*, his *half-stunned* motion to clear, a *charge*, and then carrying him, the ball and all with a *rush* into the centre of the net!" (28, my emphasis). Burke's suggestion that, at the time, football actually reproduced the conditions of front-line service (Bourke 1996: 35) is supported very well by the worrisome combination of domestic and wartime violence, athleticism and triumphant masculinity exposed in O'Casey's play.

The Great War itself is understood by the characters in two ways. On the one hand, very pragmatically, the young men's military service is a welcome source of income for those at home. It seems that Mrs. Heegan's greatest worry is not the danger of losing her son but losing the compensation payment she receives for her son's service. On the other hand, the war is obviously seen as an extension of the culture of violence at home. This becomes particularly visible at the end of Act I: The departure of Harry, Teddy Foran and their fellow comrades to the front is not a moving farewell scene of fearful Irish mothers, fathers and wives, who dread the thought of their sons and husbands risking their lives for a British cause on a foreign battlefield, but it is a rather hectic and cheerful sending-off, accompanied by the collective shout "They must go back!" (31). Going to war is obviously understood by O'Casey's Dubliners as another epi-sode – another match – in the violent competition of male bodies started at home: Simon parades the football trophy in front of the soldiers' triumphal march to the ship (32), and in the following act, the front-line soldiers receive parcels from home, one box containing a rubber ball and a note saying "To play your way to the enemies' trenches when you go all over the top" (51). As Marguerite Harkness notes, in *The Silver Tassie* "athletics are warlike, war is athletic" (Harkness 1978: 134). The play does not feature the Great War as a shocking disruption of peace, the conflict does not carry violence and dis-harmony into a peaceful civilian community – violence and disharmony are there from the start and, Ronan McDonald remarks, it even seems like "the war is a *result* of the prevailing social structure than vice versa" (McDonald 2002: 120).

However, the second act, which is set in a Red Cross hospital next to the ruins of a monastery "somewhere in France", shows that the heroism of the soldier-athlete Harry is only limited to the social structure of his Dublin milieu. Only Barney Bagnal, tied to a gun wheel for disciplinary reasons, remains as a recognisable character from Act I, while Harry and Teddy merge into the anonymous, suffering collective identity of a group of soldiers (named "1st Soldier", "2nd Soldier", etc.), underlining the notion of military service as including an erasure of individuality and war as a profoundly dehumanising experience (O'Riordan 1978: 26). Foreshadowing Harry's and Teddy's later condition of disability, Act II does not feature any actual fighting but puts emphasis on how these men have evidently lost any sense of individual agency, how they have become dependent, subject to a system of military authority that ensures that they "eat well [...] sleep well [...] whore well [...] fight well" (49). The theme of mutilation pervades the second act, bringing the traumatised and wounded bodies of the war on stage (McDonald 2002: 120). The set description mentions "heaps of rubbish, lean, dead hands are protruding" (35), the choir of the wounded on the stretchers bitterly chants "Carry on, carry on to the place of pain, / Where the surgeon spreads his aid, aid, aid" (48) and in the final moment of the act, the Staff-Wallah orders all who "can run, or can walk, even *crawl*" (56, my emphasis) to the guns. This war experience marks the beginning of Harry's downfall and the third act, set in a Dublin hospital, confirms the drastic decline of his status as an idol of strength, power and youth.

Harry has returned from the battlefield with a spine injury and has lost the ability to move his legs. The way he is perceived and treated by his environment has changed radically – the otherness of Harry the paraplegic is manifest throughout the entire rest of the play. Sylvester and Simon, once Harry's most fervent admirers, seem embarrassed and unsure about how to approach Harry, brooding in silence, numb with frustration. Preventively, they avoid too much interaction with him and discuss his fate on the quiet. For Susie Monican, in the first act a religious fanatic who desperately craved Harry's affection, now an overconfident nurse running a hospital ward, Harry has become just another damage case to be handled professionally in order to deepen his "chance in the courage and renewal of the country" (77) – he is not even referred to by name, but is reduced by her to number "Twenty-Eight", continuing the theme of de-individualisation of Act II. Harry has obviously turned from an object of admiration and desire to a "shrivell'd thing" (76), a helpless object of pity, charity and examination. His imposed passivity and powerlessness become obvious, for example, when his mother and Mrs. Foran candidly inspect his face, having to bend down to the fallen hero in his wheelchair, discussing "the hollows under his eyes" (73) as if he was not there. It is obvious that Harry has lost control over his life and that his former identity and status have become matters of the past – an agonising situation he is aware of and which he deeply detests: "It's a miracle I want – not an operation. The last operation was to give life to my limbs, but no life came, and again I felt the horrible sickness of life only from the waist up. [*Raising his voice*] Don't stand there gaping at me, man" (64).

The mutilation of Harry is also instantly connected to a maiming of his virility and manhood. Right at the start of the third act, Sylvester and Simon watch Harry in his wheelchair:

> SYLVESTER: Trying to hold on to the little finger of life.
> SIMON: Half-way up to heaven.
> SYLVESTER: And him always thinking of Jessie.
> SIMON: And Jessie never thinking of him.
>
> (59)

In the first act, the violent power and eroticism exuded by and attributed to Harry does not only earn him the awe of other men but also gives him power over women, attracting characters like Jessie Taite, a young, opportunistic and thoroughly sexualised woman, constantly in search of fame and adventure. Through Jessie, who "gives her favour to the prominent and popular" (26), O'Casey demonstrates the selective mechanisms that govern the hierarchical relations between the rivalling male bodies in the world of the play. It is, in fact, the character of Jessie and not the cherished silver trophy which functions as the "sign of youth, sign of strength, sign of victory" (26) in the community portrayed. 'Possessing' Jessie is the most explicit indicator of social and sexual power and the fact that Jessie is no longer interested in Harry underlines the painful process of his downfall. Harry is replaced by Barney Bagnal, who has won Jessie's affection after returning from the war 'decorated', in the above-mentioned sense of Bourke, with his left arm in a sling and the Victoria Cross – awarded to him, ironically, for carrying wounded Harry out of the line of fire.

Harry's injury unmistakably effecting his emasculation is an attitude shared among Harry's entire social environment. According to Teddy, who returned from the front as a blind man, "he'll have to put Jessie out of his head, for when a man's hit in the spine . . ." (73). Harry has obviously lost any means of sexual agency, which contrasts sharply with the licentiousness he exposed in the bawdy celebrations of his football triumph. Now, his impairment and the accompanying dependency on others relegate him to an asexual, quasi-infantile status, which, for example, becomes apparent when Mrs. Foran, in a failed attempt of encouragement, mentions "all the places he could *toddle* to" (73, my emphasis) with the help of crutches. Mrs. Foran also reminds Nurse Monican of the importance of hospital visits by relatives and the harm that might be done "by keeping a wife from her husband and a mother from her son" (71), unaware of the irony that the roles of wife and mother for Harry have in fact become identical – Harry has become solely an object of pity and care and has lost any sexual relevance. The realisation of this status of emasculation and powerlessness is painful and embittering and leads to the negative climax of the final act.

While the medical setting of Act III promotes emotions of pity, care and solace, Act IV puts the disability of Harry, as well as Teddy, in a different, less sheltered and understanding social context, that of the dance hall of Avondale FC, which consequently provokes different reactions to the disabled condition. From the beginning, the presence of Harry at the party is perceived as uncanny and disturbing. It is obvious that he has become an alien body:

> JESSIE: [*Hot, excited, and uneasy, as with a rapid glance back she sees the curtains parted by Harry*] Here he comes prowling after us again! His watching of us is pulling all the enjoyment out of the night. It makes me shiver to feel him wheeling after us.
> BARNEY: We'll watch for a chance to shake him off, an' if he starts again we'll make him take his tangled body somewhere else.
>
> (81)

Harry desperately attempts to challenge the rejection he experiences, which, at the beginning of the final act, he understands as a gross injustice, desperately reminding those around him that "There's medals on my breast as well as yours!" (82). He antagonises Jessie for her disloyalty and even physically attacks his successor in the role of the principal male, "wheeling his chair viciously against Barney" (82), of course without any success. Soon after, Harry himself spells out the bitter reality of his new existence: "Cram pain with pain, and pleasure cram with pleasure" (82) – a principle of segregation seen as natural and self-evident by Harry's able-bodied environment. "To carry the sick and helpless to where there's nothing but life and colour is wrong," (83) Simon notes and Sylvester agrees, pointing at the foolishness of joining "a little weakness to a lot of strength" (84).

The party at the dance hall is a social gathering celebrating the values that determine the social and sexual hierarchies of the community portrayed. The night is dedicated to masculine strength, beauty and youth, which is also indicated by the peripheral, rather observing positioning of the elderly characters in the final act. The play's celebration of masculinity, Terry Phillips argues, "goes hand in hand with a crudely exploitative sexuality" (Phillips 2010: 118) and indeed, the younger women at the event seem prepared to offer themselves to dominant men like Barney or Surgeon Maxwell: Susie Monican is "lookin' game enough to-night for anything" (90), Jessie Taite appears to be "tired of her maidenhood" (90) and Mrs. Foran is scandalised by "the way the girls are advertisin' their immodesty" (90). In this sexually charged environment, the commonly assumed inadequacy and the frustrating disconnection of the disabled become apparent. Blind Teddy describes his impression of the night:

> TEDDY: [...] In the hall the sound of dancing, the eyes of women, grey and blue and brown and black, do sparkle and dim and sparkle again. Their white breasts rise and fall, and rise again. Slender legs, from red and black, and white and green come out, go again – nothing. Strain as you may, it stretches from the throne of God to the end of the hearth of hell.
> SIMON: What?
> TEDDY: The darkness.

(89)

The memory of past moments of attraction and erotic encounters tortures Teddy, who has become a victim of the same emasculating process of infantilisation as Harry. Instead of dancing and flirting, Teddy is guided by his wife to a position at the margins of the party. Mrs. Foran, formerly a helpless victim of Teddy's violent outbursts, now is in full control of her husband, allowing him "[j]ust one glass, dear, and you'll sit down quietly an' take it in sips" (89).

As mentioned earlier, masculinity as an ideological and psychological process has been understood as relying on the rejection of otherness – in *The Silver Tassie*, rejection finally turns into blatant physical aggression. At the close of the final act, Harry's intervention against Barney's attempt to sexually abuse Jessie – an intervention, by the way, not for the sake of protecting Jessie but out of mere jealousy – means a crass affront to Barney that effects a savage confirmation of the primacy of masculine strength over emasculated weakness: "You half-baked Lazarus, I've put up with you all the evening, so don't force me now to rough-handle the bit of life the Jerries left you as a souvenir! [...] I'll tilt the leaking life out of you, you jealous, peering pimp!" (99 f.). Eventually, the two uneven fighters are separated, yet it is not Barney who is publicly embarrassed by his indecency and blamed for disturbing the party; instead, Harry is told to leave, because "[a]ny more excitement would be dangerous" (100) for him – he is simply suspected to be not strong and, consequently, not man enough for the occasion.

The transformation of Harry, as well as Teddy, from strength to weakness is a sudden and overwhelming process. Their confrontation with the new reality of disability is abrupt, which, according to Russell Shuttleworth, typically leads disabled men into a shocked state of frustration, fatalism and a sentiment of embodying defeated masculinity (Shuttleworth et al. 2012: 184) – "Life came and took away the half of life" (95), Harry sighs. Shuttleworth argues that some disabled men – however, usually men disabled from birth – succeed in accepting their disability as a part of their identity, furthermore expanding their "masculine repertoire to include and emphasise dispositions and practices that stress sensitivity and interdependence" (Shuttleworth et al. 2012: 184), thereby successfully resisting hegemonic standards. However, in the world of the play, 1916 working-class Dublin, such an integrative process of course seems impossible. Harry and Teddy cannot challenge the rules of their environment, they cannot find any other way to define and reposition themselves in the masculine hierarchy.[6]

The only option left to the disabled veterans is to resign themselves to a world of their own – a return to the cordial bonds of fate of the trenches, the homosocial spheres of soldiers, which is also indicated by Harry's return to the incantatory style of Act II (McDonald 2002: 124): "For a spell here I will stay / Then pack up my body and go – / For mine is a life on the ebb, / Yours a full life on the flow!" (93). In a final, futile gesture of defiance, Teddy announces that "what's in front we'll face like men, dear comrade of the blood fight and the battlefront!" (102), while holding on to Harry's shoulder, being led out of the dance hall along with the elderly. The play ends with a quasi-official explanation of the expulsion of Harry and Teddy. Coolly brushing away second thoughts about the treatment of the two veterans, Susie Monican declares the irreconcilability of the disabled and the able-bodied, embracing 'life' as a concept reserved for the strong, rejecting any notion of sentimentality:

> Teddy Foran and Harry Heegan have gone to live in their own world. Neither I nor you can lift them out of it. No longer can they do the things we do. We can't give sight to the blind or make the lame walk. We would if we could. It is the misfortune of war. As long as wars are waged, we shall be vexed by woe; strong legs shall be made useless and bright eyes made dark. But we, who have come through the fire unharmed, must go on living. [*Pulling Jessie from the chair*] Come along, and take your part in life! [*To Barney*] Come along, Barney, and take your partner into the dance!
>
> (103)

Sieber's aforementioned observation that the emotions of the able-bodied towards the disabled expose the idea that the disabled are practically dead is very much confirmed in *The Silver Tassie*. Despite having returned from the battlefield alive, in the eyes of their able-bodied peers, Harry and Teddy rather belong to the names on Avondale FC's "Roll of Honour" (80), which commemorates the club members killed in the war, than to the party guests in the dance hall. Harry and Teddy have left their former identities on the battlefield, "[b]ehind the trenches", "[i]n the Rest Camps", "[o]ut in France" (94) as their relatives repeat. They have become fixed forever in powerless, marginalised positions since their

---

[6] Wendy Gagen suggests that in the aftermath of the Great War disabled men continued to define themselves very much within a hegemonic masculine framework, yet, at least partly, resisted emasculation by renegotiating individually what masculinity means to them, challenging and extending the existing concepts of masculinity. See Gagen 2007.

impairment makes it impossible for them to participate in the defining contests of masculinity of their milieu, symbolised most drastically in Act IV when Harry smashes the "Silver Tassie", the trophy that temporarily signified his superior manhood, making it "[m]angled and bruised as I am bruised and mangled" (102).

Conclusion

In *The Silver Tassie* Sean O'Casey presents a domestic environment obsessed with masculine strength, built on a very narrow understanding of which bodies 'matter' – the male bodies which prevail in the violent competition with other men. In the milieu portrayed in the play, the Great War is understood simply as another facet of this competition and those who return from the distant battlefields permanently maimed are not particularly pitied and honoured for their sacrifice – their predicament is just the result of the "misfortune of war" (102), an attitude that expresses a profound sense of detachment from the realities of war. The war disabled of the play experience an erasure of their previous identity and the collapse of their social significance, which is inextricably connected to the emasculation and infantilisation that their condition entails. They come to signify an otherness that leaves them no other option than the complete withdrawal from "life", which is reserved for the strong and healthy, proceeding to an asexual realm of dependence and subordination.

O'Casey offers very little to alleviate the bleakness of the world presented in the play. For example, in contrast to earlier works like *Juno and the Paycock* or *The Plough and the Stars*, there are no level-headed, strong female characters to insist on sanity and decency (Harkness 1978: 132) – in *The Silver Tassie*, O'Casey, in fact, de-mystifies his earlier concept of female integrity (Stubbings 2000: 136). Also, Harry's final challenge to his community's fatalist acceptance of suffering, "The Lord hath given and man hath taken away!" (102), is an insight that might possibly resound among the audiences of the play, but not among Harry's peers, who, to take up Yeats's charges against O'Casey once again, have obviously not been "thwarted" by "the mere greatness of the world war", which also alludes to the problematic status of the Great War and its Irish victims in twentieth-century Ireland.

List of Works Cited

Bourke, Joanna. *Dismembering the Male. Men's Bodies, Britain and the Great War*. London: Reaktion Books, 1996.

Brown, Terrence. "Who dares to speak? Ireland and the Great War". *English Studies in Transition*. Ed. Robert Clark and Piero Boitani. London: Routledge, 1993. 226-37.

Butler, Judith. *Bodies That Matter. On the Discursive Limits of "Sex"*. New York: Routledge, 1993.

Canguilhem, Georges. *Das Normale und das Pathologische*. Trans. Monika Noll and Rolf Schubert. München: Carl Hanser, 1974.

Connell, R. W. *Masculinities*. Berkeley: U of California P, 1995.

Davis, Lennard J. "Identity Politics, Disability, and Culture." *Handbook of Disability Studies*. Ed. Gary L. Albrecht, Katherine D. Seelman and Michael Bury. London: Sage, 2001. 535-45.

Dederich, Markus. *Körper, Kultur und Behinderung. Eine Einführung in die Disability Studies*. Bielefeld: transcript, 2007.

Gagen, Wendy Jane. "Remastering the Body, Renegotiating Gender: Physical Disability and Masculinity during the First World War, the Case of J. B. Middlebrook." *European Review of History* 14.4 (2007): 525-41.

Gregory, Adrian and Senia Paseta. Introduction. *Ireland and the Great War. 'A War to Unite us All?'*. Manchester: Manchester UP, 2002. 1-7.

Harkness, Marguerite. "*The Silver Tassie*: No Light in the Darkness". *The Sean O'Casey Review* 4.2 (1978): 131-37.

Kiberd, Declan. *Inventing Ireland. The Literature of the Modern Nation*. London: Vintage, 1996.

Kosok, Heinz. *The Theatre of War. The First World War in British and Irish Drama*. Basingstoke: Palgrave, 2007.

McDonald, Ronan. *Tragedy and Irish Literature: Synge, O'Casey, Beckett*. Basingstoke: Palgrave, 2002.

McNulty, Eugene. "Incommensurate Histories: the Remaindered Irish Bodies of the Great War". *Conflict, Nationhood and Corporeality in Modern Literature. Bodies-at-War*. Ed. Petra Rau. Basingstoke: Palgrave Macmillan, 2010. 64-82.

Mitchell, David and Sharon Snyder. "Disability Studies and the Double Bind of Representation." *The Body and Physical Difference. Discourses of Disability*. Ann Arbor: U of Michigan P, 1997. 1-31.

---. "Narrative Prosthesis and the Materiality of Metaphor." *The Disability Studies Reader*. 2nd ed. Ed. Lennard J. Davis. New York: Routledge, 2006. 205-16.

O'Casey, Sean. "The Silver Tassie." *Collected Plays*. Vol. 2. London: Macmillan, 1964. 1-111.

---. *The Letters of Sean O'Casey*. Vol. 1. Ed. David Krause. London: Cassell, 1975.

O'Riordan, John. "The Garlanded Horror of War: Reflections on *The Silver Tassie*." *The Sean O'Casey Review* 5 (1978): 23-28.

Phillips, Terry. "Sean O'Casey and Radical Theatre." *Kritika Kultura* 15 (2010): 113-31.

Samuels, Ellen. "Judith Butler's Body Theory and the Question of Disability." *Feminist Disability Studies*. Ed. Kim Q. Hall. Bloomington: Indiana UP, 2011. 48-66.

Shakespeare, Tom. "The Sexual Politics of Disabled Masculinity." *Sexuality and Disability* 17.1 (1999): 53-64.

Shuttleworth, Russell, Nikki Wedgwood and Nathan J. Wilson. "The Dilemma of Disabled Masculinity." *Men and Masculinities* 15.2 (2012): 174-94.

Siebers, Tobin. *Disability Theory*. Ann Arbor: U of Michigan P, 2009.

Stocker, Susan S. "Problems of Embodiment and Problematic Embodiment." *Hypatia* 16.3 (2001): 30-55.

Stubbings, Diane. *Anglo-Irish Modernism and the Maternal. From Yeats to Joyce.* Basingstoke: Palgrave, 2000.

Tervooren, Anja. "Der verletzliche Körper. Überlegungen zu einer Systematik der Disability Studies." *Kulturwissenschaftliche Perspektiven der Disability Studies. Tagungsdokumentation.* Kassel: bifos, 2003. 37-48.

Welch, Robert. *The Abbey Theatre. 1899-1999. Form & Pressure.* Oxford: Oxford UP, 1999.

Yeats, William Butler. *The Letters of W. B. Yeats.* Ed. Allan Wade. London: Hart-Davis, 1954.

---. "On Being Asked for a War Poem." *Earth Voices Whispering. An Anthology of Irish War Poetry. 1914-1945.* Ed. Gerald Dawe. Belfast: Blackstaff, 2008. 9.

Ralf Junkerjürgen

Quantifying Desire, Qualifying Disease.
Gendered Images of Sexual Addiction in Spanish Cinema
of Pedro Almodóvar, Julio Medem, and Valérie Tasso

Sexual activity is a vital function and can hardly be considered a disease. But through its regulation of the relationship between the sexes and the possible procreation of children, each sexual act has social consequences and thus constitutes a delicate social matter. Hence society has an interest in controlling the practice of sexuality, and tends to standardize how and how often sexuality is to be performed. This norm, however, was and seems still to be deeply gendered, especially when it is broken.

In ancient medicine, based on the idea of balance and on Aristotle's principle of the "golden mean", doing not too little and not too much in everything was the key to a healthy and good life. In sexual activity too much desire was damaging and was therefore regarded as a disease, in men called *satyriasis* and in women *furor uterinus*, which much later on in the seventeenth century became known as nymphomania. Though the medical history of nymphomania has been studied in detail (Groneman 2001), it is necessary to summarise briefly the main paradigm shifts in order to understand to which tradition contemporary images of sexual addiction may belong.

The concept of nymphomania was first laid out by the French physician de Bienville in his 1771 treatise *La nymphomanie ou traité de la fureur utérine, dans lequel on explique avec autant de clarté que de méthode, les commencemens & les progrès de cette cruelle maladie*. Scientific thought on the subject did not advance much for the next 175 years. Eighteenth-century encyclopaedias like Zedler's listed a wide variety of contributing factors for nymphomania, showing that the ideas on this disease were quite heterogeneous. Various factors were held responsible for nymphomania, like the amount of *liquor genitalis* or the composition of the blood, as well as salty or bitter food, just like aphrodisiacs, the reading of romance novels and even sperm, which was thought to excite the uterus.

A major change of the medical perspective on the female body took place in the nineteenth century when male and female bodies were considered to be completely different. Now physicians believed that women were much less affected by sexual desire than men. Nymphomania was hence to be considered as a disease in comparison to satyriasis, which was just above the norm (Groneman 2001: 28).

In the beginning of the twentieth century Freud's psychoanalysis imposed a new approach to sexual deviances, claiming that they were mainly due to psychological reasons. With regard to the psychological development of female sexuality, Freud believed in a theory of transmission: after a clitoral phase pleasure had to move to the vagina; the vaginal orgasm was the "right" one and everything else represented a form of frigidity (Freud 1963: 120-123). In the light of this theory, a nymphomaniac never achieved the transference of pleasure to the vagina and was considered unable to have an orgasm, seeking insatiably for pleasure.

This theory, which is deeply marked by the physiological premises of sexuality, was substituted by other psychological approaches in the 1950s which asserted that sexual addiction was a result of a long list of conscious and unconscious causes, among them fear, incestuous desire, latent homosexuality, narcissism, etc. But no one could say how much sex was too much. The distinguishing factor for nymphomania was the compulsivity of the sexual activity and the arbitrariness in the choice of partners.

In the 1920s and 1930s the influence of hormones on sexuality was discovered (Groneman 2001: 80). Once again there was a physiological – in this case a biochemical – explanation for gender differences: behaving like a man or like a woman just depended on having more testosterone or more oestrogen. Sexual addiction was then nothing more than the result of a disorder in the equilibrium of chemical substances.

The famous Kinsey reports, *Sexual Behavior in the Human Male* (1948) and *Sexual Behavior in the Human Female* (1953), were the beginning of the end of medical nymphomania. Alfred Kinsey was the head of the Institute for Sex Research at the University of Indiana and was the first person to collect statistical material on the sexual behaviour of humans. Rates of sexual activity varied widely among individuals and there was no distinguishable point at which the frequency (or infrequency) of sex became pathological. This strictly objective empirical method provided the conclusion that nymphomania and satyriasis were not outstanding phenomena, but only a relative point on the statistical scale. In the words of Alfred Kinsey a nymphomaniac is just "someone who has more sex than you do" (Kinsey 1953: 437-38). For these researchers nymphomania did not exist anymore – having too many orgasms was just a moral assertion, not a scientific one (Groneman, 2001: 105).

Evolving views of nymphomania were reflected in the successive editions of the American Psychiatric Association's official guide to madness, the *Diagnostic and Statistical Manual of Mental Disorder* (DSM). Nymphomania was listed as a "sexual deviation" in the first DSM, published in 1951; by DSM-III

(1980) it had become a "psychosexual disorder"; in the revised third edition from 1987 the editors of DSM-III-R dropped nymphomania and its equally quaint male counterpart, Don Juanism, and replaced them with "distress about a pattern of repeated sexual conquests or other forms of nonparaphilic [nondeviant] sexual addiction." In DSM-IV (1994) even sexual addiction was abandoned (Groneman 2001: 153-54).

The development of the ideas on *satyrias* or Don Juanism did not run parallel to that of nymphomania. On the contrary, the former had mythical origins and therefore belonged much more to a literary discourse than to a scientific one. The earliest complete dramatisation is the *Burlador de Sevilla* (1630) by the catholic monk Tirso de Molina. In the play the womanizer Don Juan represents a diabolic character and is punished in the end by transcendental forces (Pennone 2005: 184-89).

The later romantic version by José Zorrilla – *Don Juan Tenorio* (1844) – has an alternative ending because Don Juan is redeemed by love. Here he no longer represents the devil, but an extreme character of romantic shape, somebody who does not care about rules and seeks his personal liberty. Numbers play an important part in establishing why Don Juan is an outcast: in one year he killed 32 men and seduced 72 women. Zorrilla's prototypical play of Spanish romanticism was an enormous success and entered Spanish popular culture because it is still traditionally performed on the first of November, All Saints' Day, supposedly to inspire women and men to moral behaviour. In the course of the nineteenth century Don Juan (like Don Quijote) becomes an autostereotype of the Spanish male national character.

The decadence of Spain and the loss of its political importance, which became obvious in the 19th century, led to several self-critical movements which aimed at reforming the country, among them the *regeneraciosmo* and the *generación del 98* (Paredes Méndez 2007; Franzbach 2007). In the light of Spanish decadence Don Juan could become problematically complex. Miguel de Unamuno, one of the heads of the *generación del 98*, described him as "bad for our people" („pernicioso para nuestro pueblo"; Unamuno 1954: 486).

In 1929 one of Spain's most prominent physicians and psychologists, Gregorio Marañon, presented a new interpretation of Don Juan in his article *Psicopatología del donjuanismo* (1924). Marañon, a follower of eugenic theory, believed that Don Juanism was detrimental for Spain's progress because it represented an unproductive masculinity. Apart from this he thought that it belonged to female behaviour because women obeyed much more to the impositions of their sexual destiny – reproduction. Though Marañon's analysis sounds anachronistic nowadays it had an important iconoclastic effect since it stated that Don Juan was a destructive autostereotype and that his masculinity was in reality a hidden feminine trait (Wright 2004: 721-38).

As we can see, in the course of the 20th century nymphomania and Don Juanism were both expunged from medical and mythical discourses and became politically incorrect concepts. But the collective desire to quantify sexual activity still remains. Overshooting an imaginary limit can obviously no longer be called nymphomania or Don Juanism and is nowadays labelled generally as sexual addiction. Though this term assumes an apparent neutrality on gender, the question remains whether the representation of sexual addiction in popular media is really unbiased between the sexes, which traditions may survive in popular knowledge and whether the scientific abandoning of the concept of sex addiction constitutes a fertile moment where new concepts may be born.

Though sexual addiction is in general a subject that is favoured by popular media and is covered by cinema, popular surveys[1] and TV-talk-shows, Spanish popular culture is of special interest, not only because Spain is Don Juan's homeland but also for the fact that until 1975 it was dominated by a regime that enforced a repressive morality which made sexuality one of the most sensitive questions of personal identity in the young democracy after the death of Franco.

Popularization of the Concept of Sexual Addiction

While Don Juan was deeply rooted in a literary and even heroic discourse and therefore omnipresent, nymphomania belonged mainly to a slim pornographic segment of popular culture. This changes at the end of the 1960s when several factors coincide: firstly, the commercialization of the contraceptive pill, which gives women the power of birth control and allows a merely pleasurable experience of sexuality, and, secondly, the sexual liberation movement combined with feminist activism and a liberal approach to pornography, which starts to become popular. Pornography was no longer banned in specialist cinemas and entered mainstream movie theatres at the beginning of the 1970s, sometimes resulting in impressive commercial successes like the 1972 movie *Deep Throat*, followed by *Behind the Green Door* and *The Devil in Miss Jones*. The formerly tabooed genre was increasingly perceived to be interesting for women as well, allowing it to also attract couples. Gender roles remained mainly misogynistic, however, and provoked a protest movement against the flourishing porn industry. Feminist theory was divided into a sex-positive and a sex-negative faction, a conflict which exploded in the so called "Feminist Sex Wars" (Villa 2012: 234-36).

It was in those years that the Franco dictatorship finally came to an end. Censorship was abolished, and sexually explicit scenes in films became possible.

---

[1] See, for example, the *FOCUS Online* test of sex addiction by Monika Preuk, http://www.focus.de/gesundheit/ratgeber/sexualitaet/tests/sexsucht/test_aid_15270.html (accessed 7 July 2012).

Between 1975 and 1982 a visible sexualisation of Spanish cinema took place, not only because pornography was celebrating its first and major phase of popularity in the history of Spanish cinema, but also because the Spanish *auteur* cinema of Bigas Luna or Almodóvar was seeking to represent repressed forms of sexuality.

A Spanish "Feminist Sex War" did not take place (Prada 2012: 133); pornography was on the contrary regarded as a sign of liberalization and is full of political statements in that respect. The first frontal nude of Spanish cinema was performed by María José Cantudo in Jorge Grau's movie *La trastienda* in the year when the dictator died and symbolized new liberty while promising individual sexual fulfilment – and this not only for men. *Las eróticas vacaciones de Stela* (Zacarias Urbiola, 1978), for example, shows striking expressions of female sexual empowerment (Kowalsky 2004: 194). Already two years after the releases of S-rated films, it was clear that directors and audiences in Spain were enthusiastically embracing softcore pornography as a distinctly Spanish film genre (Kowalsky 2004: 197). At the same time a young director coming from the margin of underground culture would soon move to the centre imposing his own sexual discourse – Pedro Almodóvar.

Iconoclasm, Irony, Utopia –
Almodóvar's Postmodern Play with Nymphomaniacs and Don Juans

Almodóvar's second motion picture *Laberinto de pasiones* (1981) tells the love story of young Sexilia (Cecilia Roth) who has been a nymphomaniac "desde niña" (since she was a child) and the homosexual Riza (Imanol Arias), the prince of fictive Tiraní, who hides himself from Islamic persecution in Madrid leading a libertine life. Both are singers in bands of the Movida, the pop-culture movement in Spain after 1975, who fall in love abandoning nymphomania and homosexuality and leave Madrid with their band for the island paradise Contadora.

Though the plot uses elements of fairy tale, it is also full of allusions to the family of Iranian Shah Mohammed Reza Pahlavi, who was overthrown by the Iranian Revolution in 1979, and who in 1980 spent some time on Contadora. The Shah's second wife, Soraya Esfandiary-Bakhtiari, is ironically portrayed in Almodóvar's infertile character Toraya who is eager to have a child and seeks the help of Sexilia's father, a world-renowned specialist in artificial conception.

The ironic manner in which these subjects are treated makes clear that Almodóvar is not interested in explicit political statements. Rather he uses the Shah's family and the Islamic persecuters merely as popular emblems and clichés to create a suspenseful plot which is nothing more than a pretext to tell a story. Indeed, the early Almodóvar was considered to be a Spanish Andy War-

hol, whose main artistic gesture relied on making a popular subject out of so-
called serious matters. This playful attitude is Almodóvar's means to break and
so "normalize" a series of taboos in each of his features, whether these taboos be
political, social or sexual.

The long dictatorship and its political alliance with the Spanish Catholic
church was especially repressive in sexual matters and linked sexuality strictly
to marriage. Apart from condemning premarital sex and adultery any lascivious
behaviour was considered sinful and homosexuality was even punished as a
crime by the change of the "Ley de vagos y maleantes" ("law of vagabonds") in
1954. It was only in 1978 that homosexuality was decriminalised and in 1979
that the last homosexuals left prison.

Almodóvar uses elements of pornography to liberalize sexual activity on the
screen and transforms the nymphomaniac into a popular character. The director
does not reinvent aspects of the genre or the character. On the contrary, the way
he deals with it is deliberately marked by convention, but in such an excessive
way that the nymphomaniac becomes an obviously postmodern ironic quotation.

Already the name of the character, Sexilia, hints at its artificiality, erecting an
ironic frame around the two serious (sexual) problems she is suffering from:
Sexilia is not only a nymphomaniac, she cannot bear the sun either.

The front credits show a pale young Sexilia with sun glasses strolling on the
Rastro, Madrid's popular open-air flea market, searching for sexual adventure
and fetishizing male genitals in the same way the cinematic "male gaze" fetish-
izes parts of the female body. In a subsequent scene we can see Riza leaving
with Patty Diphusa, a fictional porn star invented by Almodóvar, while Sexilia
organizes a party with a lot of boys, herself being the only girl. Though her
"nymphomania", as the film calls it, is not a dramatic incident, it is, however,
considered a deviance which will be cured by true love – ironically of course.
To explain the deviances of both his protagonists Almodóvar draws on psychoanalysis, the most popular of all explanations, and creates an ironic psycho-
analytical narrative which explains nymphomania as a result of emotional
deception in the childhood of his characters.

In fact, Sexilia and Riza knew each other already and were traumatized
fifteen years ago by an incident on a beach. Feeling rejected by her male friend
Riza and by her father, who is associated with the sunshine, young Sexilia seeks
attention and love in playing husband and wife with a whole group of boys
while Riza seems to feel rejected by her and consoles his sorrow with one of the
boys. The play of the children prefigures the later sexual deviance. The exaggerated use of dramatic music, however, which stands in opposition to the punk
score of the rest of the movie, shows that the staging of trauma is an ironic
quotation of the conventional psychoanalytic narrative.

This is comparable to late Buñuel, who became more and more ambivalent in his use of psychoanalysis, and in 1974 was openly mocking it in *Le fantôme de la liberté*. Adopting a self-ironic distance from his own work and from the mechanical trauma-narrative (Junkerjürgen 2011: 139-41), Almodóvar uses psychoanalysis playfully to create a story and updates it aesthetically in the context of pop art and postmodernism, dealing with nymphomania and psychoanalysis as a mere popular narrative scheme, which allows him to propagate a liberal sexual attitude within the new democratic system. The postmodern motto of "anything goes" corresponds to the two main principles of the new society: free choice for consumers and moral liberty for the citizens of democratic Spain.

The allusions to Persia's former Shah may be considered as a metaphor for the remains of the dictatorship in Spanish society. In this case the healing union of Riza, the son of the "tiranian" dictator, and Sexilia, the Spanish nymphomaniac, on the island of Contadora acquires a utopian aspect. Nymphomania and promiscuity in themselves could hence be regarded as metaphors for the sexual repression under Franco, which forced people into deviant behaviour. Though the surface of fairy tale elements deprives the film of any obvious political statements, the intertextual network and the allusive elements of *Laberinto de pasiones* allow for various political readings.

Almodóvar's struggle with sexual identities had to lead him sooner or later to the emblem of Spanish masculinity: the figure of Don Juan. His own version of the myth underpins his international breakthrough success *Mujeres al borde de un ataque de nervios* (*Women on the Verge of a Nervous Breakdown*, 1988), which made him popular in the USA and opened a new chapter of his career.

The film tells the story of Pepa (Carmen Maura), who tries to find her exboyfriend Iván (Fernando Guillén), who disappeared after having broken up with her a week ago.

On different levels the film shows how men manipulate women through lies and illusions and then search for a new one. In the opening credits one can see collages in pop-art style which show different parts of the female body, a way of showing the selective male gaze. In one picture the female attributes are surrounded by colorful butterflies which may be read as a symbol of both man's way of charming and his unsteadiness, driving him from one flower to the other. The characters work as dubbing actors and are employed to dissemble and to create illusions. In this way their lives are inseparably linked to medial representation, which tends to become a substitute for real communication.

In one of the opening scenes Pepa dreams of Iván paying compliments to a whole series of women, each representing a different cultural type. Iván, however, stands for one male type who, by the use of clichés, pleases all of them. Iván's capacity for lying and charming relies just on words and the enchantment of make-belief. By casting Fernando Guillén (1932-2013) for the part of Iván,

Almodóvar took care to choose a mature actor who emanates an appearance of paternal protection instead of sexual attraction.

The paternal Don Juan-model is shown in a short scene in the beginning of the film. Iván's ex-lover Lucía is still living with her parents and enjoys it when her father pays her compliments. She says that he knows how to lie so well and this is what she loves him for ("qué bien mientes, papá, por eso te quiero"; 13'10). As women are used to being manipulated with compliments on their beauty from early childhood on, Almodóvar does not stress the erotic part of seduction, but has a closer look at the way seduction works by make-believe. Mostly absent in the movie, Iván is represented much more by the ideas others have of him than by himself and is for some time a sort of mysterious centre of the whole story. Pepa only discovers the whole range of his cheating in the end, allowing her to distance herself. The mysterious Iván from the beginning turns out to be a coward who refuses to take responsibility. His son Carlos (Antonio Banderas) shows the same compulsive behaviour towards women, but in contrast to the paternal Don Juan type like his father, Carlos is ridiculed for his speech impediment, his glasses, and his tasteless outfit.

Pepa is not the only woman abandoned and exploited by men. There are also Lucía, the ex-lover of Iván, who has a son by him, her friend Candela (María Barranco), who was sexually exploited and then left by Shi'ite Terrorists, and Marisa (Rossy de Palma), who is left by Carlos, Iván's son, for Candela. The terrorist becomes a metaphor for Iván – "se le puede llamar así" ("one can call him like this", 49'32) – a macho who destroys love and trust and has driven Lucía to insanity.

But iconoclasm is only a part of Almodóvar's strategy to destroy a monument of a male hero, the other one consists in leaving Iván to the side and concentrating fully on the process of how Pepa becomes aware of the system of lies. Compared to Lucía she represents a younger generation who will not go insane but will seek for alternative ways of happiness. In the last scene she sits on the balcony where the virgin Marisa just awakes from a dream which made her loose her virginity.

The illusionary defloration projects a life where men are no longer necessary. Once again Almodóvar's solution includes utopian aspects. Still, not all women will be saved: for Lucía it is too late, she is taken back to a psychiatric clinic, and the naïve Candela has just fallen into the arms of Carlos.

One might say that Almodóvar does for popular culture what scientific research did before him: showing that nymphomania and the scientific discourse of psychoanalysis about it have become a case of popular entertainment. Don Juan, on the other hand, is just a coward who takes advantage of women and therefore is not an interesting subject; the film deals much more with how women try to handle this type of male terrorism called machismo in order to be happy.

Sex and Symbols in the Cinema of Julio Medem

After the iconoclasm of Almodóvar and other directors like Bigas Luna the ground of Spanish cinema was prepared for the next *auteur* generation who imposed itself in the 1990s. The political importance of sexual subjects may not have been understood abroad, but it had nonetheless become a hallmark of Spanish *auteurist* cinema. Sexual deviances as well as psychological problems play an important part in the work of one of Spain's most prominent *auteurs* of the 1990s, the Basque director Julio Medem (*1958).

In two of his movies characters are challenged with problems of promiscuity. Far away from Almodóvar's iconoclastic attitude, Medem, who studied medicine and is very interested in psychology, pursues more traditional themes, one of these being the oedipal complex. In *Los amantes del círculo polar* (1998) Medem has his male protagonist Otto pass through a period of numerous changes of sexual partners after the death of his mother. In an orthodox Freudian reading Medem suggests that Otto's promiscuity is a quest for the lost mother who cannot be found in any other woman and condemns the character to go on searching constantly.

In *Tierra* (1996), his third motion picture, Medem tells the story of schizophrenic Ángel, a character torn between heaven and earth, between disembodied and corporal spheres symbolized by two female characters: on the one side the blond Ángela, on the other the oversexed, 19-year-old nymphomaniac Mari, whose name alludes to the Basque goddess of the earth and to the telluric forces. Mari is marked by an extreme sexual capacity, which she herself considers as a problem, believing that it prevents her from falling in love:

MARI: Yo también tengo un problema [...]. Quiero cambiar de persona y de vida. Dificilísimo.
ÁNGEL: ¿Qué te pasa?
MARI: Nada, pero me excito en seguida. Tengo mucho sexo, sabes.
ÁNGEL: Pero eso no es malo, ¿no?
MARI: Ya. Pero ya estoy harta. Nunca me he enamorado. ¿Tú?
ÁNGEL: Sí. Yo sí.
MARI: Y ¿cuál es tu problema?
ÁNGEL: ¿Yo? ¿Problema? No estoy bien aquí. Estoy mal conectado. Lo mío es desdoblamiento de personalidad. Por lo visto la culpa la tiene mi imaginación que está muy excitada.
MARI: Como mi sexo.
ÁNGEL: Eso es.

MARI: Tú y yo tenemos que enamorarnos. A ti y a mí nos vendría bien quedar con otra persona.
ÁNGEL: Sí. Yo estoy terriblemente solo.
MARI: Yo necesito tener un hombre para quererle. Y olvidarme un poco del sexo.
ÁNGEL: Yo también.
MARI: Por lo menos al principio.
ÁNGEL: Yo también, yo estoy buscando a una mujer para vivir con ella y para quererle hasta la muerte.
MARI: Eso me encantaría. Pero soy gilipollas, no tengo remedio.

(*Tierra*: 01'07'00)

MARI: I have a problem as well [...]. I want to change my personality and my life. It's horribly difficult.
ÁNGEL: What happens to you?
MARI: Nothing, but I get excited immediately. I have a great sexual appetite, you know.
ÁNGEL: Well, but this is not bad, is it?
MARI: No. But I am fed up. I have never been in love. How about you?
ÁNGEL: Me. Well, I have.
MARI: So, what is your problem?
ÁNGEL: My problem? I don't feel well here. I am malfunctioning. My problem is my split personality. It seems that my imagination is responsible for that. It is always excited.
MARI: Like my sexual appetite.
ÁNGEL: True.
MARI: You and me, we should fall in love. It would be good for you and for me to be with another person.
ÁNGEL: Yes. I feel terribly lonely.
MARI: I need a man whom I can love – and to forget a bit about sex.
ÁNGEL: So do I.
MARI: At least in the beginning.
ÁNGEL: Me too, I am searching for a woman to live with and to love till I die.
MARI: That would be great. But I am stupid, I am a hopeless case.

(*Tierra*: 01'07'00, my translation)

In one of the later sequences Mari has her first sexual encounter without orgasm with Ángel, who later becomes the man of her life. Like in Almodóvar the concept of "true love" solves the problem, though with hardly any ironic undertone. In the last scene Mari and Ángel have left the countryside and are travelling to the sea, some kind of intermediate between heaven and earth, which seems to be the symbolic space of equilibrium that the two characters have finally found.

Medem has been reproached for the predominantly male perspective of his early movies by critics who regard this as a sign of an underlying machismo

(Stone 2007: 167). Indeed, Medem focuses on men who have narcissistic problems deciding between several women, but the director is quite conscious of that and always inserts a self-reflexive symbolic level in which man and woman can be read as artist and artwork. The highly symbolic charge of Medem's movies may lead sexuality itself to be considered merely as a metaphor for the artist's creative act. This allegorical reading allows, for example, for an understanding of the recurrent motif of incest in his movies (Junkerjürgen, 2012: 338-42). Still, Medem has reacted to the critical voices with his last movie, *Habitación en Roma* (2010), which stages a lesbian one-night-stand, focussing exclusively on female desire and passion.

One might conclude that even in the case of an internationally recognized *auteur*, the representation of sexual matters from the male perspective tends to be increasingly politically incorrect. This impression is confirmed by a final look at a relatively new phenomenon: the creation of pornography by women for women, which broaches the issue of sexual addiction in a different way.

Freeing Women, Incriminating Men – *Diario de una ninfómana* vs. *Shame*

Especially in the last two decades adult literature and films by women have increasingly entered the market and in some cases became extraordinarily successful, attracting enormous media attention. In France Catherine Breillat (*1948) achieved international recognition with her movie *Romance* (1999), in Germany Charlotte Roche's (*1978) novel *Feuchtgebiete* (2008) became a bestseller, and in Spain the French author Valérie Tasso (*1969), who has lived in Barcelona since 1991, sold more than 200.000 copies of her autobiographical *Diario de una ninfómana* (2003), which was made into a film in 2008.

This general development has at least three dimensions, since it has the potential to be politically, commercially, and aesthetically innovative. Politically, it is to be placed in the context of pro-sex feminist theory, which argues that pornography is an essential aspect of sex politics and that it is in the interest of women to produce their own visual code of sexual pleasure which acts as a counterpart to the stereotypes of conventional, i.e. male porn discourse. The commercial side relies on the belief that female consumers of pornography represent a market which has not yet been fully exploited (Supp 2012: 57). The aesthetic challenge, finally, consists of finding a convincing code of visualization, motives, and narrative techniques.

In Spain the Swedish director Erika Lust (*1977) published a sort of manifesto with *Porno para mujeres* (2008), which presents not only the theoretical part of the enterprise but also a history of female porn. Conceived as an introduction to the subject, the book is full of pedagogical comments on teaching the differences between male and female porn, and the way how women can use pornography effectively for their pleasure (Lust 2009: 97-217) – though the large number of sex products she proposes makes it impossible to distinguish whether Lust wants to free women by teaching them pro-sex theory or to transform them into female porn consumers.

In *Diario de una ninfómana* Valérie Tasso pursues a comparable politico-pedagogical project, declaring herself to be a feminist who wants to liberate female sexuality from male societal limits. The plot of the book can be considered a kind of sexual *Bildungsroman* in autobiographical form, which portrays the erotic quest for self-fulfilment in young Val, who is much more attracted by fleeting sexual encounters than by the idea of falling in love and having a stable relationship.

The book was adapted for the screen by Christian Molina (*1979). The script was written by Tasso herself in cooperation with Cuca Canals, who had worked successfully with Bigas Luna in the 1990s. Though the movie is full of sex scenes, the production features performances by such prestigious actors as Geraldine Chaplin or Ángela Molina, both of them icons of the Spanish *auteurist* cinema of opposition and in many instances linked to criticism of machismo. Chaplin was for many years the partner and the muse of Carlos Saura, playing, for example, the eponymous heroine in *Ana y los lobos* (1973), who is raped and murdered by three brothers who represent the three Spanish "Juans" of manhood, the military genius Juan de Austria, the mystic San Juan, and the womanizer Don Juan. Ángela Molina in turn worked with Buñuel, Gutiérrez Aragón, Borau, and Bigas Luna, and played a victim of machismo on more than one occasion: in *L'ingorgo* (Luigi Comencini; 1978), her character is raped by a group of young men, for example, while in Almodóvar's *Carne trémula* (1997) she plays a woman who is subjected to violence by her husband.

While the casting demonstrates that *Diario de una ninfómana* aspires to be a serious movie about female sexuality, by using the term nymphomania the title sounds both anachronistic and sexist. But already in the beginning the movie explains how nymphomania is to be understood. Val's grandmother (Geraldine Chaplin), whose wisdom authorizes her to define the pedagogical project of her grandchild, declares:

> Ninfomanía: un invento de los hombres para que las mujeres se sientan culpables si se salen de la norma. Cada uno es como es. Nunca renuncies a algo que realmente anhelas porque luego te arrepentirás. Para mí, lo que te pasa es que no te atreves a vivir tu vida.

> Nymphomania: an invention of men in order to make women feel guilty if they don't correspond to the norm. Everybody is like they are. Don't you ever renounce something which you really desire because you will regret it later. I believe that your problem is that you don't dare to live your life.

> (21'45, my translation)

The title thus quotes male repressive vocabulary in order to rectify it and to present a narrative manifesto for a liberalization of female sexuality. This strategy, though at first sight misleading, might be quite successful in attracting a public used to sexist stereotypes in order to break clichés and open up innovative perspectives on the subject.[2]

In order to suggest authenticity, Tasso chose the form of an autobiographical report (underlined in the book by precise locations of time and space). In the film, the action is constantly accompanied from off-screen by Val's voice, which comments or reads parts from her diary. In this sense, the movie wants to be a case study, a document which refuses to be categorized as fiction. For the part of Val the director chose Belén Fabra, an actress who looks similar to Tasso. Apart from this, Tasso has a cameo where she stands behind Fabra, implying an identification of author, actress, and character (fig. 1).

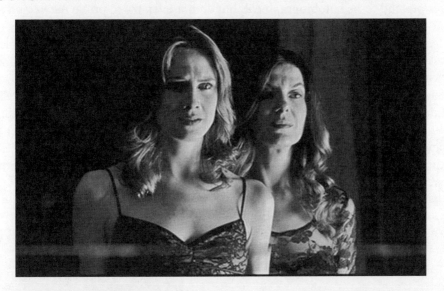

Fig. 1: Tasso's cameo blends character and author (*Diario de una ninfómana*; 1'11'50)

The character is provided with a "sensibilidad especial" (Tasso 2010: 19) and her life is marked by constant sexual arousal and a permanent change of sex partners, a life style based on a materialist philosophy which considers life a form of "pura energía" and sexuality as a way of mixing one's energies with another person's (Tasso 2010: 41).

An important part of the book and the movie talks about her time working in a brothel, a key political issue for Tasso, who tries to demystify prostitution and

[2] This is why it is quite regrettable that in the United States and the United Kingdom the film was released under the title *Insatiable – Diary of a Sex Addict*.

represents it as an important experience in her life. Val's reasons for justifying her decision to sell her body are an inextricable mixture of financial problems, curiosity, dislike of men, and lack of self esteem (Tasso 2010: 179). The representation of prostitution is in the end more positive than negative, because Val does not only earn money but leads a life full of surprises.

Tasso is not the only example for the popularization of a liberal view on prostitution. The Italian Sonia Rossi, a student of mathematics in Berlin, published a very similar autobiographical report called *Fucking Berlin* (2008), which relates how she financed her studies by working in brothels, like Tasso breaking with a lot of clichés about prostitution and stating in the end that women who decide freely to work in a brothel are not more exploited than by doing any other job. Though Rossi did not choose the form of a diary both texts are marked by the same episodic narrative rhythm. It is needless to say that both cases pretend to be autobiographical, but do not even try to prove the veracity of their reports.

Another political topic is the promotion of female masturbation. While Lust gives quite concrete advice in her manifesto how women should go about seeking pleasure (Lust 2009: 211-17), Tasso's Val recommends dildos to a friend, and even the film poster stresses the idea of independent female lust. The similarity of the film poster of *Diario de una ninfómana* and Catherine Breillat's *Romance* is not a coincidence, but part of a program (fig. 2 and 3). In fact the protagonist of *Romance* explains why she masturbates and why she does it without spreading her legs: to demonstrate that she does not need a man to feel pleasure (1'01'10).

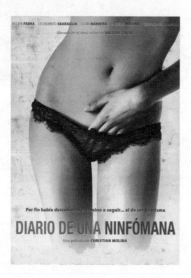 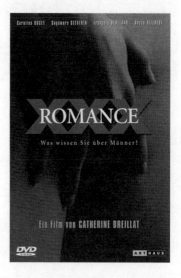

Fig. 2 & 3: Masturbation as a political message: discover yourself and free yourself from men!

Though Val feels lonely as all her attempts to have a stable relationship fail, in the end she learns to be alone and to accept the way she is. The last monologue suggests that the process of self-identification is complete:

> Soy una mujer promiscua, sí, porque pretendo utilizar el sexo como medio para encontrar lo que todo el mundo busca: reconocimiento, placer, autoestima y en definitiva amor y cariño. ¿Qué hay de patológico en eso? Si queréis ponerme un nombre, adelante, no me importa. Pero sabed que lo que soy en realidad es una nereida, una driada, una ninfa, sencillamente.

> I am a promiscous woman, yes, because I intend to use sex as a means of finding what everybody is searching for: pleasure, self-esteem and finally love and tenderness. What is sick about that? If you want to give me a name, come on, I don't care. But you have to know that in reality I am just a nereid, a dryad and a nymph.

(1'31'45, my translation)

Generally feminists agree with the idea that women should be free to live their sexuality just as they want to and that it is no longer bound to marriage or love. But one problem of the movie remains unresolved until the end – the relationship of sex and love. Val lives a sexually free and self-determined life, with the number and type of partners she wants. Though sex is – as she says in the end – a way to experience love, she does not really succeed. In the main romantic episode with Jaime (Leonardo Sbaraglia), love and sex remain disconnected themes, since Jaime is a very bad lover, but (at least in the beginning) a loving partner. The movie presents a montage sequence full of conventional images of happiness: beautiful and wealthy people, sunshine, silhouettes in front of the sea, nostalgic piano music, symbolic images like balloons which fly into the sky, etc. The conventional wish to be normal and conventional happiness both come to an end when Val discovers that Jaime is a liar and was constantly cheating on her.

The disconnection of love and sex leads to the conclusion that freeing sex from emotion also means freeing emotion from sex. The feminist journalist Natasha Walter has drawn attention to this problem and believes that this disconnection impedes emotional happiness, as it brings a new generation of young women up to regard sex as a barter trade, never experiencing real intimacy (Walter 2011: 128). The same goes for Val in the movie: In the end she is absolutely free and has found her identity – but she is still alone.

While the nymphs and dryads triumph, Don Juan seems to have disappeared completely from the scene. But it is only Don Juan's positive which has died, his negative is more alive than ever before. Direct references like *Don Juan DeMarco* (Francis Ford Coppola, 1995) carefully deconstruct the popular character by limiting his sexual activities to pure fantasy, the daydreams of a young man in psychiatric treatment, played by Johnny Depp. More recently the male sex addict has found a popular incarnation in Charlie Sheen playing Charlie Harper in one of the world's most successful television series up to date, *Two and a Half Men* (2003-2010). In the line of Almodóvar's ironical use of psycho-analysis, Harper is a character who combines a good dose of sexist humour with popular conceptions of an oedipal complex. The character overlaps with the public image of the actor, who is known for drug and alcohol problems and re-lationships with adult film actresses.

Yet another movie, the British film *Shame* (Steve McQueen, 2011), can be regarded as a perfect masculine equivalent to *Diario de una ninfómana*. It tells the story of handsome, thirty-something Brandon (Michael Fassbender), who lives and works in New York. Under the elegant and cold surface of the big city Brandon is seeking out superficial sexual contacts in the form of one-night-stands or encounters with prostitutes. While for Tasso's female character pro-miscuity is presented as a sexual quest in search of identity, Brandon's behavi-our is clearly labelled as pathological. His incapacity to form emotional bonds reduces him to superficial relationships and strikes him with impotence as soon as a relationship with a woman becomes personal. Though McQueen tries to avoid causal explanations for Brandon's sexual addiction, he hints indirectly at the impact of the big city with its impersonal and anonymous ambiance. In one of the key scenes Brandon watches a couple having sex in front of the huge window of a hotel room, a position which he will soon imitate with a prostitute, taking her from behind while he has a view over the city and the sea. This emblem of male dominance over space and the female body is everything but triumphant since Brandon's coolness turns out to be a sign of his emotional in-capacity and no more than a wall around his loneliness.

While Tasso's Val is constantly making personal remarks from off-screen and thus opens all the doors for identification, McQueen's Brandon remains distant and cold; while Val regards onanism, sex toys and even prostitution as ways of exploring herself, Brandon is a compulsive masturbator and punter, a user of internet porn sites, and a reader of porn magazines. Though it is not clear if the sex products should be regarded as a reason for, or a result of Brandon's compulsive sexual behaviour, it definitely becomes clear that he is a patho-logical case for whom both the male and the female spectator may feel pity. *Shame* turns out to be a diagnosis of and a warning against promiscuity. In contrast *Diario de una ninfómana* presents an example of a self-determined wo-man who develops a personal program of self-exploration via sex in the context of sex-positive feminist theory.

But it is not only that the male sex addicts are stigmatised, men generally appear to belong to a decadent species in these texts and movies. It is hard to find a "normal" man in Tasso, Rossi or McQueen. All of them seem to be driven by sexual instinct or hedonistic desires, unwilling to take responsibility for their wives and families. In Rossi the protagonist is married and opts for prostitution because her husband is a never-do-well who sits at home drinking beer with his friends and who is unable to find a job or to concentrate on any work (Rossi 2008: 265); most of the other men are punters who in most cases have ridiculous sexual fantasies and cannot be taken seriously either (Rossi 2008: 244). After viewing these movies and reading these books one is convinced that the male sex must be an error of evolution.

Beyond Gender: How Sex Addiction May Melt into Pluralism

The comparison of recent movies on sex addiction shows that the traditional scheme of heroic Don Juan and pathological nymphomaniac has in many cases simply been inverted. Women are entering the pornography market and proudly subscribe to sex-positive feminist theory and claim their right to promiscuity. On the contrary, the representation of male promiscuity puts men under suspicion of degrading women by treating them as objects, of being blindly driven by ego-istic desire and of urgently needing psychological help. Conventional images of male pleasure are rendered vulnerable to suggestions of being politically in-correct. This goes so far that even internationally acclaimed *auteurs* like Julio Medem are criticised for sexism.

The inversion is also observable on the aesthetic level. Female porn risks becoming as generic as conventional pornography because it has a strong ten-dency to merely exchange the archetypes of the male variant for the female: instead of male orgasm it ends with the female one, it puts cunnilingus in the place of fellatio or replaces expressions of male power fantasies with images of partnership based on emotional proximity. The first tale of Erika Lust's soft porn film *Love Life Lust* (2010) ends with declarations of love after the sexual act and the happy surprise that the woman is pregnant. Though the female variant sounds much more likeable than the male one, it hardly offers a broader panorama of motives.

The emergence of a female variant of pornography is highly welcome as a counterweight to male standards, to enrich the narrative pool, and even to edu-cate the public in female fantasies. But this should not imply the degradation of men and male fantasies. Taking a closer look at popular narratives and images has shown that the evaluation of sexual addiction, though inverted, remains deeply gendered. While women's attitude is applauded generously and associ-ated with the positive values of individualism and self-fulfilment, men's sexual addiction is primarily regarded as pathological and dangerous.

One might consider this as a backlash after thousands of years of patriarchy, but it fits too well into the current general suspicion of so-called typical male behaviour and the tendency to incriminate men. This negative andrology, as cultural studies calls it, described men as being violent and driven by instincts, while women are regarded as being the saviours of humanity (Kucklick 2008; Döge 2011).

If gender is a performative category, the movies of Tasso and McQueen work simply by inverting the schema and producing new differentiations between the genders. This can obviously not be the right way to free both sexes from oppressive or at least restrictive conventions. Maybe the path which Almodóvar followed after the flippancy of his postmodern beginnings is noteworthy in this respect. In his engagement with the question of sexual identity the director most recently entered a post-biological phase in *Todo sobre mi madre*, which corresponds to the performative theory in gender studies. Now that plastic surgery allows for the transformation of both sex and body, everyone is free to design himself and put pluralism in the place of dichotomies.

In fact the so-called post-porn movement in Spain has taken the torch, and is trying to overcome the fundamental notion that there is porn for men and porn for women. The founders of the movement in Spain – María Llopis and Agueda Bañon – fight against the concept of gender in general, which they consider to be a popular emblem for the construction of differences. Beyond gender, there is no need for male or female porn, and no need for Don Juans or nymphomaniacs, but rather space for a multiplicity of desires which can no longer be categorized (Prada 2012: 153). Instead of boys and girls, there would just be individuals, and porn as a manifestation of sex would be as varied as the people. It may be that the scenario which Llopis and Bañon sketch out and try to teach in numerous workshops has utopian facets, but it would definitively free women and men from gendered concepts, and not only of sex addiction.

List of Works Cited

Döge, Peter. *Männer – die ewigen Gewalttäter? Gewalt von und gegen Männer in Deutschland.* Wiesbaden: VS Verl. für Sozialwissenschaften, 2011.

Franzbach, Martin. "Mitos de la Generación del 98: Don Juan". *'Una de las dos Españas...'. Representaciones de un conflicto identitario en la historia y en las literaturas hispánicas. Estudios reunidos en homenaje a Manfred Tietz,* 2007. 441-46.

Freud, Sigmund. "Drei Abhandlungen zur Sexualtheorie." *Gesammelte Werke.* Vol. 5. Frankfurt: S. Fischer, 1963. 27-145.

Groneman, Carol. *Nymphomanie. Die Geschichte einer Obsession.* Frankfurt: Campus, 2001.

Junkerjürgen, Ralf. "'Quelle joie d'avoir assassiné nos enfants' – Niños y jóvenes en el cine de Buñuel". *Luis Buñuel: dos mundos. Una aportación hispano-alemana a un cine antitético.* Ed. Patricia Cavielles and Gerhard Poppenberg. Berlin: Tranvía, 2011. 125-43.

---. "Julio Medem: *Lucía y el sexo* (2001)." *Spanische Filme des 20. Jahrhunderts in Einzeldarstellungen.* Berlin: Erich Schmidt, 2012, 327-44.

Kinsey, Alfred, et al. *Sexual Behaviour in the Human Female*. Philadelphia: W.B. Saunders, 1953.

Kowalsky, Daniel. "Rated S: Softcore Pornography and the Spanish Transition to Democracy, 1977-82." *Spanish Popular Cinema*. Ed. Antonio Lázaro-Reboll and Andrew Willis. Manchester: Manchester UP, 2004. 188-208.

Kucklick, Christoph. *Das unmoralische Geschlecht. Zur Geburt der negativen Andrologie*. Frankfurt am Main: Suhrkamp, 2008.

Lust, Erika. *X-Porno für Frauen*. München: Wilhelm Heyne, 2009.

Paredes Méndez, Francisca. "Las hijas de Don Juan de Blanca de los Ríos y otros textos: Donjuanismo y flamenquismo vs. regeneración nacional." *Espéculo: Revista de Estudios Literarios* 35 (2007). n. p.

Pennone, Florence. "Aspects démoniaques de Don Juan ou les ambiguïtés d'un personnage entre comique et tragique". *Colloquium Helveticum. Cahiers Suisses de Littérature Générale et Comparée* 36 (2005) : 181-207.

Prada, Nancy. "Todas las caperucintas rojas se vuelven lobos en la práctica pornográfica". *Cadernos Pagu* 38 (2012): 129-58.

Preuk, Monika. "Sind Sie sexsüchtig?" *FOCUS Online*. Accessed 07 July 2012. http://www.focus.de/gesundheit/ratgeber/sexualitaet/ tests/sexsucht/test_aid_15270.html.

Rossi, Sonia. *Fucking Berlin*. Berlin: Ullstein, 2010.

Stone, Rob. *Julio Medem*. Manchester: Manchester UP, 2007.

Supp, Barbara. "Was will das Weib?". *Der Spiegel* 30 (2012): 57.

Tasso, Valérie. *Diario de una ninfómana*. Barcelona: Debols!llo, 2010.

Villa, Paula-Irene. "Pornofeminismus? Soziologische Überlegungen zur Fleischbeschau im Pop." *Banale Kämpfe? Perspektiven auf Populärkultur und Geschlecht*. Ed. Paula-Irene Villa et al. Wiesbaden: Springer, 2012. 229-47.

Unamuno, Miguel de. *Obras completas*. Vol. 4. Barcelona: Vergara, 1954.

Walter, Natasha. *Living dolls. Warum junge Frauen heute lieber schön als schlau sein wollen*. Frankfurt: Krüger, 2011.

Wright, Sarah. "Gregorio Marañón and The Cult of Sex: Effeminacy and Intersexuality in 'The Psychopathology of Don Juan' (1924)". *Bulletin of Spanish Studies* 81.6 (2004): 717-38.

Katharina Boehm

Gender and Medical Realism in the Poetry of Donald Hall

In his recent memoir, *Unpacking the Boxes: A Memoir of Life in Poetry* (2008), former US poet laureate Donald Hall relates the experience of his first stroke and the surgery performed on his carotid artery that followed:

> Toward the end of the procedure, Dr. Harbaugh lifted in front of me a strange object that had occluded my blood flow – it was whitish, fat as a fountain pen, maybe two inches long. I touched it; it was hard, my self-created self-destroyer. Could I take it home with me? I wanted to keep it under glass, with my collection of small antiquities from Etruscany and Greece and Phoenicia. Dr. Harbaugh refused; these carapaces go to Pathology.
>
> (Hall 2008: 180-81)

This passage, penned late in a long writing life on which illness has impacted in profound and public ways, crystallises recurring concerns in Hall's literary engagement with disease. When Hall refers to the artery plaques as "self-created self-destroyer", stringing together two hyphenated compounds which link the self to acts of creation and destruction respectively, he draws attention to the existential quality of an illness that threatens the self's integrity. However, the scene is also wryly comic: Hall's half-serious plan to conserve the plaque re-moved from his artery under glass alongside small antiquities from Europe is thwarted by the doctor's laconic comment that "carapaces go to Pathology". An object that bestows visible shape on the experience of illness – the plaque in this case – may hold significant meaning for the individual, but as this object circu-lates through the hospital apparatus, it first becomes a specimen for pathological examination and later mere waste material. Hall is conscious of this mismatch between the patient's subjective emotional investment and the hospital staff's more pragmatic stance. However, unlike many of his literary colleagues he does not admonish doctors for 'medicalising' the patient and his or her experience; instead he treats this disparity in perspective with humour and sympathy. Most importantly, Hall compares the "strange object that had occluded [his] blood flow" to a writing implement, a "fountain pen". At various times in Hall's life, but particularly so during his and his wife Jane Kenyon's cancer treatments in the 1980s and 1990s, disease staked out the conditions of Hall's writing – determining his physical and intellectual ability to work, defining the subject matter of his poetry and life writing, and triggering formal experimentation.

"Writing about cancer", Hall points out in another memoir, *Life Work* (1993), "allows me to transcend my cancer by the syntax or rhetoric of dread and suffering" (Hall 1993a: 67-68). It is an uncharacteristically grandiloquent statement for Hall, but his emphasis on "syntax" and "rhetoric" serves as an apt reminder that his translations of illness into writing, for all their diversity in style and genre, grow from disciplined attention to form.

In this essay, I offer readings of selected poems from three consecutive verse volumes – Hall's *The Museum of Clear Ideas* (1993), *The Old Life* (1996) and *Without* (1998) – to ask how the "syntax and rhetoric of dread and suffering" shapes Hall's vision of medicine, the contiguity between illness and (creative) work, and the diseased subject's relation to the social and inanimate world. An exploration of these recurring themes in Hall's poetry must take into account that both experience of and writing about illness are gendered processes. Gender is a particularly pertinent lens through which to consider Hall's poems because he writes about his own cancer – in terms that often place the illness in the context of socially constructed masculinity – as well as about Jane Kenyon's suffering and death from leukaemia. Hall was first diagnosed with colon cancer in 1989 at the age of sixty-one. Despite surgery the cancer had started to metastasise to his liver by 1992. He underwent chemotherapy and another surgery to have more than half of his liver removed. Medical prognosis was not promising for Hall, but he went into remission and the cancer has not returned to this day. Kenyon, herself an acclaimed poet, died at only forty-seven after twenty-three years of marriage with Hall. At the time of her death in 1995, she was New Hampshire's poet laureate and working on her fifth collection of poetry, entitled *Otherwise*, which was published posthumously in 1996. Kenyon was diagnosed with two different kinds of cancer – in 1985, a malignant tumour, more precisely a mucoepidermoid carcinoma, was discovered on her neck and removed operatively; in 1994, Kenyon and Hall learned that she had leukaemia. Unlike Hall, Kenyon did not write extensively about her own or her husband's cancer, and while my essay looks at Kenyon's work in passing, the principal focus is on Hall.[1] While critics such as Jeffrey Berman, Todd F. Davis and Kenneth Womack have begun to examine Hall's cancer writings with a view to the poetic enactment of grief and to "the ethics of mourning" encoded in his texts (Berman 2010: 133-56; Davis and Womack 2005: 166-78), less attention has been directed at Hall's reflections on the disease itself, on medicine and the life of the patient, and at the formal structures that contain them.

---

[1] Kenyon writes in more detail about the effects of her depression, most famously in "Having It Out With Melancholy".

"The Enchanted Grid": The Poetics of Disease, Work and Baseball

Hall's *The Museum of Clear Ideas* includes two long poems, one entitled "Baseball" and the other "Extra Innings", which frame their meditation on the place of illness in human life with an extended formal engagement with the structure of baseball games. Lines of thought begun in these texts are continued in another long poem, "The Thirteenth Inning", published in the collection *The Old Life*. Hall has called baseball "the poet's game" (Hall 1985: 57-63); he has been a baseball fan and supporter of the Red Sox his entire adult life, and he has written extensively about the sport, producing two prose books, *Dock Ellis in the Country of Baseball* (1976) and *Fathers Playing Catch with Sons* (1985), many magazine articles and some poems which deal with baseball.

"Baseball", "Extra Innings" and "The Thirteenth Inning" concentrate mostly on Hall's rather than Kenyon's illness and they locate the experience of cancer in a poetic sphere of references that is overwhelmingly male-oriented. For Hall, the cultural value of baseball derives in part from the bonds which it forges between men. He notes in an essay entitled "Baseball and the Meaning of Life" (1997), "Baseball connects American males with each other, not only through bleacher friendships and neighbour loyalties, not only through barroom fights, but most importantly through generations" (Hall 1997: 154). Hall's baseball poems build on this idea: they evoke intergenerational links between male artists and sportsmen, summoning living and deceased figures – including Henry James, Henry Moore, Kurt Schwitters and a number of famous baseball players – as interlocutors. Hall tracks his experiences with illness, ageing and the (in)-ability to work against the biographies of these male artists and athletes, while also linking his reflections on these issues to questions of poetic form. In "Baseball and the Meaning of Life", Hall observes that baseball is good to think with:

> baseball sets off the meaning of life precisely because it is pure of meaning. As the ripples in the sand, in the Kyoto garden, organize and formalize the dust which is dust, so the diamonds and rituals of baseball create an elegant, trivial, enchanted grid on which our suffering, shapeless, sinful day leans for the momentary grace of order.

(Hall 1997: 155)

Baseball's formal organisation – the "enchanted grid" which supplies "the momentary grace of order" – is the pattern on which Hall's baseball poems are structured. In professional baseball games, teams of nine players each compete for nine innings; if the score is tied after these regular innings, so-called extra innings are played to decide the match. The number nine anchors the symmetrical balance of "Baseball": the poem falls into nine sections each of which is comprised of nine numbered stanzas with nine lines of nine syllables each.

"Extra Innings" consists of three sections – "The Tenth Inning", "The Eleventh Inning" and the "Twelfth Inning" – made up, respectively, of ten, eleven and twelve numbered stanzas and corresponding numbers of lines and syllables per line. In what follows, I trace how experiences of ageing and disease impact on the "grid" – the formal constraints – of the baseball poems. Hall suggests in his poems that these experiences alter the individual's perception of time and its passing; as a result, the mathematical exactitude that we find in "Baseball" gradually gives way to the more experimental pattern of "The Thirteenth Inning".

"Baseball" touches on a variety of topics – the Connecticut of Hall's childhood, his marriage, the creative-writing industry – but its guiding theme is male old age. The speaker of the poem, Hall's alter ego "K.C.", notes: "We age past the field / so quickly; we diminish, watching / over decades, observing the young / as they dodder" (Hall 1993b: 21). K.C.'s baseball heroes – John Tudor, Dock Ellis and George 'Shotgun' Shuba – were in their prime in the 1940s and 1950s (Tudor), and the 1960s and 1970s (Ellis, Shuba), respectively. At the time of the poem's conception they are long retired or deceased. Framing his own life story within references to the biographies of these baseball stars, K.C. reveals his attraction to an older model of mid-twentieth century masculinity – one rooted in ideals of physical strength, sportsmanship and national pride – even as he wryly notes the outdatedness of this model:

> 7. All winter aged ballplayers try
> rehearsing their young manhood, running
> and throwing in Florida's sunshine;
> they remain old. In my sixtieth
> year I wake fretting over some new
> failure.
>
> (Hall 1993b: 21)

Like Hall, K.C. is a poet and he looks to other male artists when thinking about what it means to produce art in the face of death: "I dreamed // 9. of old Ezra Pound" (Hall 1993b: 18); "I felt / troubled about another old man: / Henry Moore wheelchaired at Perry Green" (Hall 1993b: 18). Hall has often described the sculptor Henry Moore as the greatest influence on his work. "Of all the older artists I've known, he's made the most difference for my own writing" (Hall, 1991: 154). In *Life Work*, Hall points out that Moore's complete absorption in his artistic labour – "Henry Moore is a model of work" (Hall 1993a: 51) – speaks to Hall's own approach to writing: "I find that work remains the matter, not only in defiance of death but in plain sight of it; it absorbs me more nearly than anything else" (Hall 1993a: 68). Fear of death and artistic failure are a constant presence in "Baseball" but K.C. suggests that both can be kept in check by disciplined "devotion" to work – be it the poet's craft or the baseball player's physical exercise – or by sexual intimacy:

> Baseball, like sexual intercourse
> and art, stops short, for a moment, the
> indecent continuous motion
> of time forward, implying our death
> and imminent decomposition.

(Hall 1993b: 35)

Time is here imagined as an incessant flow, linear and forward-moving, beyond human control and, therefore, threatening. K.C.'s notion of art as a means to stop time would seem clichéd without the poem's focus on art as craft and technique, art as "work". K.C. showcases his scrupulous attention to form throughout "Baseball": "the momentary grace of order" which the poem sets against time's unrestrainable hurtling forward is won through the careful arrangement of numbered stanzas, measured lines and syllables according to "the laboratory method / of purity, physics of nine times / nine times nine times nine" (Hall 1993b: 15). The image of Moore, the senescent workaholic in a wheelchair, from "Baseball" reappears in *Life Work*: "The work survives the worker: Henry Moore without memory sketching in a wheelchair, Henry James on the bed of paralysis speaking a senseless syntax" (Hall 1993a: 116). Hall renders the old artist who has lost part of his mental faculties but continues to be productive as a heroic figure, suggesting that it is not necessarily artistic value but craft that defies evanescence.

"Extra Innings" and "The Thirteenth Inning" shift the focus from old age to illness. Hall wrote these poems at a time in which he was suffering from colon cancer and Kenyon was recovering from her first cancer. Hall continues to use K.C.'s voice to narrate his experience with cancer in "Extra Innings": "What does K.C. stand for", asks the poem and goes on to supply a list that foregrounds cancer's impact on the identity of the male patient before dissolving into comic relief: "Kurt Carcinoma? Kid / Chumpleheart? Kitsch Champion? Kitchen Cat? Kup Cake?" (Hall 1993b: 114). K.C. describes himself as one of the already "posthumous": "We nod at each other; we / acknowledge pain, baseball, lethargy, and cracks / in the bedroom ceiling" (Hall 1993b: 107). For the "post-humous", stopping time – by means of poetic craft, sex or baseball – seems no longer possible or, indeed, desirable. Instead, K.C. turns again to baseball to articulate the therapeutic vision of an alternative temporality:

> I begin to understand what matters
> in this daily game. Listen: Baseball is types

5. of continuousness, simultaneous
hours not consecutive ones, independent
temporalities that gather ongoing
moments into a perpetual present

(Hall 1993b: 108)

"The Thirteenth Inning" continues to engage with cancer while exploring how the meaning of these "simultaneous hours" could be grasped and how they could be rendered in aesthetic terms. The poem shifts rapidly between different locales and moments in time – including the hospital in New Hampshire where Hall underwent cancer surgery, the Protestant Cemetery at Rome, Bombay and Agra, the domestic interior of John Singer Sargent's *The Daughters of Edward D. Boit* and various baseball games. A snapshot of Hall's surgery is framed by scenes that are removed both in time and space:

Dr. Sutton performed
resection. Morphine in ICU, five minute sleep
alternating with five minutes of writhing, tubes twisted
like spider legs. I remembered my friend William Trout
and Reba, who crawled into his deathbed carefully

6. to administer her warm body. For "writhing" read
"writing" throughout, as Hanuman and Ganesh appeared
bringing floral pots and intravenous nirvana.
When I woke in ICU – Abigail six days old –
I trashed among seven tubes and hoses. Unable
to speak for respiring, I punched buttons to raise up
the Red Sox playing the Orioles. Who won that game?
In the cemetery at Rome, avenues of damp
and ivied marble clutter with cats and eminent
Prostestant dead. Last year at the Whitehouse I observed
Ted Williams and Joe DiMaggio, both tall and gray,
leaning in the doorway and smiling while the awkward
president alluded to seasons fifty years past.

(Hall 2006: 286)

The morphine summons another of Hall's literary alter egos, the poet William Trout, who is "posthumous" insofar as Hall imagined him dead in "Another Elegy: In Memory of William Trout", the opening poem of *The Museum of Clear Ideas*. In Hall's vision, Trout is quickly followed by the Hindi deities Hanuman and Ganesh, here cast as morphinic muses which assist Hall in turning the experience of "writhing" among "tubes and hoses" into verse. The poem then moves on to the cemetery in Rome, which Hall and Kenyon had visited years earlier, and to one of Hall's visits to the White House. Quick succession of impressions and localities features also in "Baseball" and "Extra Innings", but it is used as structuring device in a much more radical manner in "The Thirteenth Inning". This latter work also breaks with the formal rigidness of the earlier poems, inserting a two-page long prose segment half way through the poem. The prose section expands on topics discussed elsewhere in "The Third Inning" and it groups together, apparently haphazardly, short paragraphs on the bio-graphies of Edward D. Boit's daughters, on a prolonged baseball game and on Hall and Kenyon's visit to India. The end of the prose fragment holds the key to the poem's organisation:

> The game is collage, Kurt: smells of Calcutta pasted next to shreds of a liver biopsy, Ted Williams wriggling in two dimensions on a nineteen forty-one baseball card thumbtacked with a swatch of red hair swept from Salvatore's floor, catpiss from the Protestant Cemetery, Ganesh pitching with six baseballs at once. Mary Louisa Boit in pigment, and Bill Trout drunk as dirt in the empty bleachers as the rain stops.

(Hall 2006: 288)

Hall suggests that patients who suffer from life-threatening conditions may experience time not as a linear, progressive movement but as a "collage" – a synchronic web of "ongoing moments" gathered into "a perpetual present". As cancer threatens extinction (Hall calls the poem "this last enterprise"; Hall 2006: 291), recollections of childhood and more recent family gatherings, fictional alter egos, memories of travels, professional activities and baseball games are re-lived or vividly imagined, transporting them into the present moment. In an earlier part of the poem, Hall comments on "baseball's enterprise of on-goingness, / which is the name of everything assembled together" (Hall 2006: 285). In the collage that is "The Thirteenth Inning", "everything assembled together" accumulates a force that constantly spills beyond the contours of the poem's thirteen-stanza structure, necessitating the integration of the prose fragments and a final affirmation of the "enterprise of ongoingness":

> Breathing I glue together these anthems and cutouts
> of the thirteenth inning although the game is over.
>
> 14. But not the poem. The thirteenth inning goes to fourteen
> stanzas.

(Hall 2006: 291)

Cancer Metaphors and the Ethics of Representation

The three long poems discussed above concentrate mostly on Hall's rather than Kenyon's illness. Kenyon (named "Jennifer" in the poems) speaks very rarely in these pieces. Particularly in "Baseball", K.C. takes voyeuristic pleasure in observing Jennifer's body when she is not aware of his gaze ("as Jenny pauses / by the kitchen sink and looks idly / out the window, I gaze at her ass", Hall 1993b: 223; "I stare happily at / linen that covers her slender hips / at her thighs and knees", Hall 1993b: 232). As Hall recounts in *The Best Day the Worst Day: Life with Jane Kenyon* (2005), he and Kenyon collaborated closely on their poetry, reading each other's drafts and recommending revisions. It can be assumed, then, that Kenyon did not object to the manner in which she is represented in "Baseball", but this does not necessarily make these passages less jarring. Voyeurism, like other ethically compromised representational manoeuvres, becomes exceedingly problematic in cases where sickness prevents the person represented from responding to the work of art that depicts her/his suffering (see DeShazer 2009: 215-36; Pollock 2008: 213-35). Hall's poetry about Kenyon's cancer indicates that he was conscious of these pitfalls and went to extraordinary lengths to avoid them.

Kenyon found it almost impossible to write new poems during leukaemia (although she revised a number of older poems during this period). One of only two new poems penned after the diagnosis is a short piece entitled "The Sick Wife":

> The sick wife stayed in the car
> while he bought a few groceries.
> Not yet fifty,
> she had learned what it's like
> not to be able to button a button.

                                                                    (Kenyon 1996: 221)

The woman in the poem is identified both as "sick" and as a "wife". The word "wife" immediately evokes the absent partner and the next line promptly introduces a man – referred to familiarly as "he" instead of using a name or relationship status such as "the husband". Intimacy and dependency are woven together in the poem: the sick wife is immobilised and cannot leave the car on her own, while "he" carries out quotidian tasks (grocery shopping) and, presumably, acts as her caregiver, buttoning buttons she can no longer operate.

Hall wrote many of the poems collected in *Without* by Kenyon's bedside at home and in the hospital, and he read them to her occasionally: "I believe that Jane liked it, me writing these poems. Poetry was after all the tremendous commonness between us. At least one of us was writing poems, I writing the poems that she could not write – about what she was going through" (Hall 2006: 94). The purpose of my discussion here is not to speculate about Kenyon's views on these poems, which she did not document in writing. Instead, I explore two defining features of Hall's poetry about Kenyon's leukaemia which engage with the question of how to write in an ethical manner about suffering and pain that affects another. These features are, first, Hall's engagement with traditional cancer metaphors and, second, his depiction of the relationship between the female patient and modern medicine.

The metaphors that cluster in each given cultural moment around cancer have come under close scrutiny since Susan Sontag's seminal *Illness as Metaphor* (1978) disclosed the power of metaphors in shaping not only cultural ideas about cancer but also the medical treatment and social life of patients. Sontag revealed links between two seemingly separate discourses which attach metaphors to cancer: first, the language used by medical researchers and practitioners which brims with military metaphors of war, attack, and defeat; and second, a whole range of discourses which use "cancer, and the metaphors we have imposed on it" as "vehicle for the large insufficiencies of this culture, for our shallow attitude toward death, for our anxieties about feeling, [...] for our inability to construct an advanced industrial society which properly regulates consumption, and for our justified fears of the increasingly violent course of history" (Sontag 2001: 87). Writing in the late seventies, Sontag was looking forward to a future in which the increased curability of cancer would result in the "de-mythologiz[ation]" of the illness, suggesting that "it may then be possible to compare something to cancer without implying either a fatalistic diagnosis or a rousing call to fight [...] a lethal, insidious enemy" (Sontag 2001: 87). Since the publication of Sontag's study, two particularly productive arenas for the discussion of cancer metaphors have emerged: the interdisciplinary field of narrative medicine, and the formation of a body of literary and critical texts that has become known, for lack of a better term, as 'cancer literature'. Both of these fields have their roots in the 1990s – the decade in which Hall produced the three volumes of verse discussed in this essay – and they provide a useful framework for my exploration of metaphor and cancer in Hall's poetry.

Scholars and practitioners of narrative medicine emphasise the important role of metaphor in conversations between health-care specialists and patients. In an article published in *The Oncologist*, Richard T. Penson and his co-authors come to the conclusion that "[m]etaphors help bring the patient's subjective view of illness into the forefront of the medical encounter, give meaning to the experience, and allow the doctor and patient to strengthen the therapeutic alliance around a shared vision" (Penson et al. 2004: 715). Carola Skott, in an ethnographic study of cancer ward narratives, describes cancer metaphors as semantic nodes "in which social and cultural factors are interwoven with experiences from the medical sector and medical language" (Skott 2002: 234). While both Penson and Skott note the continued prevalence of military cancer metaphors, they also highlight the positive impact of an increasingly varied spectrum of cancer images which patients can appropriate and mould according to their own experience. Surprisingly, Penson and Scott do not link the availability of this broader range of metaphors to the rapid growth of a market for "cancer literature" since the 1990s.

Today, amazon.com lists "cancer" as a genre fiction subsection (no other disease has received this distinction on the website of the online retailer) with 12,161 titles – almost as many titles as are linked to "aging" (12,834) and significantly more than "diet & weight loss" titles (1,098). Authors of all genres and audiences – from experimental drama to young adult literature – have made cancer the subject of their writing. In the thirty-odd years following Sontag's statement that "[c]ancer is a rare and still scandalous subject for poetry; it seems unimaginable to aestheticize the disease" (Sontag 1978: 20), a growing number of poets, including Philip Hodgins (e.g. *Dispossessed* (1994) and *Things Happen* (1995)), Marilyn Hacker (*Winter Numbers* (1994)), Sandra Steingraber (*Living Downstream* (1994)) have published acclaimed collections with a focus on cancer. Mary K. DeShazer and Werner Senn have noted that the work of these and other poetic contemporaries of Hall features innovative metaphors that move beyond the stereotypical images of war, journey, quest and challenge (DeShazer 2005: 14-20; Senn 2008: 239).

While medical practitioners, scholars of narrative medicine and poets of the 1990s found fruitful new applications for cancer metaphors, Hall's poems about Kenyon's illness are wary of metaphorising cancer. "The Tenth Inning", a section of "Extra Innings", deals with Hall and Kenyon's first encounter with cancer when surgeons removed the tumour on her neck in 1985. While they await the biopsy results, Hall is plagued by nightmares in which garden vegetables (associated with Kenyon and Hall's love for country life on Eagle Pond Farm) shrivel and disintegrate on the vine, oozing poisonous liquids, including "corrupt lymph": "I dreamt of a garden / where tomatoes sagged erupting black juice, / where squash lapsed softly drooling corrupt lymph / 6. And seed, where Kentucky Wonders curled up, / cankered, and dropped from derelict vine" (Hall 1993b: 104). Uncharacteristically for Hall's sparse and often ironic verse, this overwritten passage brims with unnecessary adjectives and pushes assonance and consonance to almost comic excess, climaxing in the lines on the Kentucky Wonders: "curled up, cankered, / and dropped from the derelict vine". The nightmarish quality of the scene described here is also rendered through the awkward metaphorical excess of the poem's language itself – a conscious rhetorical manoeuvre on Hall's part, I believe, to mock an overreliance on clichéd metaphors in popular and literary writing on cancer.

Hall notoriously has little patience with sloppy metaphors: "The practice I deplore", he writes in a critical essay, "Hall's Index" (2009), "is the unwitting use of DMs [dead metaphors] in the pursuit of poetic effect: the unrealized comparison as false colour" (Hall 2009). Throughout this essay, Hall demonstrates the weaknesses of dead metaphors by example, drawing particular attention to the language of disease: "Illness provides ten thousand wounds DM to the language, which Hall's Index would nurse DM back to health DM. The dead metaphor is a cancer DM in the poem's language, which only revisionary scrutiny can cut out DM. We are crippled DM when we use crippled, except in its literal sense" (Hall 2009). "The Tenth Inning" ends with a call from the hospital's pathology department, and both the nature of the medical message and the literalness of its language come as a relief:

> Pathology telephoned its words: "a
> muco-epidermoid carcinoma,
> the size of a grape, intermediate
> in virulence, encapsulated in
> the membrane of the salivary gland" –
>
> 10. with no likelihood of metastasis
> and little for recurrence. Next morning,
> we woke alert in the pink-and-green dawn,
> aware of joy at waking
> […]
> Routine was paradise – walking the dog,
> newspaper, coffee, love, rye toast, work, grape
> juice

(Hall 1993b: 275-76)

The medical diagnosis is cited verbatim, the interjection of the physician's voice highlighted by the quotation marks, but it is also fitted neatly into the poem's strict syllabic metre of ten syllables per line. As a result, the medical register does not jar the reader, and the factual language of the doctor is balanced in the last stanza by Hall's plain enumeration of mostly mono-syllabic nouns, "newspaper, coffee, love, rye toast, work, grape / juice" – objects which represent his and Kenyon's return to their cherished routine. Like the doctor's diagnosis, Hall's list foregrounds language's referential power. It contrasts starkly with the ornate cancer-garden passage discussed above, and it indicates that in writing about another person's cancer – a disease that has been thoroughly mythologised over the centuries – resistance to metaphor may in itself constitute an ethical act.

Much more so than in texts about his own cancer, Hall uses exact diagnostic and medical terms in his poems about Kenyon's leukaemia. In a review of *Unpacking the Boxes*, Peter Stevenson calls Hal "the reluctant bard of prednisone, Cytoxan and bone marrow" (Stevenson 2008) – a fitting moniker for a poet whose writing about pharmaceutical drugs and medical paraphernalia is not always immediately accessible to lay readers. When Hall published "Without" (included in *The Old Life*), one of his most famous poems about Kenyon's disease, he appended an explanatory note to help readers with little known words:

Unfamiliar words are mostly chemicals infused to initiate or sustain remission from
leukemia. Petechiae are red marks on the skin that indicate a deficiency of platelets in
the blood; platelets help with clotting. PCP is a form of pneumonia common to people
with compromised immune systems, like sufferers from AIDS or ALL (acute lympho-
blastic leukemia). Herpes zoster: shingles.

(Hall 1996: 134)

"Without" is concerned with the language of cancer and it tests a range of metaphors, some conventional and some more inventive, to articulate the existential
distress felt by the patient.

artillery sniper fire helicopter gunship
grenade burning murder landmine starvation
the ceasefire lasted forty-eight hours
then a shell exploded in a market
pain vomit neuropathy morphine nightmare
confusion the rack terror the vise

vincristineara-c Cytoxan vp-16
loss of memory loss of language losses
pneumocystiscarinii pneumonia bactrim
foamless unmitigated sea without sea
deliriumwhipmarks of petechiae
multiple blisters of herpes zoster

(Hall 1996: 128)

The poem introduces military images, arguably still the most dominant class of
cancer metaphors (Penson et al. 2004: 715), only to dismiss their capacity to say
something meaningful about the experience of cancer. The beginning of the
stanza quoted above strings together military terms without conjunctions or
punctuation, a structure that is then repeated in lines 5, 7 and 9 where Hall lists
chemotherapy drugs and diagnostic terms. However, the semantics of these two
groups of words are fundamentally different: while the military terms are
densely metaphorical (each word is seemingly introduced to express an aspect of
cancer), the medical terms, like the medical diagnosis and the list of nouns in
"The Tenth Inning", are purely referential. Indeed, their referential character is
reinforced by Hall's inclusion of the explanatory footnote cited above. The
clinical terms demand the reader's attention – their very structure ("ara-c
Cytoxan vp-16") is unfamiliar and will send the majority of Hall's audience to
the annotations. Because these words are not part of the everyday lexicon, they
have not accrued metaphorical meanings; cancer here signifies only itself. The
title of the poem, "Without", lends itself to many readings, including the notion
that writing about another person's cancer demands to do so "without" the
conventionalised tools of poetic language.

Cancer, Gender and Medical Realism

A commitment to a form of 'medical realism' also pervades Hall's "Her Long Illness", a long poem on Kenyon's leukaemia interspersed between the other poems that make up the volume *Without*:

> Following the protocol
> for ALL, now the doctors began
>   the Fourth Intensification –
> two weeks of infusions, shots, and nausea.
>   Already, since Ara-C,
> Jane used a walker, slept fourteen hours,
>   and believed that they lived
>   on the Newport Road of her childhood.

(Hall 1999: 14)

This passage is characteristic of other parts of "Her Long Illness" which depict medical treatments, controlled by doctors, which render the female patient vulnerable and mentally and physically exhausted. While Hall worked on the poems that are collected in *Without*, a number of feminist thinkers published studies on the medicalisation of the female subject and body in biomedical discourses. Works such as Anne Oakley's *Essays on Women, Medicine and Health* (1993), Margrit Shildrick's *Leaky Bodies and Boundaries* (1997) and Jackie Stacey's *Teratologies: A Cultural Study of Cancer* (1997) criticised medical practices and cultural narratives which perpetuate the (long-standing) gendering of the spheres of professional medicine and science on the one hand, and of illness and bodily/mental weakness on the other. Female patients, they argued, can be victimised by discourses which place the power to control their allegedly "disorderly" or "horrific" bodies in the hands of modern medicine, constructed as masculine, rational and objective. "Given that the devaluation of corporeality [...] has been a dominant feature of masculinist knowledge," Shildrick points out, "my contention is that a resistant feminism must seek to explore the body anew [...] both the material body and the female as positioned as other to the transcendent subject and denied expression in ethical paradigms" (Shildrick 1997: 9). These feminist interventions provide a fruitful foil for Hall's poems about Kenyon's illness. As we shall see in what follows, Hall's depiction of the relationship between modern medical technology and the female patient leaves dichotomous conceptions of male and female gender largely intact. Yet his writings about Kenyon's cancer often break down other hierarchies – between patient and medical authority, rational science and embodied empathy – which Shildrick, Stacey, Oakley and other feminists also wish to eradicate.

Occasionally, Hall portrays doctors as an anonymous mass that administers agonising treatments ("As they killed her bone-marrow again / she lay on a gurney alone"; Hall 1999: 20), but more often his poems depict physicians and nurses as individualised, sympathetic human beings. Hall frequently includes the full names of doctors and caregivers – we meet Kenyon's haematologist Letha Miller, her nurse Maggie Fisher, as well as the surgeon who performed Hall's liverectomy, Dr. Sutton, and hear their voices:

> Jane's haematologist Letha Mills sat down,
>   stiff, her assistant
> standing with her back to the door.
>   "I have terrible news,"
> Letha told them. "The leukaemia is back.
>   There's nothing to do."
> The four of them wept.

(Hall 1999: 35)

In depicting this final turning point in Kenyon's long struggle with cancer (she died eleven days after this meeting), Hall does not zoom in on Kenyon's or his own response to Mills's diagnosis. Instead, his restrained verse suggests that Mills and her assistant participate in his and Kenyon's pain and respond to it with physical and emotional empathy: "The four of them wept". As a female cancer patient, Kenyon is not – in Shildrick's words – "denied expression in ethical paradigms". In this moment of Kenyon's greatest vulnerability, Mills and her assistant abandon their roles as authoritative health care specialists and their sympathetic involvement bears humane witness to Kenyon's suffering.

"The Ship Pounding", another poem included in *Without*, discusses the patient's dependency on medical technology even if the curative powers of this technology may be limited. Hall compares the patients to "passengers" on a sea voyage who wear "masks or cannulae / or dangled devices that dripped / chemicals into their wrists" (Hall 1999: 15).

> Each morning I made my way
> among gangways, elevators,
> and nurses' pods to Jane's room
> to interrogate the grave helpers
> who tended her through the night
> while the ship's massive engines
> kept its propellers turning.

(Hall 1999: 15)

While Laura E. Tanner suggests that the poem encapsulates "expulsion from the narrative world of the present" (Tanner 2006: 242), Davis and Womack note that Hall's representation of "chilling technology" (Davis and Womack 2005: 167) speaks to his frustration with a medical apparatus that enables the continuation of Kenyon's life and suffering but no longer holds out the promise of recovery. The poem's last lines speak of Jane's "readmission to the huge / vessel that heaves water month after month", and their alliterative structure – "without leaving / port, without moving a knot, / without arrival or destination, / its great engines pounding" – conveys a strong sense of the depression of stasis, of being adrift without direction. Still, I believe that the poem's portrayal of the relationship between patient and medical technology can be understood in more ambivalent terms when read alongside "Her Long Illness".

In "The Ship Pounding", the image of "the vessel" points to something more complex than the idea that patients are at the mercy of an institutionalised and increasingly mechanical health care system. Rather, Hall figures the vessel or ship as an assemblage of embodied human experience, inanimate medical machines and equipment, and a discourse of suffering and medical care. My use of "assemblage" here deliberately evokes Janet Bennett's recent work, following Gilles Deleuze and Felix Guattari, on assemblages. For Bennett, assemblages are "ad hoc groupings of diverse elements, of vibrant materials of all sorts. Assemblages are living, throbbing confederations that are able to function despite the persistent presence of energies that confound them from within" (Bennett 2010: 23-24). Placed in relation to Hall's poem, Bennett's concept of assemblage also invites us to think about Hall's portrayal of illness and care as distributed phenomena that go far beyond the sick individual and draw into affective contact a group of formerly separate human and non-human agents. The boundaries of the human body, for instance, are no longer stable in "The Ship Pounding": bodies and machines interpenetrate as IV lines and cannulae are inserted through the skin into a vein, and oxygen masks help patients breathe. Indeed, the immobile "vessel" can be seen both as the terminally ill body and as the medical apparatus that keeps this body alive; it is the body's physical deterioration that halts progress, and it is the machines' work that precludes (at least temporarily) collapse. The notion of the assemblage also allows for a more positive reading of the ship's suspended movement. The temporality of the assemblage is simultaneity, or a continuous present, rather than chronology – a concept of time which links the depiction of the vessel to the celebration of "ongoingness" in "The Thirteenth Inning" and prompts us to read "The Ship Pounding" as a continuation of Hall's experiments with the different temporal modes of sickness that he had begun in this earlier poem.

Hall explains that once but not any more "I believed that the ship / traveled to a harbour / of breakfast, work, and love" (Hall 1999: 15). The vessel, then, is also formed by Hall's feelings about the future and by the daily routines of care-giving that he performs alongside the "grave helpers" – the ambiguously named group of doctors and nurses who oversee, with kindness and respect, a course of treatments that will not avert Kenyon's death. Hospital staff, patients (referred to in the plural when Hall calls them "passengers"), and caregivers like Hall are the vessel's principal constituents – they form a community into which inanimate machines and medical paraphernalia are also admitted. Thus, Hall's image of the vessel describes Kenyon's experience as cancer patient as traumatic but not alienated: her suffering is shared by other patients, and empathetically observed by Hall, the hospital staff and even – in a symbolic sense – by medical appliances.

Animate medical objects play an important role in "Her Long Illness". Untitled sections of this poem are scattered throughout *Without*. The first section, placed at the very beginning of the volume, gives an account of Kenyon's time in hospital before the bone marrow transplant:

> When it snowed one morning Jane gazed
>   at the darkness blurred
> with flakes. They pushed the IV pump
>   which she called Igor
> slowly past the nurses' pods, as far
>   as the outside door
> so that she could smell the snowy air.
>
> (Hall 1999: 1)

Calling an object by a human name, assigning gender even, is an act of anthro-pomorphisation that draws an object into human community and acknowledges the extent to which things share our lives. This is one of the central insights of thing theory, which holds that our exchanges with and emotional investment in objects always exceed their commodity status (see Brown 2003; Freedgood 2006). In "Her Long Illness", medical appliances mediate rather than complicate the relationship between Hall and Kenyon. In their writings and joint interviews, Kenyon and Hall described their marriage as close and loving. Each acted as caregiver for the other during their respective struggles with cancer. "Her Long Illness" includes a retrospective glimpse at Hall's liverectomy:

> When he roiled in Recovery
> after the surgeon cut out half his liver
>   two years earlier,
> Jane pushed the morphine bolus.
>   She brought him home,
> a breathing sarcophagus, then rubbed his body
>   back to life with her hands.
>
> (Hall 1999: 12)

Jane's prosaic operating of the morphine bolus is described as much as an act of love as her esoteric rubbing "his body back to life with her hands". In another section of "Her Long Illness", Hall describes the technicalities of his own daily routine of caring for Jane: "He counted out meds / and programmed pumps to deliver / hydration, TPN, / and ganciclovir" (Hall 1999: 24). Hall writes in *Life Work* that the physical intimacy of these acts of caregiving heightens his experience of bodily empathy: "I have come so close to Jane that I feel as if I had crawled into her body through her pores – and, although the occasion of this penetration has been melancholy, the comfort is luminous and redemptive" (Hall 1993a: 123). The intimacy of medical care is more central to "Her Long Illness" than the intimacy of sexuality, which occupies an important place in much of Hall's other writings. However, instead of suggesting that one form of physical closeness replaces the other, Hall imbues medical and other objects with sexual life to suggest in humorous tones that Kenyon's and his sexual relationship finds a continuation of sorts in the object world that surrounds them.

Kenyon, who mourns the loss of her sexuality in another passage of "Her Long Illness" ("Jane burst into tears / and cried: 'No more fucking. No more fucking!'"; Hall 1999: 40), observes that the conglomerate of medical gown, hat, latex gloves and boots which Hall wears when he visits her after intense radiation looks like "a huge condom" (Hall 1999: 22). Hall himself frames his attempts to assemble the tubing for Kenyon in a humorous sexual conceit: "He needed to learn [...] how to assemble the tubing, to insert / narrow ends into / wide ones. 'From long experience,' Maggie [the nurse] / told him, 'I have learned to distinguish "male" from "female"'" (Hall 1999: 12). In "The Porcelain Couple", also included in *Without*, Hall vividly evokes some of the keepsakes of his and Kenyon's married life:

> All day, while I ate lunch or counted out pills,
> I noticed the objects of our twenty years:
> a blue vase, a candelabrum Jane carried on her lap
> from the Baja, and the small porcelain box
> from France I found under the tree one Christmas
> where a couple in relief stretch out asleep,
> like a catafalque, on the pastel double bed
> on the box's top, both wearing pretty nightcaps.
>
> (Hall 1999: 10)

Taken out of context, the porcelain sculpture is a sentimental kitsch commodity, but Hall puts it to complex use. The porcelain couple's marriage bed brings to mind the iconic "painted bed" that Kenyon and Hall shared and that is featured in many of Hall's poems. The couple, sleeping with their nightcaps on, is depicted in an intimate and humorous manner, but the "catafalque" gives the impression that this image has been recorded after the couple's death. Porcelain freezes a moment in time – bodies intact, happiness remembered – but it is also eminently breakable. The porcelain box 'stores' Hall and Kenyon's relationship: it serves as a mnemonic object that brings to mind memories of their life together, and it gives external shape to Hall's hopes and fears regarding their future.

The porcelain sculpture has been part of Hall and Kenyon's household for much longer than the medical equipment that enters it when Hall and Kenyon develop cancer. Yet Hall's poetry suggests that, just like the porcelain box, medical objects like "Igor" (the IV pump) can also offer a certain amount of comfort by inviting emotional relationships with the humans who interact with them. He does not gloss over the fact that some of the treatments which Kenyon receives cause intense pain ("mucositis / from the burn of Total Body Irradiation / frayed her mouth apart / cell by cell, peeling her lips and tongue"; Hall 1999: 22). However, he refrains from presenting medical objects as demonic agents of Kenyon's suffering and instead focuses on the ways in which these objects are bound up with and add new dimensions (not all of them negative) to his interactions with Kenyon.

Scholars in the medical humanities have described *Without* as "a touchstone for people who've lost a life partner and health care professionals whose work is with the dying and their survivors" (Childress 2007: 5). Poems from *Without*, but also from other volumes of Hall's poetry, are now widely taught in modules on narrative medicine and medical humanities in American medical schools and residencies. Hall holds readings more rarely today, but in the 2000s he gave a number of talks for patients and medical professionals in medical institutions and cancer centres. As I hope to have shown in this essay, Hall's poetry on cancer is rich and varied in form: it accommodates reflections on the experience of male and female cancer patients, on the perspectives of caregivers and medical professionals, on the hospital environment and medical technology, and on the impact of illness on the patient's perception of time and the object world. In envisioning cancer and cancer therapy as distributed phenomena, Hall's poems can serve as a common ground for readers who are patients, doctors or caregivers. They provide a forum – literal in the case of readings and discussion groups, or imagined when read alone – where these different groups can meet and enter into conversation.

List of Works Cited

Bennett, Jane. *Vibrant Matter: A Political Ecology of Things*. Durham, NC: Duke UP, 2010.

Berman, Jeffrey. *Companionship in Grief: Love and Loss in the Memoirs of C.S. Lewis, John Bayley, Donald Hall, Joan Didion, and Calvin Trillin*. Amherst: U of Massachussetts P, 2010.

Brown, Bill. *A Sense of Things: The Object Matter of American Literature*. Chicago: Chicago UP, 2003.

Childress, Marcia K. "Ethics and the Humanities: Review of Without". *Medical Ethics* 14.2 (2007): 5.

Davis, Todd F. and Kenneth Womack. "Reading the Ethics of Mourning in the Poetry of Donald Hall." *Response to Death: The Literary Work of Mourning*. Ed. Christian Riegel. Edmonton: U of Alberta P, 2005. 166-78.

DeShazer, Mary K. "Cancer Narratives and an Ethics of Commemoration: Susan Sontag, Annie Leibovitz, and Daniel Rieff". *Literature and Medicine* 28.2 (2009): 215-36.

---. *Fractured Borders: Reading Women's Cancer Literature*. Ann Arbor: U of Michigan P, 2005.

Freedgood, Elaine. *The Ideas in Things: Fugitive Meaning in the Victorian Novel*. Chicago: Chicago UP, 2006.

Hall, Donald. "The Art of Poetry: Interview". Interviewed by Peter A. Stitt. *The Paris Review* 33.120 (1991): 154.

---. "Baseball and the Meaning of Life", *The Complete Armchair Book of Baseball*. Ed. John Thorn and David Reuther. Edison: Galahad, 1997. 152-55.

---. *The Best Day the Worst Day: Life with Jane Kenyon*. New York: Houghton Mifflin, 2005.

---. *Dock Ellis in the Country of Baseball*. New York: Coward, McGann & Geoghegan, 1976.

---. *Fathers Playing Catch with Sons: Essays on Sport, Mostly Baseball*. San Francisco: North Point Press, 1985.

---. "Hall's Index". *Narrative Magazine*. Spring 2009. http://www.narrativemagazine.com /issues/spring-2009/hall's-index.

---. *Life Work*. Boston: Beacon Press, 1993.

---. *The Museum of Clear Ideas*. New York: Ticknor & Fields, 1993.

---. "Telling Suffering: A Brief Interview with Donald Hall". Interviewed by Marcia D. Childress. *Hedgehog Review* 8.3 (2006): 93-99.

---. *Unpacking the Boxes: A Memoir of Life in Poetry*. Boston: Houghton Mifflin, 2008.

---. *White Apples and the Taste of Stone: Selected Poems 1946-2006*. New York: Houghton Mifflin, 2006.

---. *Without*. New York: Houghton and Mifflin, 1999.

Kenyon, Jane. *Otherwise: New and Selected Poems*. Saint Paul, MN: Graywolf, 1996.

Oakley, Ann. *Essays on Women, Medicine and Health*. Edinburgh: Edinburgh UP, 1993.

Penson, Richard T. et al. "Cancer as Metaphor". *The Oncologist* 9.6 (2004): 708-16.

Pollock, Griselda. "Dying, Seeing, Feeling: Transforming the Ethical Space of Feminist Aesthetics". *The Life and Death of Images: Ethics and Aesthetics*. Ed. Diarmuid Costello and Dominic Willsdon. Ithaca, NY: Cornell UP, 2008. 213-35.

Scott, Carola. "Expressive Metaphors in Cancer Narratives". *Cancer Nursing* 25.3 (2002): 230-35.

Senn, Werner. "Voicing the Body: The Cancer Poems of Philip Hodgins". *Bodies and Voices: The Force-Field of Representation and Discourse in Colonial and Postcolonial Studies*. Ed. Merete Falck Borch et al. Amsterdam: Rodopi, 2008. 237-49.

Shildrick, Margrit. *Leaky Bodies and Boundaries: Feminism, Postmodernism and (Bio)ethics*. London: Routlegde, 1997.

Sontag, Susan. *Illness as Metaphor and AIDS and Its Metaphors*. London: Picador, 2001.

Stacey, Jackie. *Teratologies: A Cultural Study of Cancer*. London, Routledge: 1997.

Stevenson, Peter. "Intimacy and Solitude: Review of Unpacking the Boxes". *New York Times*. 7 November 2008. http://www.nytimes.com/2008/11/09/books/review/Stevenson-t.html.

Streznewski, Marylou Kelly. "Thinking with Muscle and Tongue: The Poetry of Donald Hall". *Wild River Review* 3.3 (2006).

Tanner, Laura E. *Lost Bodies: Inhabiting the Borders of Life and Death*. Ithaca, NY: Cornell UP, 2006.

Anita Schilcher

Ein richtiger Indianer?
Kranke Jungen in der Kinder- und Jugendliteratur

Kranke oder sterbende Kinder werden nicht nur während politischer und humanitärer Krisen instrumentalisiert, um an das Mitleid der Welt in Kriegen, Hungersnöten und bei anderen Grausamkeiten zu appellieren. Kein Regime und keine Organisation verzichtet darauf, uns medial Kinder vorzuführen, die unter den Angriffen des Gegners oder unter Naturkatastrophen leiden oder sterben. Dies zeigt, dass Kinder in der westlichen Welt – und vermutlich nicht nur dort – zu den ranghöchsten Werten unserer Gesellschaft zählen.

Auch in der Literatur verschiedener Epochen wird deutlich, dass die Darstellung kranker Kinder meist mit Zusatzbedeutungen aufgeladen wird. So gehört der „Erlkönig" mit seiner Darstellung eines sterbenden Kindes zu den bekanntesten Balladen der deutschen Literatur. Auch wenn der Vater das Kind warm und sicher hält, gelingt es ihm nicht, dem Sohn mit seinem aufklärerischen Gestus („in dürren Blättern säuselt der Wind") die Angst vor dem bedrohlichen Erlkönig zu nehmen und den Knaben zu retten. Wilhelm Tell dagegen, der sich zunächst weigert, sich dem Freiheitskampf seiner Landsleute anzuschließen, wird zum Helden des Aufstandes, nachdem er sich an Geßler für den „Apfelschuss" gerächt hat, der ihn gezwungen hat, sein eigenes Kind einer Todesbedrohung auszusetzen. Als „Beschützer der Familie" wird er zum Sinnbild der Befreiung. Söhne – so lässt sich an unzähligen Beispielen der Literaturgeschichte zeigen – spielen in der Wahrnehmung der Väter eine besondere Rolle: Als Stammhalter oder Ebenbild verkörpern sie oft die Hoffnung auf ein besseres Leben oder den Fortbestand des ihrer Werte und Normen

Diese besondere Stellung, die Söhne gesellschaftlich wie literarisch eingenommen haben, lässt sich in der Literatur funktionalisieren, so dass der Tod oder der anderweitige Verlust des Sohnes oft als Verlust des ranghöchsten Wertes die Ideologie des Textes besonders markant unterstreicht. Gerade in der Literatur des 19. Jahrhunderts lässt sich zeigen, dass die Texte selten Zweifel an der Schuld des Vaters oder der Eltern lassen, wenn ein Sohn erkrankt oder gar stirbt. Entweder überfordert der Vater den Sohn mit seinen Ansprüchen oder der Gesundheitszustand des Sohnes steht zeichenhaft für die krisenhafte Beziehung der Eltern. Beispielhaft kann das in folgenden Texten verdeutlicht werden:

1. In *Aquis submersus* von Theodor Storm steht der Tod des Jungen zeichenhaft für die Schuld der Eltern, die sich durch eine nicht standesgemäße und nicht-eheliche Beziehung über die Konventionen der Zeit hinwegsetzen. Als der Maler Johannes seine ehemalige Geliebte Katharina als Ehefrau eines Pfarrers wiedertrifft und es wieder zu einer Annäherung der einst Liebenden kommt, ertrinkt der gemeinsame Sohn im nahen Teich.

2. In Conrad Ferdinand Meyers *Das Leiden eines Knaben* stirbt der Sohn an der Überforderung des Vaters: „Geradeheraus: entweder hat der Marschall einen kurzen Verstand, oder er wollte sein gegebenes Wort mit Prunk und Glorie selbst auf Kosten seines Kindes halten" (Meyer 1968: 265).

3. In den *Buddenbrooks* scheitert der einzige Sohn Hanno an den übersteigerten Anforderungen des Vaters, der ihn gegen seine Natur zu einem Kaufmann erziehen will. Sein Tod steht zudem sinnbildlich für das Ende der Dynastie der Buddenbrooks und für die gescheiterte Ehe der Eltern. Interessant sind die Wendungen, mit denen der Tod Hannos beschrieben wird: Er verschließt sich der „Stimme des Lebens". Sein fehlender Lebenswille lässt ihn Zuflucht nehmen „auf dem Weg, der sich ihm zum Entrinnen eröffnet hat" (Mann 1974: 754). Nicht mehr nur die Rache des Schicksals dient hier als Motiv, sondern auch das Scheitern des Individuums an seiner Umwelt, die Erkenntnis das zugedachte Leben nicht leben zu wollen.

4. Auch in *Brennendes Geheimnis* von Stefan Zweig kränkelt der Sohn analog zur Beziehung seiner Eltern. Und hier thematisiert der Text die Bedeutung von Krankheit im Gesamtzusammenhang: „Kinder sind immer stolz auf eine Krankheit, weil sie wissen, daß Gefahr sie ihren Angehörigen doppelt wichtig macht" (Zweig 1913: 10).

5. Krankheit und Tod stehen dabei stets für die persönliche Katastrophe im Leben der Eltern, etwa in Theodor Storms Gedicht „Geh nicht hinein":

> – Und ein Entsetzen schrie aus seiner Brust,
> Daß ratlos Mitleid, die am Lager saßen,
> In Stein verwandelte – , er lag am Abgrund;
> Bodenlos, ganz ohne Boden. – »Hilf!
> Ach Vater, lieber Vater!« Taumelnd schlug
> Er um sich mit den Armen; ziellos griffen
> In leere Luft die Hände; noch ein Schrei –
> Und dann verschwand er.

Dort, wo er gelegen,
Dort hinterm Wandschirm, stumm und einsam liegt
Jetzt etwas; – bleib, geh nicht hinein! Es schaut
Dich fremd und furchtbar an; für viele Tage
Kannst du nicht leben, wenn du es erblickt.

(Storm 1978: 193)

Das Entsetzen über den Tod eines Kindes steigert sich gesellschaftlich bis heute und wird in der medialen Inszenierung (und vermutlich auch in der Realität) zur schlimmsten persönlichen Katastrophe, die erwachsenen Figuren widerfahren kann.

Krankheit und Tod werden dabei in der Literatur verschiedener Epochen unterschiedlich funktionalisiert, etwa indem sie mit „Schuld" korreliert werden, den Ausnahmestatus einer Figur am Rande des normalen bürgerlichen Spektrums signalisieren oder als Schicksalsschlag das Ausgeliefertsein des Helden thematisieren.[1] Dies verdeutlicht, dass Literatur – auch bei Vorspiegelung einer größtmöglichen Realitätsnähe – nie die gegebene soziale Wirklichkeit abbildet: „In ihr spiegeln sich vielmehr die Vorannahmen ihrer Autoren über die gesellschaftliche Realität, mithin bestimmte, für den Schreibprozeß konstitutive Deutungsmuster und Weltbilder" (Kaulen 1999: 126f.).

Gerade dann, wenn die hochrangigsten Werte einer Gesellschaft verhandelt werden, wie das beim Thema des kranken, manchmal vom Tode bedrohten, Kindes der Fall ist, kann man davon ausgehen, dass dieses Thema bewusst gewählt wurde. Kranke Kinder, oft kranke Jungen, tauchen nicht unbeabsichtigt oder nebensächlich in der Literatur auf. Krankheit, Behinderung und Tod geben als ideologisch hoch bewertete Topoi Aufschluss über das in der Literatur vermittelte Normen- und Wertesystem. Sie werden also sowohl in der Allgemeinliteratur wie auch in der Kinder- und Jugendliteratur oft zeichenhaft zur Untermauerung expliziter wie impliziter Ideologien benutzt. Stephens beschreibt den Zusammenhang von Fiktionalität und Normativität in der Kinder- und Jugendliteratur folgendermaßen:

Fiction presents a special context for the operation of ideologies, because narrative texts are highly organized and structured discourses whose conventions may either be used to express deliberate advocacy of social practices or may encode social practices implicitly. They may both, as when a desired ideological significance is grounded in specific social practices at story level. A text may overtly advocate one ideology while implicitly inscribing one or more other ideologies.

(Stephens 1992: 43)[2]

---

[1] Vgl. z.B. Anz 1989.
[2] Vgl. dazu auch: „Literarische Texte zeichnen sich immer wieder dadurch aus, daß der hegemoniale Diskurs gebrochen wird durch eine gegenläufige Textbewegung, die ihn in Frage stellt" (Spinner 2000: 83).

Dem „narrativen Diskurs" liegt damit ein spezieller Gebrauch von Sprache zugrunde, durch den eine Gesellschaft ihre vorherrschenden Werte und Haltungen ausdrückt und kundtut, und zwar unabhängig von der Absicht des Verfassers (vgl. Stephens 1999: 20f. und Reese 2007: 167). Gerade implizite Werte und Normen können ein wirksames Vehikel für eine Ideologie sein, da die

> Reproduktion von Überzeugungen und Annahmen, deren sich Autor(inn)en und Leser/innen weithin nicht bewußt sind, die Ideologie unsichtbar macht und folglich implizierte ideologische Positionen dadurch legitimiert, daß sie sie als natürlich erscheinen läßt. Mit anderen Worten: Ein Buch, das ein Leser für ideologiefrei hält, wird ein Buch sein, das weitgehend mit den eigenen unbewußten Annahmen dieses Lesers übereinstimmt; und das Erkennen solcher Ideologien wird es oft erforderlich machen, die Sprache und den narrativen Diskurs des Textes sehr genau zu lesen.

(Stephens 1999: 21)

Dies trifft auch – und gerade – für die Auseinandersetzung mit Krankheit und Tod zu. Verschiedene Untersuchungen zu Krankheit oder Behinderung in der Kinder- und Jugendliteratur zeigen, dass sich epochenspezifische Ideologien bei der Analyse größerer Textkorpora zu den Themen Krankheit und Behinderung aufdecken lassen. So zeigen etwa Farber und Reese, dass Behinderung je nach zeitgeschichtlichem Kontext bestimmten Strickmustern und Stereotypen folgt.[3] Das kann zum einen durch die Figurenzeichnung geschehen, die den Behinderten oder Kranken sympathisch oder unsympathisch erscheinen lässt. Hierbei finden sich neben dem sanften und duldsamen „Musterkrüppel", der „Tyrann", der „Held" und der in die Phantasie Fliehende (vgl. Reese 2010: 4). Auch die vorherrschend dargestellten Behinderungen und Krankheiten unterliegen Modewellen. Bis zur Mitte des 20. Jahrhunderts ist Blindheit die dominanteste Behinderung in der Literatur, was zu einer deutlichen Überrepräsentation führt (vgl. Reese 2007: 167). Blindheit eignet sich nach Reese in besonderem Maß für die Erregung von Mitleid oder Bewunderung, weil ihr der Reiz des „Andersartigen" und „Heroischen" anhaften kann. Blindheit ist bereits in der griechischen Mythologie als schwere Strafe aber auch als Vehikel für die Gabe der Erkenntnis und Prophezeiung funktionalisiert (vgl. Teiresias, Ödipus oder Polyphem). Zum anderen lassen sich Werte und Ideologien aber auch durch den Handlungsverlauf und -ausgang vermitteln. So wird in der Aufklärung – die erste Epoche, in der intentionale Kinder- und Jugendliteratur als eigenes Subsystem entsteht – die Darstellung von Krankheit vor allem dazu instrumentalisiert, „rationale" Belehrung und „Vernunftkontrolle" (Farber 1991: 315) zu legitimieren. Als Beispiel kann Christian Gotthilf Salzmanns *Moralisches*

---

[3] Vgl. Farber 1991 und Reese 2007.

Elementarbuch (1783) dienen, in dem ein mahnendes Abschreckungsszenario entworfen wird:

> Nach etlichen Jahren spürte man eine sehr merkliche Abnahme an Wilhelms Kräften. Sein Wachstum hörte auf, seine Wangen wurden bleich, er bekam blaue Ringe um die Augen, ja man merkte sogar deutlich, daß seine Geisteskräfte abnahmen: indem er auch die leichtesten Sachen nicht begreifen konnte. Rudolph hingegen wuchs empor und wurde schlank, wie eine junge Tanne; sein Gesicht blühte wie eine Rose; jedermann bewunderte seinen Verstand. [...] Im zwanzigsten Jahre nun schrumpfte Wilhelm gar zusammen, und starb unter großen Schmerzen. Und Rudolph wurde ein gesunder und schöner Mann. Er erfuhr nun auch, daß Wilhelm durch heimliche Sünden seinen Leib geschwächt und seine Gesundheit zerstört habe, und daß er von diesen Sünden ebenfalls angesteckt worden sey, wenn ihm der Vater erlaubt hätte, den elenden Knaben zu besuchen.
>
> (Salzmann 1783, zit. nach Ewers 1980: 263)

Wie Reese zeigt, ist die Darstellung von Behinderung als Bestrafung von der Aufklärung bis ins 19. Jahrhundert hinein als Strickmuster literarischer Texte für Kinder und Jugendliche durchaus üblich (vgl. Reese 2007: 143). Das ausgehende 19. und das beginnende 20. Jahrhundert nutzen die Darstellung kranker und behinderter Kinder zur Harmonisierung, zur Hinlenkung zum religiösen Glauben (vgl. ebd.) und zur Aufwertung einer naturnahen Lebenswelt. Zimmermann spricht mit Bezug auf einen der bekanntesten Klassiker – *Heidi* (1880/81) von Johanna Spyri –, in dem der duldsame und sanftmütige „Musterkrüppel" Klara durch die natürliche Umgebung auf der Alm gesundet, vom „Heidi-Syndrom" (Zimmermann 1982: 172). Ähnliches gilt auch für *The Secret Garden* (1909) von Frances Hodgson Burnett, in dem sich der ans Bett gefesselte „Tyrann" Colin durch die Begegnung mit seiner Cousine Mary und dem Spiel im geheimen Garten zu einem gesunden Kind entwickelt. Rollstuhl und Korsett stehen hier für die (physische) „Verstümmelung" des Kindes. Erst die unmittelbare Naturbegegnung heilt sie und ermöglicht ihnen ein lebenswertes Leben.

In der nationalsozialistisch geprägten Kinderliteratur können anhand des Themas Krankheit indes vorbildliches Verhalten, Tapferkeit und Gehorsam in einem moralisierenden und repressiven Erziehungsstil vermittelt werden (vgl. Farber 1991: 315). Murken zeigt in seinem Überblick über die Themen Krankheit und Krankenhaus im Kinder- und Jugendbuch diesen präventiven Charakter der in den 30er-Jahren entstandenen Kinderbücher (Murken 2004: 23). In diesen wird Krankheit verteufelt und muss durch richtiges Verhalten vermieden werden, was in Titeln wie Rudolf Ernst Schenkes „Was allen Kindern hilft und nützt und sie vor böser Krankheit schützt" (1936) zum Ausdruck kommt (Murken 2004: 2).

Nach dem zweiten Weltkrieg stehen anknüpfend an die Literatur der Vorkriegszeit Wertvorstellungen wie Tugend, Frömmigkeit, guter Wille und

Bescheidenheit im Mittelpunkt der Darstellung, während sich ab den sechziger Jahren im Rahmen der sich stärker durchsetzenden soziorealistischen Kinderliteratur eine aufklärende Haltung etabliert (Farber 1991: 315). Diese differenziert sich im Laufe der siebziger Jahre aus, so dass Kinder im Rahmen der Lektüre einen vertieften Einblick in einzelne Krankheitsbilder gewinnen. In der erzählenden Literatur der 70er-Jahre wird *Das war der Hirbel* (1973) von Peter Härtling zu einem paradigmatischen Text, der in der Folge die Darstellung von Krankheit und Behinderung nachhaltig prägt. Während das Nachwort aufklärerisch und sachlich gehalten ist, ermöglicht die Erzählweise Härtlings einen Blick in das subjektive Erleben des geistig schwer behinderten Protagonisten. Bis heute dominiert dieser Tradition folgend in Texten der Kinder- und Jugendliteratur eine Erzählweise, die versachlichte Darstellung und Innenperspektive kombiniert. Reese konstatiert, dass bei der Darstellung von Behinderungen eine Verschiebung zu geistigen Behinderungen und sprachlichen Beeinträchtigungen stattgefunden hat: Blindheit und fehlende Gliedmaßen werden heute weit seltener thematisiert (vgl. Reese 2010: 7). Bei den Krankheiten dominieren nun – wie weiter unten noch gezeigt werden wird – Tumorerkrankungen und psychische Krankheiten.

Wieso aber spielen gerade Krankheit und die Bedrohung durch den Tod als deren Folge in der Kinder- und Jugendliteratur angesichts der vielen aktuellen Bücher zu diesem Thema eine so wichtige Rolle, während diese Themen im gesellschaftlichen Diskurs eher verdrängt werden? Zunächst muss berücksichtigt werden, dass Kinder- und Jugendliteratur hinsichtlich ihrer Adressierung eine Besonderheit aufweist: Sie richtet sich zwar „offiziell" – wie der Begriff schon sagt – an Kinder und Jugendliche, allerdings bedarf es, je jünger die intendierten Adressaten sind, einer stärkeren Auswahl durch entsprechende Vermittlungsinstanzen, damit ein Buch auf den Buchmarkt gelangen bzw. auf diesem bestehen kann. Kinder- und jugendliterarische Kommunikation ist damit eine vor allem über Dritte vermittelte literarische Kommunikation (Ewers 2000: 101): Die erwachsenen Vermittler – Eltern, Bibliothekare, Lehrer und Pädagogen – wirken bei ihrer Auswahl entscheidend mit. In der Regel sind sie es, die das Angebot zuerst prüfen, um dann die in ihren Augen geeigneten Texte weiterzuempfehlen. In der Kinderliteraturforschung hat sich für diesen Umstand der Begriff der „Doppeltadressiertheit" etabliert, der impliziert, dass erst die erfolgreiche Kommunikation mit den Vermittlern den Zugang zu den intendierten Lesern eröffnet (vgl. Ewers 200: 103). Dies verdeutlicht, dass Texte über das Thema „Krankheit" nicht nur die Funktion haben, die Kinder als Leser zu informieren sowie Mitgefühl und Verständnis zu evozieren, sondern eben auch den erwachsenen Mitlesern geeignet erscheinen müssen, um Kindern dieses gesellschaftlich weitgehend tabuisierte Thema nahe zu bringen.

Da literarische Texte als „symbolische Repräsentation ästhetisch-fiktionaler (Als-ob-) Weltauffassungsentwürfe" (Kaulen 1999: 258)[4] zu verstehen sind, stellt sich gerade bei der Auseinandersetzung mit Kinder- und Jugendliteratur die spannende Frage, inwieweit diese mit den gesellschaftlich relevanten Diskursen übereinstimmen oder von ihnen abweichen. Dies kann zu interessanten Ergebnissen und Funktionshypothesen führen, da Kinderliteratur eben nicht nur literarische Ambitionen verfolgt, sondern auch erzieherische Zielvorstellungen. Auch Shavit weist auf die enge Verknüpfung der Kinderliteratur mit anderen kulturellen Diskursen hin:

> Children's literature, more than any other literary system, results from a conglomerate of several systems in culture, among which the most important are the social, the educational and the literary. If one is interested in studying such complex relationships in culture, if one is interested in the mechanism of culture and its dynamics, children's literature is the most promising area of research. No other field equals children's literature in the immense scope of the cultural parameters involved. Children's literature is the only system I know of that belongs simultaneously and indispensably to the literary and the social-educational system. It is the only system whose products have always purposefully addressed two antithetical audiences, catering to the needs and expectations of both.
>
> (Shavit 1994: 4)

Lotman definiert die Funktion eines Textes als seine „soziale Rolle", als die Fähigkeit und Eignung des Textes, „bestimmte Bedürfnisse der ihn umgebenden Gemeinschaft zu befriedigen" (Lotman 1981: 34). Kinderliteratur kann dabei sowohl Bedürfnisse der Kinder befriedigen, aber auch die der sie produzierenden bzw. vermittelnden Erwachsenen. Während z.B. mit *Heidi* oder *The Secret Garden* den Kindern der Wert des freien Spiels, der Freundschaft und der Wert der Natur nahe gebracht werden sollen, indem zahlreiche Tätigkeiten mit Freunden in der Natur dargestellt werden, prallen innerhalb der erwachsenen Figuren Diskurse über die richtige Erziehung von Kindern aufeinander. Während die einen das einengende bürgerliche Leben als „gesundheitsschädlich" vermitteln, plädieren die anderen für eine strenge Erziehung hin zu bürgerlichen Tugenden oder für eine Abschottung und allumsorgende Pflege des kranken Kindes. Der Ausgang der Handlung verstärkt das „richtige" Wertesystem und bestätigt eine bis heute wirksame Erziehungsideologie, nämlich, dass Kinder sich am besten entwickeln, wenn sie sich ohne Einengung durch erziehende Erwachsene in der freien Natur aufhalten.

---

[4] Vgl. auch Titzmann: „‚Literatur' ist das Produkt kulturellen – mentalen und nicht-mentalen – Handelns und kann zu kulturellem Handeln führen: insofern ist sie Teil des faktischen Sozialsystems. Sie entwirft Modelle der ‚Realität': insofern ist sie Teil des kulturellen Denksystems" (1991: 413).

Bis in die aktuelle Kinder- und Jugendliteratur hinein spielen dabei auch Geschlechterrollenideologien eine zentrale Rolle. Während sich aus einem einzelnen Text kaum Aussagen über Darstellungsmuster eines literarischen Subsystems treffen lassen, ist ein Blick auf ein größeres Korpus lohnenswert, um Aussagen über die Beziehung von „Geschlecht und Krankheit" treffen zu können. Farber etwa kommt bei ihrer Analyse von 235 Kinder- und Jugendbüchern von 1845 bis 1985 zu dem Ergebnis, dass der Anteil von weiblichen Kranken innerhalb ihres Korpus mit fast 55% überwiegt (Farber 1991: 312). In einem Überblick über zentrale Texte zum Thema „Krankheit" oder „Behinderung", die seither entstanden sind, fällt auf, dass es nun überwiegend Jungen sind, die als Protagonisten eine Krankheit durchleiden.

Im Folgenden sollen zwei exemplarische Textkorpora diesbezüglich einer genaueren Analyse unterzogen werden: Die Kinderliteratur der 1990er Jahre und die Jugendliteratur seit 2000. Die Auswahl ist nicht erschöpfend für die in dieser Zeit entstandenen Kinder- und Jugendbücher, aufgrund der Vielzahl an Texten können jedoch durchaus Trends bestimmt werden.

Im Kampf gegen vorgegebene Rollenbilder:
Die Kinderliteratur seit den 1990er Jahren

Gerade für die Literatur des 19. Jahrhunderts und der ersten Hälfte des 20. Jahrhunderts ist das typische Mädchen eher schwach und wenig autonom. Protagonistinnen wie *Alice im Wunderland* (1865) von Lewis Carroll oder *Der Trotzkopf* (1885) von Emmy von Rhoden lassen erste abweichende Darstellungen von Mädchenfiguren erkennen, zeigen aber auch, dass am Ende wieder eine weitgehende Assimilation an das bürgerliche System gelingt. Dieses Bild ändert sich in der zweiten Hälfte des 20. Jahrhunderts: In der Folge von Texten wie *Pippi Langstrumpf* (1945) von Astrid Lindgren oder *Die rote Zora* (1941) von Kurt Held werden Mädchen zunehmend als starke, autonome Heldinnen dargestellt, die sich vorherrschenden Normen widersetzen. Im Gegensatz dazu nimmt die Darstellung schwacher Jungen zu. In der soziorealistischen Literatur der 1990er-Jahre gibt es vermehrt zentrale Jungenfiguren, die nicht dem Schema des starken Abenteuerhelden entsprechen, sondern eher ängstlich und zurückgezogen sowie körperlich unterlegen dargestellt werden (vgl. Schilcher 2001: 58-63). In vielen dieser Texte wird jedoch thematisiert, dass Jungen einem starken Erwartungsdruck der Umwelt ausgesetzt sind und Scham darüber empfinden, dem internalisierten (idealen) Rollenbild nicht zu entsprechen. Im Gegensatz zu den meisten Mädchenfiguren wehren sich die Jungen aber nicht aktiv gegen die an sie herangetragenen Erwartungen, sondern übernehmen diese unreflektiert in ihr Selbstkonzept („Ein richtiger Junge muss…"). Da diese Jungen im Kontext der Handlung jedoch immer positiv besetzt werden – also als ‚diskursmächtige

Figuren' auftreten und letztendlich in ihrem Verhalten durch Erfolg und Akzeptanz bei Gleichaltrigen belohnt werden – werden die vorgegebenen Rollenerwartungen als irrelevant für das Gelingen ihres Lebens gesetzt und entwertet. Ideologisch könnte man daher die Aussage der Texte wie folgt zusammenfassen: Jungen sind eben auch dann akzeptabel und wertvoll, wenn sie nicht dem herkömmlichen Klischee entsprechen. Die Darstellung von kranken Jungen ermöglicht es deshalb, die Diskrepanz zwischen der rollenklischeehaften Stärke und der Realität der Jungenfiguren besonders augenfällig darzustellen. Das könnte erklären, warum es in der Literatur der 90er-Jahre zu einer Kulmination von Büchern mit kranken Protagonisten kommt – wie folgende Beispiele anschaulich demonstrieren:

1. Hannes in Regina Ruschs *Zappelhannes* (1996) leidet an einer minimalen cerebralen Disfunktion,

2. Simon in Renate Welshs *Eine Krone aus Papier* (1992) zwinkert ständig, wenn er aufgeregt ist und hat Minderwertigkeitsgefühle,

3. Till in Dagmar Chidolues *Der Schönste von allen* (1995) ist auf einem Auge blind und könnte vollständig erblinden,

4. Annes Bruder in Renate Welshs *Drachenflügel* (1988) ist schwer geistig behindert,

5. Lars in Peter Härtlings *Lena auf dem Dach* (1993) ist Diabetiker, so dass sich seine Schwester mütterlich um ihn kümmert, als sich die Eltern trennen,

6. Leander in Doris Meissner-Johannknechts *Leanders Traum* (1994) leidet an schlimmen Allergien und Asthmaanfällen.

Die auffällige Häufung kranker und behinderter Jungen verstärkt den Kontrast ‚erwartete Rolle' versus ‚Realität der dargestellten Welt' und macht somit noch klarer deutlich, dass eine Erfüllung der traditionellen Erwartungen von vielen Jungen nicht geleistet werden kann und die Vorstellung vom „starken Jungen" aufgegeben werden muss. Interessanterweise sind es gerade die Väter, die die Krankheit oder Behinderung ihrer Söhne nicht akzeptieren können:

Als Papa den Sattel losläßt, reißt Hannes blitzschnell die Füße von den Pedalen und stützt sich breitbeinig auf dem Boden ab. Gerade noch rechtzeitig. Sonst wäre er umgefallen. „Stell dich doch nicht so dämlich an", sagt Papa verärgert. Hannes legt den Kopf auf den verrosteten Lenker und beginnt zu schluchzen. „Was ist eigentlich so schwierig daran?" fragt Papa. Die Tränen schießen Hannes in die Augen. Papa tritt einen Schritt zurück.

(Rusch 1996: 36)

„Jetzt steh nicht so schisserig da!" schnauzte sein Vater. Er brüllte fast, vielleicht wegen des Windes, der auf der Höhenterrasse pfiff. Die Leute schauten sich um.
„Lass den Jungen", sagte Oma.
„Nun guck doch bloß, wie der dasteht! Der macht sich ja gleich in die Hose!" [...]
„Na los, nimm die Hände vom Geländer. Mein Gott, was bist du bloß für eine Memme!"

(Gutzschhahn 1993: 26)

Der Vater als Repräsentant der vorhergehenden Generation fordert ein „jungenhaftes" Verhalten ein, er wird jedoch vom Text als unsympathisch, kalt und wenig verständnisvoll dargestellt; vor allem dann, wenn der Text deutlich macht, dass die Söhne durch Krankheit oder Behinderung beeinträchtigt sind, erscheint der Vater, der dies nicht erkennt und akzeptiert, als besonders herzlos. Die Mütter hingegen akzeptieren ihre Söhne meist als Individuen und unterstützen ihre Entwicklung. Krankheit oder Behinderung werden bei ihnen zu einer individuellen Facette des Kindes, die berücksichtigt werden muss. Im Gegensatz zu früheren Epochen steht die „Heilung" oder Bekämpfung der Krankheit nicht mehr im Fokus. In der Kinder- und Jugendliteratur der 1990er-Jahre werden Ängste oft vor allem genau dann überwunden oder abgebaut, wenn die Umwelt sie als Teil der Persönlichkeit akzeptiert. Damit wird implizit Kritik geübt an dem sozialen Druck, einem bestimmten Ideal zu entsprechen, der dazu führt, dass Ängste und Ticks entstehen oder sich vertiefen.

Krankheit, so meine These, dient in diesen Texten dazu zu zeigen, dass Jungen schwach und abweichend sein dürfen und dass sie daran auch nichts ändern können. Im Sinne der Doppeltadressiertheit enthalten diese Texte sowohl die Aufforderung an die Jungen sich nicht dem gesellschaftlich geforderten Männlichkeitsstereotyp zu unterwerfen, während sie den erwachsenen Mitleser auffordern, Geschlechterrollenstereotype aufzugeben. Krankheit als individuelles Schicksal wird von den Texten instrumentalisiert, um Vorstellungen von richtiger Erziehung und einem kindgerechten Leben zu „transportieren".

Die Kinderliteratur der 1990er-Jahre war, wenn auch ideologisch „korrekt", gerade bei den Jungen als Lesestoff nicht beliebt. Befragungen wie die Erfurter Studie (2001) oder die Untersuchung Gattermeiers (2003) zeigen, dass gerade Jungen soziorealistische Literatur ablehnen, dagegen Fantasy-, Abenteuerliteratur und Kriminalromane bevorzugen, in denen der starke Held nach wie vor den Normalfall darstellt. Der Buchmarkt hat sich diesem Bedürfnis in den letzten Jahren angepasst: Die dargestellten Jungen sind zwar nicht mehr die klassischen, unbesiegbaren Helden vergangener Jahrzehnte, sie werden jedoch wieder zu Helden, die – meist Seite an Seite mit tapferen Mädchen – Abenteuer bestehen und Ängste überwinden, wie etwa *Der kleine Ritter Trenk* (2006) von Kirsten Boie, *Die tollkühnen Abenteuer von JanBenMax* (2008) von Zoran Drvenkar oder Arthur in *Potilla* (1992) von Cornelia Funke.

Autonomie trotz Krankheit: Die aktuelle Jugendliteratur

Im Gegensatz dazu findet sich in der Jugendliteratur – gerade auf den Bestsellerlisten – in den letzten Jahren eine fast unüberschaubare Menge an Titeln, in denen kranke Jungen die Hauptrolle spielen.[5] Wirft man einen genaueren Blick auf die Texte, so lassen sich auch hier Thesen zu den impliziten Ideologien der Texte aufstellen und auch dazu, warum sich männliche Geschlechtsrollenentwürfe hierfür besonders eignen.

Zunächst ist zu konstatieren, dass sich die Bücher auf wenige Krankheiten fokussieren: Der überwiegende Teil der Jungen erkrankt in den Texten an Leukämie oder einer anderen Krebserkrankung, gefolgt von Autismus und Depression. Diese Krankheiten zeichnen sich gerade nicht durch „Visibilität" aus, einem Merkmal, das bei der hohen Anzahl an blinden Protagonisten und solchen mit fehlenden oder geschädigten Gliedmaßen im 19. Jahrhundert entscheidend war, um die Andersartigkeit des Protagonisten zum Ausdruck zu bringen und dadurch dem Rezipienten Distanzierung zu ermöglichen (Reese 2007: 167). Den Protagonisten in den aktuellen Jugendbüchern sieht man ihre Erkrankung oft nicht an[6] und die überwiegend als Ich-Erzählung vermittelten Texte konfrontieren den Rezipienten mit intensiven Innenperspektiven, die zeigen, dass es sich hier um einen Jugendlichen mit normalen Wünschen und Bedürfnissen handelt. Auch die zentralen Themen dürften dem jugendlichen Rezipienten nicht fremd sein. Sie betreffen selten die Auseinandersetzung des Protagonisten mit der Krankheit selbst, sondern die Möglichkeit, ein „normales" und intensives Leben trotz Krankheit zu führen. Nicht mehr der duldsame „Musterkrüppel" oder „Musterpatient" stehen hier im Zentrum, sondern die ungeduldigen, fordernden, oft zynischen Pubertierenden. Themen sind dabei der pubertäre Kampf um Autonomie, Selbstbestimmung und Selbstverantwortung, die sich an kranken Jungenfiguren besonders eindringlich zeigen lassen, weil die Sorge der Eltern hier besonders gut nachvollziehbar ist und die Interessenskonflikte eine dramatische Zuspitzung erlauben. Die untersuchten Texte zeigen durchweg positive Mutterfiguren (und oft hilflose Vaterfiguren), die nichts unversucht lassen, um die kranken Jungen zu unterstützen, gleichzeitig jedoch scheitern müssen, weil sie damit den in der Pubertät verständlichen Willen zu einem

---

[5] Es finden sich auch Titel mit kranken Mädchen, überwiegend stehen jedoch Jungen im Fokus.

[6] Auch in *Das Schicksal ist ein mieser Verräter* (2012) von John Green ist es die weibliche Hazel, deren Sauerstoffschläuche auf den ersten Blick sichtbar sind, während sich Augustus' Prothese nur durch den schiefen Gang erahnen lässt.

autonomen Leben behindern. Jeder der dargestellten Jungen muss sein „Problem" am Ende alleine lösen, unabhängig von den Eltern oder umsorgenden Erwachsenen (zum Teil auch Klinikpersonal).

In Sally Nicholls *Wie man unsterblich wird. Jede Minute zählt* (2008; dt. 2010) möchte der elfjährige Ich-Erzähler Sam trotz seiner Leukämie-Erkrankung ein möglichst normales Leben führen, in dem seine Krankheit nicht im Zentrum steht. Alles, was ihn hindert, die Krankheit zu vergessen, stört:

> Ich zog mein T-Shirt hoch, damit sie an meinen Hickman-Katheter kam.
> Das ist eine Art langes dünnes Röhrchen, das in meinem Brustkorb steckt. Dadurch kann sie mir Blut entnehmen und mir auch irgendwelches Zeug einflößen. Es ist keine große Sache, aber es nervt trotzdem, weil es immer da ist und einen nie vergessen lässt, dass man krank ist.
>
> (Nicholls 2010: 38f.)

Da Sam um die ernste Lage seines Gesundheitszustandes weiß, stellt er eine Liste mit Dingen auf, die er gerne vor seinem Tod verwirklichen möchte, z. B. ein Mädchen küssen, ein berühmter Forscher werden, Rolltreppen verkehrt rum hoch- und runterlaufen, ein Teenager werden, typische Teenager-Sachen machen, wie rauchen und trinken und Freundinnen haben, mit einem Luftschiff fahren. Zusammen mit seinem 13-jährigen, krebskranken Freund Felix versucht er, seine Wünsche in die Realität umzusetzen. Das Buch zeigt, dass das Wichtigste für Sam der enttabuisierte Umgang mit seiner Krankheit ist. Das Schweigen und Verleugnen seines Vaters sowie die Überbesorgtheit der Mutter gefährden den Wunsch, weiterhin in das normale Familienleben integriert zu sein. Als Sam am Ende stirbt, tut er dies im Kreis der Familie und mit der Genugtuung, dass er sich einen Teil seiner Wünsche erfüllen konnte.

Auch Augustus *(Das Schicksal ist ein mieser Verräter)* möchte sich die Reise nach Amsterdam mit Hazel nicht verbieten lassen, obwohl er einen Rückfall hat:

> Während wir auf das Haus zugingen, hörten wir plötzlich, wie drinnen jemand weinte. Ich dachte gar nicht daran, dass es Gus sein könnte, weil es nicht wie das tiefe Brummen seiner Stimme klang, aber dann hörte ich eine Stimme, die eindeutig eine verzerrte Version von seiner war: „WEIL ES MEIN LEBEN IST; MOM: ES GEHÖRT MIR."
>
> (Green 2012: 129)

Den Kampf um ein normales, d.h. in die Gesellschaft integriertes Leben trotz Behinderung führt auch Colbert mit seinem geistig schwer behinderten Bruder „Simpel" (*Simpel* von Marie-Aude Murail, 2006; dt. 2007), als er mit ihm in eine Pariser Studenten-WG zieht, um Simpel nicht in das verhasste Heim geben zu müssen. Während die Mitbewohner zunächst befremdet und verärgert auf Simpel reagieren und ihn als Störfaktor ihres normalen Lebens empfinden, wird er mehr und mehr zu einem „normalen", selbstverständlichen Mitglied der WG. Durch seinen kindlich-unverstellten Blick bringt Simpel oft Wesentliches auf den Punkt und eröffnet manchem „normalen" Mitbewohner einen unverstellten Blick auf die Realität. Als Colbert resigniert und bereit ist, seinen Kampf um ein normales Leben für Simpel aufzugeben und deshalb einen Heimplatz organisiert, erhält er Unterstützung durch die anderen Mitbewohner. Gemeinsam vereinbaren sie einen Betreuungsplan für Simpel, so dass dieser Teil des täglichen WG-Lebens wird.

Der autistische Held Christopher in *Supergute Tage oder die sonderbare Welt des Christopher Boone* (2003, dt. 2005) von Mark Haddon ringt nach dem Tod des Nachbarhundes und der Entdeckung, dass seine vom Vater für tot erklärte Mutter noch lebt und versucht hat, mit ihm Kontakt aufzunehmen, um eine Wiederherstellung einer berechenbaren Alltagsroutine, die ihm ein angstfreies Leben ermöglicht. Da Christopher jedoch nicht über den Betrug des Vaters hinwegkommt, bricht er aus seiner schützenden, im wörtlichen Sinn berechenbaren Lebenswelt aus und macht sich auf den Weg nach London, um seine Mutter zu finden. Eindrücklich schildert der Text die Ängste, Schwierigkeiten und Verunsicherungen seines Protagonisten. Trotzdem betont das Ende des Textes, dass Christophers Zukunft ein „möglichst normales Leben" sein soll. Trotz seiner Behinderung entwirft er ein optimistisches Bild seiner Zukunft:

> Ich werde den Test bestehen und bestimmt wieder eine Eins bekommen. Und in zwei Jahren kann ich dann mein Physik-Abitur machen, auch wieder mit einer Eins.
>
> Und wenn ich das geschafft habe, werde ich in einer anderen Stadt eine Universität besuchen. [...] Dann kann ich in einer Wohnung leben, die einen Garten und eine richtige Toilette hat. Und ich werde Sandy und meine Bücher und meinen Computer mitnehmen können. Und dann mache ich ein Prädikatsexamen und werde Wissenschaftler.
>
> Ich weiß, dass ich das schaffe, weil ich tapfer war, ganz allein nach London gefahren bin.
>
> (Haddon 2005: 278f.)

Auch der 16-jährige Ben in *Ben X* (2009) von Nic Balthazar leidet unter Autismus. Das Leben in der Schule wird für ihn zur Hölle, zwei seiner Mitschüler traktieren und demütigen ihn. Jede Abweichung vom gewohnten Tagesablauf ängstigt Ben und lässt ihn in Panik geraten. Nur im „Chat" mit „Barbie" und im Computerspiel findet Ben Zuflucht. Seine Mutter und seine Lehrer versuchen ihn zu beschützen, es gelingt ihnen jedoch nicht.

> Nein Ben ging nicht gern in die Schule, aber das hatte auch mit anderen Dingen zu tun. Nirgendwo fühlte er sich sicher. Überall bekam man irgendein Papierkügelchen an den Kopf geworfen, oder es piekste im Rücken. Täglich gab es mindestens einen Anschlag. Und nichts war schlimmer als ein Lehrer, der einen davor beschützen wollte. Auch

jetzt gab es wieder so einen Samariter, der es nicht lassen konnte: „Jungs, lasst Ben in Ruhe! Ben ist ein bisschen anders als ihr. Sonst nichts. Versucht mal ein bisschen Respekt dafür aufzubringen." Eine Verurteilung zum Tode wäre nicht weniger grausam gewesen. Denn am Ende der Stunde, als der Lehrer nach draußen gockelte, stolz auf die gute Tat, konnte man davon ausgehen, dass Dumm und Jerry, wie Ben sie manchmal nannte, mit Sicherheit der Meinung waren, sie wären nun wieder am Zuge.

(Balthazar 2009: 12)

Am Ende inszeniert Ben den eigenen Selbstmord, um seinem schulischen Lebensumfeld zu entkommen. Der Text zeigt damit zum einen die Schwierigkeiten eines Lebens mit Autismus, unterstreicht jedoch den Wunsch nach einer selbstbestimmten Lebensführung. Letztlich kann sich Ben nur selbst befreien, ebenso wie Christopher Boone seine Mutter allein finden muss.

In Ned Vizzinis *Eine echt verrückte Story* (2006) kämpft der 14-jährige Craig mit einer schweren Depression, die ihn an den Rand des Selbstmordes treibt. Als er sich schließlich freiwillig in eine psychiatrische Klinik begibt, deren Station für „Teenager" bezeichnenderweise gerade renoviert wird, so dass er in die Erwachsenenpsychiatrie eingewiesen wird, gewinnt er Autonomie und überwindet (im Erwachsenwerden) seine Depression. Gleichzeitig wird der Roman nicht müde, die „Normalität" von psychischer Krankheit zu betonen. Sowohl Craig als auch die anderen Patienten der psychiatrischen Abteilung leiden unter ihren Lebensumständen, ihre Reaktionen auf diese sind jedoch durchaus nachvollziehbar, so dass sie dem Rezipienten nur wenig fremd erscheinen und Identifikationspotential bieten.

Eine andere Perspektive auf das Thema Krankheit nimmt Jordan Sonnenblick in seinem Roman *Wie ich zum besten Schlagzeuger der Welt wurde – und warum* (2004) ein. Hier geht es um die Bewältigung der Leukämieerkrankung des kleinen, 5-jährigen Jeffrey, der einen 13 Jahre alten Bruder namens Steven hat. Um sich ein Stück eigene, unabhängige Lebenswelt zu bewahren und sich gleichzeitig der Krankheit des Bruders stellen zu können, flieht Steven in sein Schlagzeugspiel. Was zunächst Flucht ist, gibt ihm zunehmend die Stärke, sich mit der Krankheit auseinanderzusetzen und den kranken Bruder als wichtigen Teil seines Lebens zu akzeptieren – nachdem er ihn zunächst verschweigt, um wenigstens in der Schule ein „normaler" Junge zu sein. Dieses lässt ihn reifen und zu einem wichtigen Bezugspunkt für Jeffrey werden. Am Ende konstatiert sein Vater stolz: „Vielleicht habe ich es noch nicht gesagt – aber ich bin wirklich sehr stolz auf dich. Du bist ein echt guter Mann" (Sonnenblick 2004: 178).

Krankheit wird damit in einer modernen, weitgehend gefahrlosen Lebenswelt zu einem der letzten existentiellen Themen, zu einem Auslöser für den Kampf um Autonomie und Eigenverantwortung, der den jugendlichen Protagonisten zum Mann reifen lässt. Ist der Held vom Tod bedroht, spielt Erotik meist eine wichtige Rolle. So will der 11-jährige Sam (*Wie man unsterblich wird. Jede Minute zählt*) trotz seines jungen Alters noch ein Mädchen küssen, Donalds (*Superhero*, 2006; dt. 2007) intensivster Wunsch ist es trotz seiner Leukämieerkrankung mit einem Mädchen zu schlafen und auch August und Hazel *(Das Schicksal ist ein mieser Verräter)* erleben trotz (oder wegen) der lebensbedrohlichen Erkrankungen eine leidenschaftliche Liebesbeziehung.[7] Krankheit und Behinderung tragen damit auf unterschiedliche Weise dazu bei, das Leben zu intensivieren und Autonomie zu erlangen. Während es bei den lebensbedrohlichen Krankheiten darum geht, sich von der Krankheit intensive (erotische) Erfahrungen nicht nehmen zu lassen, überwinden die autistischen Helden die Beschränkungen, die ihnen durch ihre Behinderung auferlegt sind.

Darüber hinaus tragen diese Texte gerade in der Jugendliteratur dazu bei, Normalitätsgrenzen auszuweiten.[8] Immer wieder betonen die Protagonisten in ihrer Figurenrede, aber auch durch ihr Verhalten im Verlauf der Handlung den Wunsch nach „Normalität", d.h. nach einem normalen Leben in Familie und Freundeskreis, nach normalen Liebesbeziehungen und nach einer Teilnahme am normalen sozialen Leben. Gesellschaftliche Heterotope wie Heime für Behinderte, Krankenhäuser oder durch die Eltern behütete und überwachte, private Lebensräume werden entgrenzt und die Protagonisten durchbrechen die Schranken, die ihnen das Leben mit Krankheit oder Behinderung scheinbar auferlegt. Damit partizipiert die aktuelle Jugendliteratur an den Fragestellungen der modernen[9] Literatur, die sich für Randcharaktere, Marginalisierungen, irreversible Denormalisierungen sowie „Aus- und Rückfahrten" über Normalitätsgrenzen interessiert (vgl. Link 1997: 60). Durch die Darstellung von Rand-Charakteren, randständigen und extremen Lebensweisen und -situationen werden in der Jugendliteratur Normalitätsgrenzen auch hinsichtlich des Themenspektrums erweitert: Krankheit, Behinderung und Tod werden zunehmend zu normalen Themen, wie das Angebot an Büchern zeigt. Dass diese Literatur damit auch die Grenzen im Sinne des *crossreading* und *crosswriting* zur Allgemeinliteratur

[7] Diese Thematik wird auch in Filmen der letzten Jahre aufgegriffen: In der international erfolgreichen und mit renommierten Preisen ausgezeichneten belgischen Jugendkomödie *Hasta la Vista – Pflücke das Leben* (Geoffrey Enthoven, 2011, dt. 2012) wird sie auf die Spitze getrieben: Die drei behinderten Freunde Lars (aufgrund einer fortschreitenden Krankheit an den Rollstuhl gefesselt), Philip (vom Hals abwärts gelähmt) und Jozef (fast ganz blind), die alle Mitte zwanzig und noch immer Jungfrauen sind, flüchten eines Tages aus der Obhut ihrer überfürsorglichen Eltern und brechen mit einem weiblichen Ex-Häftling als Busfahrerin in einem Kleinbus nach Spanien auf, um dort in einem Bordell speziell für Behinderte ihr erstes Mal zu erleben. Durch diese Kombination aus Freundschaft, Autonomie, Naturerkundung und sexuellen Erfahrungen erlangen die Protagonisten im Rahmen ihrer abenteuerlichen Reise neuen Lebensmut.

[8] Zum gesellschaftlichen Normalitätsdiskurs vgl. Link, Jürgen. *Versuch über den Normalismus. Wie Normalität produziert wird*. Opladen: Westdeutscher Verlag, 1997.

[9] Link nennt hier Autoren wie Musil, Proust, Kafka, usw.

überschreitet, zeigt ihr Erscheinen auf Nominierungs- und Bestsellerlisten beider literarischer Subsysteme (z.B. wurde *Das Schicksal ist ein mieser Verräter* sowohl für zahlreiche Jugendbuchpreise nominiert, war aber auch monatelang auf der *Spiegel*-Bestsellerliste in der Sparte Belletristik vertreten).

Kriegsmetaphorik: Der Kampf gegen die Krankheit

Ein Phänomen, das sich an den Texten beobachten lässt, irritiert durch die Vielzahl seines Auftretens, nämlich die Verwendung von Kriegs- und Kampfmetaphorik für das alltägliche Leben:

> Der Bus kam täglich um 7.27 Uhr. Darauf konnte man zählen. Das war sicher. Das war gut. Danach war *Krieg*. Danach galt es zu *überleben*. Jeden Tag. Denn jeden Tag wurden die Spielregeln verändert.
>
> (Balthazar 2009: 7, Hervorhebung A. S.)

Der Kampf um ein normales und selbstbestimmtes Leben wird als Krieg deklariert, nichts verläuft vorhersehbar, von allen Seiten sind Angriffe auf die Alltagsroutinen zu erwarten, auf die Ben angewiesen ist. Am Ende schafft er es jedoch, sich durch das Verlassen der Opferrolle aus seiner Lage zu befreien und sich ein Stück Normalität zu erkämpfen.

Besonders auffällig ist die Kriegsmetaphorik in Anthony McCartens *Superhero* (2006; dt. 2007). Hier zieht sie sich durch den gesamten Text und wird auch den unterschiedlichen Figuren zugeschrieben, nicht nur – wie dies in anderen Texten der Fall ist – dem Protagonisten.

> Es ist schwer für Renata, mit ihrem Sohn zu sprechen, wenn dabei eine tragbare Travenol-Pumpe auf dem Boden neben seinem Bett über einen Schlauch und durch den Permaport an der Schulter Chemikalien in seinen Körper transportiert. [...] Was es so schwer, ja gerade unmöglich macht, ist das Wissen, dass die Travenol-Pumpe in diesem Augenblick, in dem sie vor sich hinplappert, die *abscheulichsten Gifte* in ihren geliebten Sohn befördert, die ein menschlicher Körper überhaupt aushalten kann, ein *chemotherapeutischer Ansturm*, der die gesunden wie die wuchernden Zellen *zerstört*, der ohne Unterschied *tötet*, bis nichts mehr von ihrem Sohn übrig ist [...].
>
> Sie weiß also ganz genau, dass ihr Junge in diesem Augenblick *umgebracht* wird, Zelle für Zelle, im Mikrokosmos, immer in der Hoffnung, dass sich so das Ganze retten lässt: *stalinistische* Medizin, die ganze *Völker opfert*, damit die Idee des Staates Bestand hat.
>
> (McCartens 2007: 28, Hervorhebung A.S.)

> Aber was kann sie machen? Sie ist erschöpft von den Versuchen, in ihm das Bewusstsein für seine Krankheit zu wecken, den Versuchen, ihn zum Mitmachen im *großen Kampf* zu bewegen. Er hat ausgezeichnete Chancen, die Krankheit zu *besiegen*, aber er selbst trägt nichts dazu bei.
>
> (McCartens 2007: 29, Hervorhebung A. S.)

JIM: Er wehrt sich nicht. Kein *Kampfgeist*.

(McCartens 2007: 42, Hervorhebung A. S.)

Doch die Innenperspektive Donalds zeigt, dass es sich aus seiner Sicht um keinen Krieg handelt, der im traditionellen Einzelkampf gewonnen wird, sondern dass die „Waffen" (siehe unten), die er als „Patient" (als Erleidender) verwenden muss, ebenso tödlich sind (oder so erlebt werden) wie die Krankheit:

> Dann um die Mittagszeit ein kleiner Ausflug zur Radiologie, eine Art Mittagspause auf dem *Atomwaffentestgelände* [...].
> Als Donald aus *Hiroshima* zurückkehrt, von der Radiologie [...].

(McCartens 2007: 173f., Hervorhebung A.S.)

Adrian, Donalds Psychotherapeut, versucht Donald über die Comics, die dieser zeichnet, näher zu kommen und ihn zu verstehen. Donald wehrt sich jedoch anfangs dagegen, da er annimmt, dass Adrian ihn ebenso wie seine Mutter beschützen und zum aktiven Kampf animieren möchte.

> ADRIAN: MiracleMan – das ist ein guter Name.
> DONALD: Hm…
> ADRIAN: Ein Superheld. Interessant.
> Donald hat nicht die Absicht, sich in ein Gespräch verwickeln zu lassen.
> ADRIAN: Er furzt. [*Pause*] Interessant.
> DONALD: Er ist echt. Leute furzen eben. Na, Sie wahrscheinlich nicht.
> ADRIAN: Er ist echt – aber unverletzlich. [*Schweigen*] Und über wen triumphiert MiracleMan?
> DONALD [*starrt ADRIAN eindringlich an*]: Arschlöcher. [*Schweigen*]
> ADRIAN: Und …nichts kann ihn umbringen?
> DONALD: Nichts. Das ist es doch, was unverletzlich heißt.
> ADRIAN: Mir ist aufgefallen, dass er manchmal Frauenleichen ausgräbt und Sex mit Ihnen hat. Warum tut er das?
> DONALD: Es bleibt ihm nichts anderes übrig. Die Mädchen wollen ihn nicht.
> ADRIAN: Warum nicht?
> DONALD: Weil er furzt.
> ADRIAN: Warum gibst du deinem MiracleMan so eine Eigenschaft?
> DONALD: Hab ich doch gesagt. Weil er echt sein soll. Ich hab die Nase voll von bescheuerten Superhelden.
> ADRIAN: Aber Superhelden sind nicht echt.
> DONALD [*kühler Blick*]: Sind sie da jetzt grade draufgekommen?
> ADRIAN: [*reicht ihm den Comic zurück*]: Sein Erzfeind – Gummifinger? Ein Chirurg, der immer mit einem schnappenden Laut seine Handschuhe anzieht?
> DONALD: Das ist cool.
> ADRIAN: Du magst keine Ärzte?
> DONALD: Hätten Sie nicht gedacht, was? Kann ich jetzt gehen? Ich krieg heute Nachmittag noch Strahlen.

(McCartens 2007: 50)

Die Szene verdeutlicht, wie Donald versucht, seine Realität in einem selbst entworfenen Comic zu verarbeiten. Hier zeigt sich auch, dass Donald weniger an der Krankheit selbst verzweifelt, sondern daran, dass sie ihn aus dem „normalen Leben" ausschließt. Sein größter Wunsch, vor seinem Tod noch Sex zu haben, ist aus seiner Sicht aufgrund seiner Krankheit unerfüllbar. Während seine Mutter will, dass er gegen die Krankheit kämpft, setzt sich Donald dafür ein, das Leben, das ihm noch bleibt, auszukosten. Als es ihm schließlich mit Hilfe Adrians, der seinen Wunsch versteht, gelingt, verändert sich auch das Leben seines Helden – er hat eine Beziehung und stirbt am Ende versöhnt mit seinem Schicksal:

> Ein GIFTPFEIL steckt in seinem HERZEN. Ungerührt zieht er ihn heraus. Vorn steckt eine lange Nadel daran. Seine Stimmung ändert sich nicht. Er ist bereit, sein Schicksal anzunehmen. Er seufzt und mit einem LÄCHELN wirft er den Giftpfeil fort.

> (McCartens 2007: 293)

Der Giftpfeil, der mit der Nadel auf den medizinischen Kontext verweist, kann leichter ertragen werden, sobald der „Held" sein Leben gelebt hat. Nun ist er bereit, sein Schicksal anzunehmen. Die Medizin wird im Text daher äußerst ambivalent gesehen. Sie verlängert zwar das physische Leben, verhindert aber gleichzeitig das emphatische Leben, das sich Donald wünscht. Erst als er sich sowohl über die Verbote der Eltern wie auch seiner Ärzte hinwegsetzt und nachts aus der Klinik flieht, erreicht er das ersehnte Glück und nimmt – wie sein Held – sein Schicksal an. Obwohl Donald eben nicht gegen die Krankheit, sondern für ein emphatisches Leben kämpft, erlebt seine Umwelt sein Sterben als Kampf. Interessanterweise ist es am Ende unter anderem der Priester, der wiederum zur Kriegsmetaphorik greift:

> Die Trauerreden konzentrieren sich darauf, wie *tapfer* er am Ende *gefochten* hat, als keine Hoffnung mehr war, und jeden, der ihn kannte, damit überrascht hat. Der Priester spricht von einer *„letzten entscheidenden Schlacht"*.

> (McCartens 2007: 261, Hervorhebungen A. S.)

In *Das Schicksal ist ein mieser Verräter* entlarven die beiden Protagonisten die Kriegsmetaphorik als hohle Phrase, die den Außenstehenden hilft, den Kranken zu ermutigen.

> „Du kannst gegen den Krebs kämpfen", sagte ich. „Das ist dein Kampf. Und du wirst weiterkämpfen", sagte ich. Ich hasste es, wenn Leute versuchten mich aufzubauen, mir Kampfgeist einzuflößen, und trotzdem tat ich das gleiche mit ihm. „Du... du... du

musst dein bestes Leben heute leben. Das ist jetzt dein Krieg." Ich hasse mich für die abgedroschenen Sprüche, aber was bleibt mir anderes übrig?

„Toller Krieg", sagte er sarkastisch. „Gegen wen führe ich Krieg? Gegen den Krebs. Und woraus besteht der Krebs? Aus mir. Die Tumoren gehören zu mir. Sie gehören genauso zu mir wie mein Gehirn und mein Herz. Es ist ein Bürgerkrieg, Hazel Grace, ein abgekarteter Bürgerkrieg, bei dem der Sieger feststeht."

(Green 2012: 198)

Als Augustus stirbt und ein Freund auf seiner Facebook-Pinnwand von einem „legendären Kampf gegen Krebs" (Green 2013: 243) schreibt, verwehrt sich Hazel gegen die Bezeichnung. John Greens Text zeigt durchgehend, dass die Kriegsmetaphorik dem Erleben der Kranken nicht gerecht wird.

Etliche Texte bedienen sich jedoch des Bildes nach wie vor unreflektiert. In Ned Vizzinis *Eine echt verrückte Story* (2006; dt. 2007) ist es bezeichnenderweise ein imaginärer Army-Officer, mit dem Craig (Selbst)gespräche führt. Schon durch die Wahl des Gesprächspartners liegt eine Kampf- und Kriegsmetaphorik nahe:

Ich hab nur ein einziges Mal mit ihr gesprochen.

Sie mag dich, Junge, und wenn du das nicht erkennen kannst, wirst du im *Krieg* kein *Gewehr* von einer *Spielzeugpistole* unterscheiden können.

Von was für einem Krieg reden wir jetzt?

Von dem, den du in deinem Kopf austrägst.

Wie kommen wir voran?

Du machst Fortschritte, *Soldat*, siehst du das nicht selbst?

(Vizzini 2007: 215, Hervorhebungen A. S.)

Auch hier wird der Kampf gegen die Krankheit als Krieg bezeichnet. Das Leben, das in den westlichen Gesellschaften kaum mehr von Krieg bedroht ist, wird selbst zum Krieg stilisiert, vor allem dann, wenn die Helden krank sind. Die Korrelation von Krieg und Krankheit bietet auch eine Erklärung dafür, warum die Protagonisten überwiegend männlich sind. Durch die Koppelung der Themen Krieg und Kampf mit lebensgefährlichen Krankheiten gewinnen die Bücher eine existentielle Dimension, die es erlaubt, Männlichkeitsstereotypen weiterzuführen, aber auch zu hinterfragen: Es sind keine wehleidigen Helden, die sich in den Romanen finden. Viele haben einen zynischen, distanzierten Blick auf die Welt. So gesehen generieren diese Texte aus Rezipientenperspektive durchaus „bewundernswürdige Heldenfiguren". Damit unterscheiden sich die Kinderfiguren aus den Texten der 1990er-Jahre deutlich von den Texten mit modernen männlichen Jugendlichen. Bei letzteren wird Krankheit nicht zum Zeichen für Hilflosigkeit und Schwäche, sondern sie steht für die Widerstände und Schicksalsschläge, die das Leben mit sich bringt und die den Protagonisten reifen lassen.

Gleichzeitig zeigen die Texte aber auch, dass es wenig Sinn hat, in den Krieg zu ziehen, wenn ein Kampf nicht gewonnen werden kann. Vielmehr lohnt sich dann die Konzentration auf das, was das Leben lebenswert und sinnvoll macht. Und dafür lohnt sich auch der Kampf gegen diejenigen, die „nur" helfen wollen. Krankheit und Tod dienen damit als Katalysatoren, um die Bedeutung eines emphatischen, intensiven Lebens besonders hervorzuheben. Um ihr Leben auch dann auskosten zu können, wenn es bedroht ist, brauchen die Protagonisten Autonomie und Gestaltungsfreiheit. Somit geht es im Kern um die Themen der Jugendliteratur im Allgemeinen, intensiviert dadurch, dass „jede Minute zählt".

Literaturverzeichnis

Anz, Thomas. *Gesund oder krank? Medizin, Moral und Ästhetik in der deutschen Gegenwartsliteratur*. Stuttgart: Metzler, 1989.

Balthazar, Nic. *Ben X*. Frankfurt: S. Fischer, 2009.

Bontrup, Hiltrup. *„… auch nur ein Bild": Krankheit und Tod in ausgewählten Texten Theodor Fontanes*. Hamburg: Argument, 2000.

Ewers, Hans-Heino. *Kinder- und Jugendliteratur der Aufklärung. Eine Textsammlung*. Stuttgart: Reclam, 1980.

---. „Kinder- und Jugendliteratur zwischen Pädagogik und Dichtung. Über die Fragwürdigkeit einer angeblichen Schicksalsfrage." *Kinder- und Jugendliteraturforschung 1999/2000. Mit einer Gesamtbibliographie der Veröffentlichungen des Jahres 1999*. Hrsg. Hans-Heino Ewers, Karin Richter und Ulrich Nassen. Stuttgart: Metzler, 2000. 98–114.

Farber, Astrid. *Krankheit im Kinder- und Jugendbuch von 1945 bis 1985*. Herzogenrath: Verlag Murken-Altrogge, 1991.

Goethe, Johann Wolfgang von. „Der Erlkönig." *Poetische Werke*. Bd. 1. Berlin: Aufbau Verlag, 1960. 115-16.

Green, John und Sophie Zeitz. *Das Schicksal ist ein mieser Verräter*. München: Hanser 2012.

Gutzschhahn, Uwe-Michael. *Der Sog*. München: dtv, 1996.

Haddon, Mark. *Supergute Tage oder die sonderbare Welt des Christopher Boone*. München: cbt, 2006.

Henzler, Rosemarie. *Krankheit und Medizin im erzählten Text. Eine Untersuchung zu Wilhelm Raabes Spätwerk*. Würzburg: Königshausen & Neumann, 1990.

Kaulen, Heinrich. „Vom bürgerlichen Elternhaus zur Patchwork-Familie. Familienbilder im Adoleszenzroman der Jahrhundertwende und der Gegenwart." *Familienszenen. Die Darstellung familialer Kindheit in der Kinder- und Jugendliteratur*. Hrsg. Hans-Heino Ewers und Inge Wild. Weinheim: Juventa, 1999. 115-27.

Link, Jürgen. *Versuch über den Normalismus. Wie Normalität produziert wird*. Opladen: Westdeutscher Verlag, 1997.

Lotman, Jurij M. *Die Struktur literarischer Texte*. München: Fink, 1986.

Mann, Thomas. *Buddenbrooks*. Frankfurt: S. Fischer, 1974.

McCarten, Anthony. *Superhero*. Zürich: Diogenes 2007.

Meyer, Conrad Ferdinand. „Das Leiden eines Knabens." *Sämtliche Werke*. Bd. 1. München: Winkler, 1968. 252-300.

Murken, Axel Hinrich, Christiane Kretzschmar und Christa Murken-Altrogge. *Kind, Krankheit und Krankenhaus im Bilderbuch von 1900 bis 1982*. Herzogenrath: Murken-Altrogge Verlag, 1982.

Murken, Axel Hinrich. *Kind, Krankheit und Krankenhaus im Kinder- und Jugendbuch*. Troisdorf: Burg Wissem – Bilderbuchmuseum der Stadt Troisdorf, 2004.

Nicholls, Sally und Birgitt Kollmann. *Wie man unsterblich wird. Jede Minute zählt*. München: DTB, 2012.

Reese, Ingeborg. *Behinderung als Thema in der Kinder- und Jugendliteratur*. Hamburg: Kovač 2007.

---. „Strickmuster und Stereotypen. Die Darstellung von Behinderung im Kinder- und Jugendbuch." *JuLit* 20.1 (2010): 3–8.

Rusch, Regina. *Zappelhannes*. Kevelaer: Anrich, 1988.

Schilcher, Anita: *Geschlechtsrollen, Familie, Freundschaft und Liebe in der Kinderliteratur der 90er Jahre. Studien zum Verhältnis von Normativität und Normalität im Kinderbuch und zur Methodik der Werteerziehung*. Frankfurt: Lang, 2001.

Shavit, Zohar. *Poetics of Children's Literature*. Athens: U of Georgia P, 2009.

Spinner, Kaspar H. „Kinder- und Jugendliteratur im Spannungsfeld zwischen pädagogischer Autorität und literarischer Subversion." *Kinder- und Jugendliteraturforschung 1999/2000. Mit einer Gesamtbibliographie der Veröffentlichungen des Jahres 1999*. Hrsg. Hans-Heino Ewers, Karin Richter und Ulrich Nassen. Stuttgart: Metzler, 2000. 82–85.

Stephens, John. *Language and Ideology in Children's Fiction*. London: Longman, 1992.

---. „Analysing Texts for Children: Linguistics and Stylistics." *Understanding Children's Literature. Key Essays from the International Companion Encyclopedia of Children's Literature*. Hrsg. Peter Hunt. London: Routledge, 1999. 56–68.

Storm, Theodor. „Geh nicht hinein". *Sämtliche Werke*. Bd. 1. Berlin und Weimar: Aufbau Verlag, 1978. 192-94.

Titzmann, Michael. „Skizze einer integrativen Literaturgeschichte und ihres Ortes in einer Systematik der Literaturwissenschaft." *Modelle des literarischen Strukturwandels*. Hrsg. Michael Titzmann. Tübingen: Niemeyer, 1991. 395–438.

Vizzini, Ned. *Eine echt verrückte Story*. München: Heyne, 2013.

Zimmermann, Rosmarie. *Behinderte in der Kinder- und Jugendliteratur*. Berlin: Verlag Volker Spiess, 1982.

Zweig, Stefan. *Brennendes Geheimnis*. Leipzig: Insel-Verlag, 1913.

Barbara Oettl

Picturing Disease (♂) – Performing Disease (♀)

> [Art] can cure you, heal you or something. It is probably better than medicine. I think art is pretty good, it is pretty important.
>
> (Damien Hirst, quoted in Cicelyn 2004: 111)

Given the fact that science has proven that there are diseases related to gender and also that in most cases medical practice, remedy and relief cope with disease on a gender-based level, we will also agree on the very simple fact that every human being – be it male or female – is afflicted with disease and in the very end overtaken by death. Disease and death, two of the most frightful threats to mankind, do not spare us by trying to be politically correct or arguing about who is who in the contemporary race of equal opportunities of the sexes. Thomas Hobbes' words taken from *Leviathan* are distressful and, at the same time, helpfully frank in this context: "And the life of man, solitary, poore nasty, brutish, and short" (Hobbes (1651) 1909: §12). This may sound quite appalling; however, does it not at the same time offer some relief concerning the gender-based debates on disease, healing-methods and the death of likewise men *and* women? For it goes without saying that this Hobbesian macro-structure of life can equally be applied to both the sexes, to every race, nationality, class or age.

Still, the micro-structures of life force us to think as individuals. Thus, death is naturally a major concern of every single one of us in his and her uniqueness. The stubborn fact of our lives ending on the one side and the physiological overlap of data between all humans on the other, causes us to not only seek help on a medical and scientific basis. We are rather thrown back on our mental and intellectual abilities in the matter. This is certainly the reason why topics such as death and disease have always occupied an important position in the thought of philosophers and anthropologists, sociologists and psychologists, writers and poets, and, last but not least, among artists.

In fine arts – as in any other discipline – the interpretation of a work of art can be based on gender-related arguments. For the last few centuries we can attest very clear-cut and conservative role models in the production of art which Amelia Jones classifies thus: "Conventionally speaking, men act and women pose" (Jones 1998: 153). Beginning with the second half of the twentieth century, namely during the 1960s and 70s, art history registered a change in these traditional role models, as well as in art production. While the contents remained the same, concepts, genres, movements and styles have undergone a major transformation: painting the image of a body is replaced by painting *with* the body, sculptural art is superseded by installations and environments and artists are adding new forms of theatrical expression through performances, Fluxus and the Happening. Also, the range of artistic material in use is expanding and, in fact, the material used is apt to become the form and content of a piece of art. This is precisely what is happening in the case of Body Artists and the body in art: in the end the body has become the subject *and* the object of art.

In the face of all these developments it may have remained undetected by the impartial beholder that the prescribed role models of male activity and female passivity are not sustainable anymore. The strategies in the art world have gone into reverse.[1] In conjunction with the body, its diseases, vulnerabilities and the final termination of the flesh, at the turn of the 21st century this means that in contemporary art men are *picturing* disease while women are *performing* the subject.

This argument is in the following exemplified on the male side by two of the so called Y(oung) B(ritish) A(rtists), Marc Quinn and Damien Hirst, who came to fame through the much-discussed and infamously renowned *Freeze* show at London's docks in 1988 and *Sensation* in London (1997) and New York (1999), and on the female side by two illustrious women performers, Marina Abramović and ORLAN, both of whom started their art practices in the 1960s when Body Art was still in its early stages.

The male protagonists are looking at death as the "fundamental flaw in the planet", something that "seems kind of rude." However, Damien Hirst has to admit that this is "a very western way of looking at the world." (Cicelyn 2004: 164) He and Marc Quinn try to solve the mystery of life and death and they apply artistic as well as scientific means to do so, as both – art and science – can

---

[1] If this may sound like an exaggerated generalization it needs to be referred to in the context of debates which have persisted ever since the emergence of Action Painting, which is commonly known to be a primarily male-dominated art practice. The inversion of male and female role models in subsequent styles in the art world – such as Pop Art, Op Art, Minimal Art, Land Art, Body Art and performative art practices – have been widely discussed and confirmed by notable, conservative, as well as, progressive art critics and historians in the light of the preceding developments in the art world. We have to acknowledge a basic agreement on the reciprocal paradigm of the female being modeled versus female modeling which can be considered more than just a tendency but rather an obvious and sought-after trend.

For further reading on the subject of female and male role models in the arts compare the following selection of authors: Simone de Beauvoir, Judith Butler, Michel Foucault, Michael Fried, Clement Greenberg, Amelia Jones, Hilton Kramer, Rosalind Krauss, Jacques Lacan, Kathy O'Dell, Andrew Perchuk, Donald Preziosi, Barbara Rose, Harold Rosenberg, Calvin Tomkins, et al.

complement one another: "Like science, art attempts to understand what it means to be a living, material being" (Marc Quinn quoted in Groninger Museum 2006: 21). In fact, Quinn and Hirst interlace scientific and artistic practices in equal measure in their works, thus demonstrating that art can be a main contributor to solve the riddles of human life and death: the metaphysical solution, so to speak, that is nonetheless based on attestable fact.

In order to illustrate Marc Quinn's perspective, I would like to draw attention to his self-portraits, which the artist started to produce in 1991: *Self*[2] is cast from 4.5 litres of the artist's blood – which equals the average amount of blood of an adult male person – and which Quinn had provided over a period of five years. Hence, the meticulous medical process of harvesting his own life-giving bodily fluid enables the artist to mould his head in a recurring cycle every five years. It goes without saying that the handling of blood in an artistic context is nevertheless in need of a clinical surrounding: To prevent haemorrhage Quinn's counter-image is coated in silicone. Also, the casts of his head have to be kept at a permanent temperature of -70 °C and are, for that purpose, protected from melting atop a stainless steel appliance, behind a transparent showcase housing a special cooling-system. This artificial machinery, therefore, implies the sudden death of an artwork in case the temperature should rise or the power supply be cut off. Quinn ponders on his transient allegory on life:

> *Self* is a frozen moment on life-support. Every five years I make a new cast of my head, using ten new pints of my frozen blood. Each is displayed in its own refrigerated cabinet. Like a living person, if the power is cut, the sculpture turns into a pool of blood, you can't say where the form has gone, just that it was there and now it's not. This, to me, is a profound metaphor in the language of sculpture for the elusive and preciousness of life.
>
> (Groninger Museum 2006: 40)

Quinn's *Self* might even outlive us all; however, only with the help of a life-sustaining machine. His portraits stay "alive" just the way blood-reserves do for a later extraction, recovery, re-production or even re-animation. Thus, Quinn has created a self-portrait that is more complete than the tradition of art history has offered so far: the artistic and bodily material – with the blood constituting a unipotent ancestral or stem cell – will be able to serve as a memory map for an eventual reconfiguration of the immortal artist.

Let us now turn to the apparently classical sculptural art works within Quinn's oeuvre. In 2005 the artist took life-size casts from several people. In their outer form, composition and technical execution these resemble statues redone in a traditional Greek style. This semblance is due to the polymeric wax

[2] Since some of the art works discussed in this article are of an explicit nature it was decided to abstain from illustrating the text altogether.

material which makes the figures look like they have been cut from white marble. However, contrary to the cold and polished finish of a marble statue the surface of the nude bodies represented here feels warm and soft to our touch, just like real skin. All of them appear to have been taken down from the plinths that used to elevate them just a moment ago, lying on the floor on their backs, waiting to be lifted up again in order to be repositioned on their pedestals. However, as an installation the casts remain splayed out on the floor, some of them in awkward, uncomfortable-looking cramped positions, some of them like fallen angels, fast asleep, floating just above the ground.

The whole group of models laid out there on the floor of the museum bears the title *Chemical Life Support*. The chemicals the title is hinting at are blended into the material used for the casts and consist of the different medications the depicted persons, whose full names are added in the title as well, have to take in real life in order to survive. Each polymer-medication mixture for each single cast, therefore, needs to be an individually-created cocktail of a daily dose of medicines to fight diseases such as AIDS, lupus or diabetes, to keep someone alive after organ transplantation, allergic shock reactions or a heart attack. This way, the lifeless casts come to be replicas of the living individuals depicted, including their distinct course of disease, medical histories, and probable life expectancy. However, their apparent uniformity – immaculate, white, hovering above the floor, ideal in proportion – lacks any visual basis for differentiation and makes them appear disturbingly generic. The disease as such, the abnormities of the body that would make them victims of discrimination if rendered visible, are inscribed into this outer perfection of the imagery and the uniformity of the installation. In every respect, the hidden differences guarantee the survival of the whole group.

Amidst this environment, the artist has displayed his baby son. Quinn describes this self-referential act as follows:

> In 2003, my son Lucas had a severe anaphylactic reaction to the first bottle of formula milk he was given. His allergy was so severe that milk and wheat were life-threatening for the first three and a half years of his life. Apart from his mother's breast milk he could only drink Neocate, a food powder made in the lab which the body does not recognize as milk. This inspired me to make the sculpture *Innoscience*, a sculpture of him at eight months asleep, cast in a special high-melt polymer wax mixed with Neocate milk powder. It was like a chemical equivalent for the changes in his body and a celebration of science and medicine. After making this piece I became interested in other conditions which could be kept in check by taking a drug or compound.

(Groninger Museum 2006: 86)

The title of the cast *Innoscience* points to the innocent, but diseased baby boy and at the same time refers to the scientific remedies of the medicated status quo his son had to be in as a life-saving action.

The medicated status quo of our bodies is at its best able to prolong our lives. The boundaries of this possibility are demonstrated by Damien Hirst's artistic work. Titles of art works such as *The Physical Impossibility of Death in the Mind of Someone Living,* which Hirst gave to his infamous shark displayed in a transparent showcase filled with formaldehyde solution in 1992, or *The Existence of Nothing Causes Nothing*, one of his medical cabinets from 2001, pose the perpetual and unvarying questions about our lives and deaths and what happens in between; in a nutshell, *Where Are We Going? Where Do We Come From? Is There a Reason?*[3] (2000-2004). In Hirst's repertoire of artistic expression art is intertwined with science[4] and religious concepts engage with human medicine and psychology, always assigning new trains of thought and opening up new pathways for solutions. The objects he accumulates in his works of art frequently consist of medical and pathological equipment, hospital and morgue settings, drugs and medicine containers, skeletons and carcasses. His art reeks of disease and death. But its outer appearance is shiny, new, showcased in a clinical fashion in transparent glass and polished stainless-steel containers. Therein creation and decay are repeated in close intervals by Hirst's art.

In 1989 Damien Hirst started a twelve-piece series of medicine cabinets[5] for a group exhibition at London's *Building One* titled *Modern Medicine*. The objects consist of glass vitrines, each shelf of which is filled to the brim with bottles, vials and boxes of medicine and drugs. All empty, by the way. As every single one of these chemicals, fluids and pills offers relief to certain organs and parts of the body, the medication on display is arranged in a way to represent the whole human body and mind, including its obsessions, starting with the head (upmost shelf), going over the heart and belly all the way down to the feet (lowest shelf). When asked whether the names and types of the drugs, the pharmaceutical company or the packaging were also of any importance for the composition, Hirst answered:

> I toyed with all that. I chose the size and shape of the cabinet like a body. I wanted it to be kind of human, like with an abdomen and a chest and guts. […] Then I played

---

[3] This is another one of Hirst's quite literary titles, in this case of a stainless steel and glass cabinet containing numerous animal skeletons of seemingly prehistoric creatures.

[4] Hirst employs over 30 people, on the one hand, to carry out the major part of his artworks, and on the other hand to market his trade name and art. The company's name is *Science*.

[5] The cabinets are named after the twelve songs of the *Sex Pistols'* 1977 album *Never Mind the Bollocks*.

around with the idea of putting the drugs for your head at the top and those for your feet at the bottom […]. I started trying to find out what all the drugs were.

(Cicelyn 2004: 105-106)

However, these prescription drugs are not exhibited in order to expose one specific person and his or her special needs as is the case in Quinn's casts in *Chemical Life Support*. Hirst's packaging and bottles are rather sorted out in a formal way which is likely to make a real physician wonder as the artist realised at such an encounter:

I remember being in an exhibition when there was a doctor looking at it going "Oh, yeah! Strange". I said, "What do you mean?" He said "I would never put these drugs with these drugs." You can work out the personality of the doctor. If you were a GP you can work out what his patients' problems are, because he is obviously using a lot of those drugs […].

(Cicelyn 2004: 106)

Thus, the medicine cabinets do not interfere with the confidential medical communication as it is protected by the law. The cabinets do not talk; no personal chronicle is given, but an old dispute among artists is prioritised: the dispute between form and colour. Thus, the arrangement of the cabinet's contents allows free associations of one product with another on a purely aesthetic basis. Hirst claims that "[…] la cosa che mi si presenta per prima è l'aspetto formale – gli scaffali con le medicine sono tutti disposti in base al colore, per esempio. La gente mi dice: 'Perché li hai disposti in quell modo?'. Ed è sempre la solita antiquate risposta da artista: colore, forma"[6] (Stolper 2006: 5). In the end, the geometric rigor and calculated colour chart of the cabinets cannot hide the fact that we are confronted with containers that commonly contain everything from life-saving medication to pain killers. To emphasise their outer appearance at the cost of the actual pharmaceutical ingredient reflects the fact that what the medicine cabinets offer has limits. A detail the artist is perfectly aware of: "You can only cure people for so long and then they're going to die anyway. You can't arrest decay, but these medicine cabinets suggest you can" (Dannatt 1993: 63).

At the same time Hirst began to manipulate the actual packaging of medication. His art work *The Last Supper* (1999) is an ironic comment on our medical consumerism. *Last Supper* intermingles art and sciences with the well-nigh religious belief in medical help promised by doctors, hospitals, and phar-

[6] "[…] the thing that I am occupied with primarily is the formal aspect – the medicine cabinets, for example, are all arranged in terms of color and form. People ask me: 'Why do you arrange them this way?' And it's always the same old story as an artistic response: color, form" [my translation].

macies. A typical mixture of British staple foods, such as steak and kidney pie, beans, corned beef, liver, bacon and chips, are now written out on the labels of the medication, the brand names of which have all been changed into *DamienHirst*. Only at a second glance do we realise this alienation of otherwise perfectly normal drug containers as suggested by the typical colouring, design, the components of the medication and other data printed on them. And only through expert knowledge are we able to identify the pharmaceuticals which include substances against severe and typically fatal illnesses such as AIDS or heart disease. Especially perfidious is the box inscribed *Omelette*, which in a subtitle hints to the chemical ingredient *ondansetrone*, which is usually given to cancer patients undergoing chemotherapy as a remedy against nausea and vomiting. This bitter sarcasm leads us back to the title of Hirst's work *The Last Supper*, which insinuates that the patient is fated to die in the end in a religious as well as a therapeutic sense.

Keeping all this in mind, we have to admit that at some point of everyone's life we will be *Standing Alone on the Precipice and Overlooking the Arctic Wastelands of Pure Terror* (1999-2000), another one of Hirst's glass showcases, this time filled with over 6.000 single tablets in different shapes and colours. This pill cabinet makes us catch a glimpse of the wastelands of disease and the follow-up of the inevitable, repetitive and detached drug therapies of always the same and yet always different remedies. In order to obtain this impression on a formal level Hirst keeps over 20 assistants occupied with the manual fabrication and arrangement of the artificial pills. These have to fulfil certain standards of a minimal and puristic look:

> If you have a problem you can step back from it in order to see it. There is no limit to how far you can step. Things look different from very far away. [...] like a molecular structure or something, or like looking under the microscope. I guess that it has a kind of scientific look. On a superficial level they are just a matrix of lots of little elements. I always notice loads of references or crossovers in works. I arrange things in a very formal way, just colour or something like that, Hans Hoffman. I spend a long time working out the meaning and metaphorical elements just to get myself in a position where I can do a very playful colour thing. [...] When you say, which pills go next to which pills in the cabinet, it is just colour. I say, toss out those green ones, put that blue one over there. You are just doing that colour thing that artists do.

(Cicelyn 2004: 227)

However, doing a "colour thing that artists do" with over 6000 pills means taking on an obsessive character – if not for the artist, then for the beholder who is promised and hopes for unlimited chances of cure.

That these are welcomed with open arms in our contemporary society is proven by Hirst's *Pharmacy*, a project that started out as a space created by the artist, which over the years turned into a real restaurant where people could wine and dine. In 1992, when *Pharmacy* was initiated as an art work, people entered the galleries that had been rearranged and presented in a very clinical and hygienic look. The seemingly commercial space of a pharmacy had had a reception desk added to it, onto which the artist had put mysterious looking testtubes filled with similarly unidentifiable fluids in primary colours. The dominant colour of the furniture is kept to white and the entire walls are covered with shelves holding all kinds of boxes with medicines. In these surroundings, art and medicine become an entity, intruded on only by the electric fly killer hanging down from the ceiling at the centre of the installation. Life and death are apparently closely aligned and the purified space in all its obsessive sterility cannot belie the fact that our body's contamination through age, drugs, medication, and other seductions is an irreversible process.

Over time, the *Pharmacy's* artistic environment turned into a professional restaurant for people to dine in, to have drinks from glasses decorated with the Aesculapius snake, to sit on stools in the shape of aspirin tablets and to be attended by waiters wearing lab coats and scrubs designed by Prada. Nothing seemed more natural in this context and thus the factual and mental gap of picking up medicine from a pharmacy in the afternoon, attending an exhibition opening at a gallery in the evening and going out for dinner afterwards all become one within the context of Hirst's installation, which can be positioned somewhere in between life and its opposite. In all of Hirst's works we can find this fusion of a daily routine with the exceptional circumstances of sickness, an intermingling of hope and resignation, the alternation of safety and anxiety. In addition to that, Hirst's sterile cabinets with titles derived from a medical background stress the fragility of our bodies in metaphorical images: "I want [people] to go away having experienced something and leaving richer on some level. I want to give you the energy to go away and think about your life again. To pose some questions. They may be uncomfortable questions but they need to be asked. To make people think again about what they know" (Cicelyn 2004: 238).

Like in Marc Quinn's oeuvre, most of Hirst's objects come in glass and stainless steel containers. On the one side, these offer protection to the enclosed environments and keep up the clinically hygienic surroundings the artists are eager to create for their biotopes. On the other side, the containers generate a strict threshold that cannot be transgressed. Hirst's and Quinn's works detach themselves from the beholder, not only physically but especially through their cool and aesthetic outward appearance. Within the framework of the sober and reserved museum context, in which art works present themselves on a formal basis, these works do not hold back with regard to contents which are fit to enter our lives and thoughts in a most shocking and intense way, however. This male view is without any doubt an appropriate depiction of disease.

Let us now turn towards the contemporary female point of view on disease and examine how two of the protagonists, namely Marina Abramović and ORLAN, express their thoughts in performative ways. These highly-structured and precisely-choreographed performances carefully follow pre-determined strategies in order to exemplify psychological and physical pain caused by the sickness and discontentment of our society. Their strategies also rely on the effect that the factual representation of physical pain consciously evokes aversion, antipathy and disgust in the beholder. In her book *Regarding the Pain of Others*, Susan Sontag adds the following thought to this aspect: "But the spectacular is very much part of the religious narratives by which suffering, throughout most of Western history, has been understood" (Sontag 2003: 80). To utilise this clash of two value systems and to illustrate the psychological as well as physical pain of the human being at the beginning of the twenty-first century therein is part of Abramović's and ORLAN's aspirations. After all and this is the way ORLAN puts it, "Art is not meant to decorate our apartments. That's what we have aquariums, plants, curtains and furniture for" (ORLAN 1995: n.p., my translation).

According to Marina Abramović's diary in note form, it was the year 1972 when she assigned her body as the artistic material she would be working with from then on: "'72 I start using my body as material, blood, pain, watching major operations in hospitals. Pushing my body to its physical and mental limits" (Biesenbach 2008: 34). Abramović is one of the pioneers in Body Art, using her body as a means of visual as well as mental communication. Abramović is also known for extreme action that can cause pain to her body on a physical and at the same time psychological level. For the artist, experiencing pain and putting herself in dangerous situations is not a crazy thing to do, as the Western world is likely to believe it to be. In fact, most of the time, Abramović gives herself over to pain and mental stress in a very passive way in order to experience non-western belief-systems. It is well known that, for example, native tribes and aboriginals deliberately seek out dangerous and painful situations in order to generate self-healing qualities. Near-death experiences are pushed to their limits to broaden the mind and to obtain secret knowledge on life and death as the artist intends to "enter through the pain into that other space" (Biesenbach 2008: 22). Still, Abramović *does* make a difference between self-inflicted pain, which she considers to be useful, and the unintentional pain sickness imposes on us without asking. She describes the latter as unimaginable and uncontrollable, something that cannot be shared as an experience with others. The pain she examines is a conscious one that can be subdued by performing it:

> Every ceremony, every ritual from ancient times until now, including Catholic Church or Orthodox Church, stages rituals that include pain. When you are sick, when it's something inflicted without your will, it's a different story. Torture is not something you want to go through. Neither is the pain of being sick. This kind of pain is another thing. When you stage the pain we are talking about how to actually understand how the mind and the body work and what pain exactly is.
>
> (Biesenbach 2008: 22)

From 1973 to 1974 Abramović underwent a countdown of performances titled *Rhythm*, staging eleven scenes which contain painful actions, either in a self-inflicting manner or pain inflicted upon her by the beholder. Starting in 1973 with *Rhythm 10* in which the artist used knives to stab the space in between the fingers of her own hand that she had placed on the floor in fast and repeated succession, the countdown ended with *Rhythm 0* in which the artist invited everyone in the gallery to apply 72 objects she had put on a table to her body. This last performance within the context of *Rhythm* left the artist mutilated and physically in pain as she was cut and whipped by the audience and when, as a final act, someone put a loaded gun against her throat the performance was put to an end by a person who called the police. This last one of Abramović' *Rhythm* performances recalls the famous Stanley Milgram experiment that had been published a few months before the artist's last action was performed, probably not coincidentally. Both Milgram and Abramović were able to give evidence to the fact that cruelty wins over ethical objection.

However, for the purpose of the subject in question, gender and disease, I want to focus on *Rhythm 2* (1974), a performance in which Abramović intertwines pain and disease, on the one hand, as well as medicine and healing, on the other, through the means of self-inflicted suffering. In the Galerija Suvremene Umjetnosti in Zagreb, Abramović used her body for an experiment. She took two different types of psychoactive medication that are used to treat catatonia and schizophrenia in patients who have been hospitalised. Influenced by these drugs that caused unpredictable reactions, the artist would nevertheless try to report on what she experienced, physically and mentally. Patients with schizophrenia are afflicted by a mental disorder that leads to a breakdown of thought processes and a poor emotional responsiveness. In the case of Abramović, taking the medication against schizophrenia in a perfectly healthy state led to a severe contraction of her muscles, which she was not able to control anymore. By contrast, when the artist took the medicine for the treatment of catatonia, a state of neurogenic motor immobility and behavioural abnormity manifested by stupor, Abramović's body started to cramp, causing her to sit in the same posture for six hours: "I was feeling cold, then I lost consciousness, forgot, who and where I was" (Warr 2005: 124, my translation). The typical characteristics of the actual disease – rigidness of the body, the lack of critical cognitive functions, unresponsiveness due to a lack of consciousness, showing reactions only in the case of physical pain – were developed by Abramović as a counter-reaction to the otherwise helpful drugs.

The at first sight uncontrollable situation the artist had put herself in – to give up self-control over her bodily functions and her mind, this condition of utmost vulnerability in front of an audience – was only experienced in this way by the members of the audience, who were unable to interfere and were restricted to the role of mere observers. Abramović describes the significance of her action as follows: "[The idea] was about time, but the other was really about consciousness and unconsciousness. I could not accept that a performance would have to stop because you lost consciousness. I wanted to extend the possibility [...] in which the performance continues even if the performer is unconscious. I didn't accept the body's limits" (Biesenbach 2008: 14). In *Rhythm 2* the artist had once again wanted to master a painful and dangerous situation that anybody else would try to avoid. By taking this risky action onto herself there is no need for the audience to do likewise. For by being present, the audience is able to be in the same space, time and circumstance together with the artist through *Einfühlung* and cathartic empathy, thus perceiving and feeling comparable sensations. At the very end, the mental limits are extended and even transgressed by both the artist and – through her – by the audience in equal measure. As is the case with all of her performances, this one has also been chronicled via photographs the artist had commissioned: "[...] I knew I wanted to have documentation. I was in control of it, and this is how I wanted it to be" (Biesenbach 2008: 16).

Similar actions and re-actions are to be expected when we turn from the usage of internal psychotropic drugs in the case of Marina Abramović to the appliance of external surgery in an artistic context in the case of ORLAN. Beginning her oeuvre in the 1970s, her multimedia works consist of body works, sculpture and *tableaux vivants* as well as video- and performance pieces most of which are quoting a Jewish-Christian iconography. With the enactment of her famous and frequently cited long-term performance of *The Re-Incarnation of St. ORLAN*, also known as *Omniprésence* (1990-1993), ORLAN began to call her works Carnal Art, as a radicalisation from Body Art. For the purpose of my argument, this performance in the form of plastic surgery will serve as an example and metaphor for the subject of gender and disease because – and this is how ORLAN puts it: "I am the first female artist to introduce surgery as a medium in order to persuade plastic surgery to abandon its purpose of beautification and rejuvenation" (ORLAN 1995: n. p., my translation). Yet, this is precisely what ORLAN has decided to do to herself and in 1990 she initiated a complete metamorphosis of her outer appearance through plastic surgery over the period of three years. For *The Re-Incarnation of St. ORLAN* the artist's studio was replaced by the hospital's operating room furnished and decorated at ORLAN's will and design and the artist acts as the stage director of her own re-placement of skin, fat and facial structures, as well as her flesh and facial bones being put into new shapes. Paralleling this rearrangement of her body parts ORLAN worked together with psychoanalysts in order to re-shape her personality.

The optical change the artist went through is not without precedent. If we think of the famous Greek painter Zeuxis of Heraclea, for example, who in his time applied a rather eclectic mode of painting when he was asked to depict the ideal woman. For that purpose, he had invited the most beautiful women to his studio to select from each of them the ideal parts of their faces and bodies and had thus re-constructed an ideal female concept. Such is the method that was applied by ORLAN. For the re-making of her face in the course of seven operations, she picked the chin of Botticelli's Venus, the nose of Psyche in the way she was depicted by Gérôme, the lips of François Boucher's Europe, the eyes of Diane from a painting done by the French school of Fontainebleau and the high forehead of Leonard da Vinci's *Mona Lisa*. In order to give a rough impression of the expected changes ORLAN offered a computer animation of her new self in advance of the first operation. However, linked to the optical changes according to the female ideals listed above are certain features of personality of the ladies in question that ORLAN accordingly wanted to include into her new personality: Venus as the lascivious Goddess of fertility, love and creativity, Psyche representing the soul and Diane as an aggressive and active counterpart to men, to just briefly mention some of the features aspired to. Consequently, the cuts the artist chose to have done to herself go deeper than just below skin: this operational transfiguration leaves marks on more than just one level as it does not only refer to the optical changes in progress but also concerns the changes of the artist's and the audience's psyche.

Before we come to the latter we will have to take a closer look at the orches-trated staging of the scene in the operating room where the artist undergoes the transformation. This also includes an increased risk for the patient as ORLAN insists on mere local anaesthesia in order to be able to perform during the sur-gery. The epidural block allows the artist to read texts, for example by Michel Serres, that are contextualised with her changing image and the operating theatre is arranged accordingly, depending on the nature of the theme for each oper-ation. Moreover, the artist's and the surgery staff's costumes are created by re-nowned designers for the particular occasions and the rest of the set is elaborately equipped with fruit still lives. Additional props, musicians and dancers support ORLAN's act following her script. The whole performance is recorded on video and is then transmitted live via satellite to the public in Tokyo, New York, Paris, Toronto, Hamburg and other cities. The conversation between ORLAN and the audience is kept up through fax machines and videophone for everyone to witness and the whole procedure is translated into sign language as well.

The purpose of this interactive play is to profane the surgical invasion, so that in the end this private occasion would become a public and transparent event. (ORLAN 1995: n. p.) As already mentioned above, ORLAN's performances derive from a very traditional background. On the one hand, they mirror the bloody affairs of martyrdom and sainthood as well as practices we can find in the context of the Catholic Church. On the other hand, she alludes to a recent tradition persistent in contemporary TV-shows such as *E(mergency) R(oom)*, *House, M. D.* and other productions that have by now obtained cult status and that count on the audience's appetite for and fascination with medical settings, rituals and the beauty frenzy of actors and patients alike. The iconic typology in both cases inspires ORLAN's re-incarnation as a saint, as well as her canonisation according to the requirements of the Catholic Church. In addition, she sells photographs, videotapes and even relics of her body to help finance her follow-up performances. The vials containing blood, fat or the artist's flesh, and the bloody gauze remains from the surgery are framed and sealed the way fan articles are merchandised, all of them being certified by ORLAN with the inscription "This is my body, this is my software". ORLAN has already managed to create her post-human persona today.

The question remains why the artist undergoes this change of identity in such a radical and, for most witnesses, disgusting act. In the age of plastic surgery, medical omnipotence and stem cell research, ORLAN is addressing a legal and at the same time ethical issue: firstly, she legally obtains a new identity and therewith raises the question how far we are allowed to go in terms of an identity change that has become a medical possibility in the age of plastic surgery. The same set of problems is evoked by leaving behind DNA-material of her body, thus implying the eventuality of an after-image and after-life in the age of the scientific clone. Secondly, ORLAN's new super-natural look and identity invites the unsettling moral question of how much medicine should be able and allowed to interfere in who we are and for how long? This holds especially true for women undergoing plastic surgery in order to satisfy the male dictates of female perfection. Amelia Jones addresses this particular matter:

> ORLAN's work points to the fact that plastic surgery, rather than allowing us to gain control over our bodies, exacerbates our subordination to their vulnerabilities and morality – a subordination all the more dangerous for women, due to its long precedent in Western representation and thought. The more we attempt to reverse the signs of aging

or supposedly misbegotten facial and bodily features, the more obviously we are
obsessively driven by our corporeality (specifically, its visual appearance as psychi-
cally incorporated into our senses of self).

(Jones 1998: 227-228)

To make sure that this message is an absolutely believable one, ORLAN uses
herself as a crass example of mutilation to illustrate the unattainability of perfection and the horrible processes involved in this effort. Thus, the confrontational clash between art and surgery goes along with the confrontational colli-
sion of what the audience perceives and cherishes as art and what the audience
shies away from as an impertinence to the eye and mind likewise:

> I am sorry to make you suffer, but remember, I am not suffering, except like you, when
> I look at the images. There are very few images that cause most of us to close one's
> eyes: death, suffering, the cutting-open of the body, certain types of pornography, and
> for others giving birth. The eyes become black holes that swallow up these images.
> Whether you like it or not these images vanish in this abyss and strike the bottom
> where it hurts without going through the usual filters. Just as if the eyes were not
> connected to the brain anymore.
>
> (ORLAN, 1995: n. p.)

Watching surgery being carried out on the artist's body and face makes our own
muscles twitch and we feel the urge to cover our eyes. And still we feel the urge
to watch from behind our splayed fingers. And ORLAN wants us to watch as a
reminder that the reforming instruments of the medical sciences have gone
beyond biological limitations. For this very same reason she is also convinced
that a successful justification of such actions can only work in the context of art:

> For me, art which is interesting is related to and belongs to resistance. It must upset our
> assumption, overwhelm our thoughts, be outside norms and outside of the law. It
> should be against bourgeois art; it is not there to comfort, nor to give us what we
> already know. It must take risks, at the risk of not being accepted, at least initially. It
> should be deviant and involve a project for society. And even if this declaration seems
> very romantic, I say: art can, art must, change the world, for that is its only justifi-
> cation.
>
> (Weintraub 1996: 83)

In performing their subject, the female point of view on disease and medical
salvation takes on a radical expression compared to the male counterparts as
highlighted above. Though based on only a few examples, the result may be
regarded as symptomatic in art history. Whereas the male perspective adopts a
detached perspective that privileges the aesthetic qualities of the art works over
a clear-cut positioning of viewpoints as regards content, the female artists tend

to get involved personally by taking the action out on themselves, exploiting their own bodies and minds.

Yet, an instance of union between the sexes exists: in her latest project ORLAN is distributing her DNA all over the globe in order to create the possibility of an eventual re-birth of her persona when the time is ripe and science as well as the law will be ready to allow the process of human cloning. Consequently, the artist is "[b]ypassing both natural and unnatural conception" as "ORLAN performs the ultimate creative act by willing her own rebirth" (Weintraub 1996: 79): "My work is a struggle against the innate, the inexorable, the programmed nature, DNA (which is our direct rival as artists of representation) and God! My work is blasphemous" (quoted in Weintraub 1996: 81). Again, the artist is taking up a stance against our intent to control organic processes and to rely on technology, medicine and science in order to interfere with the human matrix predetermined by nature.

This leads us back to the case of Marc Quinn, who, beginning in the year 2000, produced genomic portraits as works of art. One of these was commissioned by the London National Portrait Gallery and contains the genomic information of Sir John Sulston, winner of the Nobel Prize for the decoding of DNA. Quinn's portrait does not show the usual external features of the former director of the Sanger Institute, but only his bacteria culture gained from Sir John Sulston's sperm. The collaboration between the artist and the scientist is described by Quinn in the following: "The sequencing of the genome is a profound moment in human history; we are the first people to be able to read the instructions to make ourselves. What was interesting to me in the results of sequencing of the human genome was that we share 99.9 % of our genome with everyone else and in fact most of it with every living thing on the planet, both animals and plants" (Groninger Museum 2006: 66). This overlap between all humans is the reason why the DNA material of Sir John Sulston is presented in a glass container, reflecting the recipient in its mirror-like structure. The apparently abstract portrait gains its utter realism on a second glance and it predicts the fact that mankind will go beyond crisis point given the opportunities and legal setting.

List of Works Cited

Biesenbach, Klaus, Chrissie Iles and Kristine Stiles (eds.). *Marina Abramović*. New York: Phaidon, 2008.

Cashell, Kieran. *Aftershock. The Ethics of Contemporary Transgressive Art*. New York: I. B. Tauris, 2009.

Cicelyn, Eduardo, Mario Codognato and Mirta D'Argenzio (eds.). *Damien Hirst. The Agony and the Ecstasy. Selected Works from 1989-2004*. Naples: Electa, 2004.

Dannatt, Adrian. "Damien Hirst. Life's Like This. Then It Stops." *Flash Art* 169 (1993): 63.

Hobbes, Thomas. *Leviathan or the Matter, Form and Power of a Commonwealth Ecclesiastical and Civil.* 1651. Oxford: Clarendon Press, 1909.

Jones, Amelia. *Body Art. Performing the Subject.* Minneapolis: U of Minnesota P, 1998.

Marc Quinn. Recent Work – Recent Sculpture. Groningen: Nai Publishers, 2006. [Exhibition catalogue of the Groninger Museum, Groningen]

ORLAN. "Intervention d'Orlan". *Suture – Phantasmen der Vollkommenheit.* Salzburg: Symposium Salzburger Kunstverein, 1995. 33-50.

Sontag, Susan. *Regarding the Pain of Others.* New York: Picador, 2003.

Stolper, Paul (ed.). *Damien Hirst. New Religion.* Bologna: Damiani, 2006.

Warr, Tracy (ed.). *Kunst und Körper.* Berlin: Phaidon, 2005.

Weintraub, Linda. *Art on the Edge and Over. Searching for Art's Meaning in Contemporary Society, 1970s-1990s.* Litchfield: Art Insights Publishers, 1996.